HEALTH AND CITIZENSHIP: POLITICAL CULTURES OF HEALTH IN MODERN EUROPE

STUDIES FOR THE SOCIETY FOR THE SOCIAL HISTORY OF MEDICINE

Series Editors: *David Cantor*
                      Keir Waddington

TITLES IN THIS SERIES

Forthcoming Titles

HEALTH AND CITIZENSHIP: POLITICAL CULTURES OF HEALTH IN MODERN EUROPE

Edited by

Frank Huisman and Harry Oosterhuis

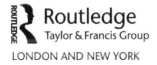

Routledge
Taylor & Francis Group

LONDON AND NEW YORK

First published 2014 by Pickering & Chatto (Publishers) Limited

Published 2016 by Routledge
2 Park Square, Milton Park, Abingdon, Oxfordshire OX14 4RN
711 Third Avenue, New York, NY 10017, USA

First issued in paperback 2015

Routledge is an imprint of the Taylor & Francis Group, an informa business

BRITISH LIBRARY CATALOGUING IN PUBLICATION DATA

Health and citizenship: political cultures of health in modern Europe. – (Studies for the Society for the Social History of Medicine)
1. Medical policy – Europe – History – 20th century. 2. Medical policy – Europe
– History –21st century. 3. Public health – Europe – History – 20th century.
4. Public health – Europe –History – 21st century.
I. Series II. Huisman, Frank editor of compilation. III. Oosterhuis, Harry editor
of compilation.
362.1'094'09045-dc23

ISBN-13: 978-1-138-66298-8 (pbk)
ISBN-13: 978-1-8489-3432-0 (hbk)

Typeset by Pickering & Chatto (Publishers) Limited

CONTENTS

ACKNOWLEDGEMENTS

It is a great pleasure to finally see this volume go to print. Its foundations were laid during an Anglo-Dutch-German Wellcome Workshop on the History of Medicine which took place in Maastricht, The Netherlands, from 23 to 25 June 2005. The workshop was organized by Harold Cook and Anne Hardy (then Wellcome Trust Centre for the History of Medicine at UCL), Hilary Marland (University of Warwick), Robert Jütte and Martin Dinges (Robert Bosch Foundation, Stuttgart) and Frank Huisman and Harry Oosterhuis (Maastricht University). It was supported by the Wellcome Trust, the Robert Bosch Stiftung, the Netherlands Organisation for Scientific Research (NWO), the Huizinga Institute and the Faculty of Arts and Culture of Maastricht University.

Almost half of the contributions to this volume were commissioned after the workshop and were meant to introduce a new approach to the topic and a new structure to the book. The text of Anne Hardy's contribution is taken from the second chapter of her forthcoming book *Salmonella, Infections, Networks of Knowledge, and Public Health in Britain, 1880–1975*, the argument being modified for the theme of the current volume. Many people helped to shape this volume. We are indebted to Logie Barrow, Harold Cook, Roger Cooter, Martin Dinges, Dagmar Ellerbrock, Sylvelyn Hähner-Rombach, Thorsten Halling, Robert Jütte, Christopher Lawrence, Hilary Marland, Thorsten Noack, Hasso Spode, Claudia Stein, Gunnar Stollberg, Mathew Thomson, and Jörg Vögele. The Studies for the Society for the Social History of Medicine series editor at Pickering & Chatto, David Cantor, has been very stimulating from the start, and we would like to thank him for his encouragement. Above all, we are grateful to the contributors to this volume for their continuing intellectual engagement, their hard work and their patience; and to Anne Hardy for her meticulous correction of the English.

LIST OF CONTRIBUTORS

Rosemary Elliot is a lecturer and researcher in the School of Social Sciences and the Institute of Health and Well-being, University of Glasgow. Her research focuses on the social and medical history of late nineteenth-century to present-day Britain and Germany, particularly in relation to addictive behaviours, gender and public health. The research discussed in this volume is part of a project looking at smoking and health in post-war East and West Germany, funded by the Wellcome Trust.

Larry Frohman received his PhD from the University of California, Berkeley with a dissertation on the German philosopher Wilhelm Dilthey, and he is currently an associate professor of history at the State University of New York at Stony Brook. His first book, *Poor Relief and Welfare in Germany from the Reformation to World War I* was published in 2008 and he has published several articles relating to various aspects of the welfare state. He is currently working on a project entitled 'Surveillance, Privacy, and the Politics of Personal Information in the Federal Republic of Germany'.

Anne Hardy was on the academic staff of the Wellcome Institute for the History of Medicine and its successor the Wellcome Trust Centre for the History of Medicine at UCL, from 1990 to 2010. She is currently Honorary Professor at the Centre for History in Public Health, London School of Hygiene and Tropical Medicine. Her book *Salmonella Infections, Networks of Knowledge and Public Health in Britain, 1880–1975* will be published by Oxford University Press in 2014.

Klasien Horstman, trained in historical sociology, philosophy and science and technology studies, studies the relationship between medical expertise and technology and society. She was Professor of Philosophy of Bioengineering at the Technical University Eindhoven, the Netherlands (2001–9) and in 2009 she was appointed Professor in the Philosophy of Public Health at Maastricht University, the Netherlands. She published, besides many international articles, *Public Bodies, Private Lives. The Historical Construction of Life Insurance, Health Risks and Citizenship in the Netherlands 1880–1920* (2001) and *Genetics from Laboratory into Society. Societal Learning as an Alternative to Regulation* (2008).

Frank Huisman is Professor in the History of Medicine. He teaches in the History Department of Maastricht University and at the University Medical Center Utrecht. He is also Past President of the European Association for the History of Medicine and Health. He has published on medical historiography, quackery and the cultural authority of medicine and is the author of *Stadsbelang en standsbesef. Gezondheidszorg en medisch beroep in Groningen 1500–1730* (1992), a local case study of early modern Dutch health care. He has co-edited, with John Harley Warner, *Locating Medical History. The Stories and their Meanings* (2004). He is now working on a book exploring the transformation of the Dutch health care system between 1880 and 1940.

Harry Oosterhuis teaches history at the Faculty of Arts and Social Sciences of Maastricht University. His research focuses on the cultural and social history of psychiatry and mental health care, of sexuality and gender, of health and citizenship and of bicycling. He is author of *Stepchildren of Nature: Krafft-Ebing, Psychiatry, and the Making of Sexual Identity* (2000), co-author of *Verward van geest en ander ongerief: Psychiatrie en geestelijke gezondheidszorg in Nederland (1870–2005)* (2008) and co-editor of *Psychiatric Cultures Compared. Psychiatry and Mental Health Care in the Twentieth Century: Comparisons and Approaches* (2005).

Evert Peeters is a cultural historian. He has published on the history of science, medicine and the body. In particular, he has studied medical discourses on urbanization and the spread of new sorts of body culture since the twentieth century. Currently, he is working on psychological expertise and labour performance during the interwar period. He has also been exploring patriotic cultures of the past. His books include *Beyond Pleasure. Cultures of Modern Asceticism* (co-edited with Leen Van Molle en Kaat Wils, 2011) and *De beloften van het lichaam. Een geschiedenis van de natuurlijke levenswijze, 1890–1940* (2008).

Martin Powell is Professor of Health and Social Policy at the University of Birmingham. He has research interests in the history and evaluation of health services in Britain, and has received grants from the Economic and Social Research Council, the National Institute for Health Research and the Wellcome Trust. He has published over seventy articles and ten books on areas including British voluntary and municipal hospitals, evaluating health reforms and health inequalities policy in Britain. His latest book is a co-edited text entitled *Shaping Health Policy: Case Study Methods and Analysis* (2011).

Matthew Ramsey teaches history at Vanderbilt University, where he served as founding director of the Center for Medicine, Health and Society. His main research interests are in the history of medicine, medical practice and public health in Europe, with an emphasis on modern France. His current work deals with the history of therapeutics, including the medicinal uses of now taboo substances, such as excrement and human body parts and their elimination from the pharmacopoeia in the eighteenth and early nineteenth centuries.

Ine Van Hoyweghen is Research Professor at the Centre for Sociological Research (CeSO) at KU Leuven. Her work focuses on the societal, regulatory and ethical dimensions of biomedicine. In particular, she is interested in the ways in which science and politics constitute each other, and how they interact with understandings of humanness, sociality and citizenship. She is a member of the Young Academy of the Royal Flemish Academy of Belgium for Science and the Arts (KVAB).

Kaat Wils is Professor of History at KU Leuven and head of the Research Group Cultural History since 1750. Her research deals with the intellectual history of the humanities and the biomedical sciences in the nineteenth and early twentieth century. Among her publications are *De omweg van de wetenschap*, on positivism and intellectual culture in Belgium and the Netherlands between 1845 and 1914 (2005) and, co-edited with Evert Peeters and Leen Van Molle, *Beyond Pleasure. Cultures of Modern Asceticism* (2011).

THE POLITICS OF HEALTH AND CITIZENSHIP: HISTORICAL AND CONTEMPORARY PERSPECTIVES

Harry Oosterhuis and Frank Huisman

At the end of the Second World War, health was defined as a universal human right. The Preamble to the Constitution of the World Health Organization, drafted in 1945, states that '(t)he enjoyment of the highest attainable standard of health is one of the fundamental rights of every human being without distinction of race, religion, political belief, economic or social condition'.[1] And article 25 of the *Universal Declaration of Human Rights*, proclaimed by the United Nations in 1948, reads: 'Everyone has the right to a standard of living adequate for the health and well-being of himself and of his family, including ... medical care'.[2] In the course of the twentieth century health and disease became a matter for the state in most Western countries as well as in the former communist world. The provision of medical care is considered not just as a favour or a commodity, but as a civil right – no matter whether such rights are explicitly laid down in constitutions, in social security laws or in the administrative regulations of the welfare state.

The notion of health care as a civil right can historically be traced back to the enlightened human rights discourse based on natural law, the principles of the American *Declaration of Independence* (1776) and the *Déclaration des droits de l'homme et du citoyen*, issued by the revolutionary French National Assembly in 1789. In the past two centuries this ideal gradually materialized: more and more, medicine and politics became mutually entwined. Next to poverty, ill health was the first social issue targeted by the emerging intervention-state in the nineteenth century. Following the principle of a fair allocation of resources to meet basic needs, many countries introduced collective funding of health care in the course of the twentieth century in order to share costs equitably. Apart from inevitable biological distinctions between individuals, equal access to health care is an aspect of democratic citizenship.

All of this may be understood as the logical outcome of growing humanitarianism and democratization in combination with scientific and technological progress. However, collective health care arrangements were also supported by

authoritarian and totalitarian regimes. Also, there have always been counter
movements that seriously doubted the idea of scientific progress in medicine.
The relation between health and citizenship is far from self-evident and uncontested; it is fraught with complications and ambiguities. The idea that health care
is a civil right is easily formulated in the abstract, but practical implementation
is another matter. Unlike freedom of speech or religion, universal suffrage or fair
trial, health cannot be construed as an absolute, legally enforceable right. Not
only are individual health and illness to a large extent still a matter of nature and
fate, but the realization of health as a civil right also requires resources (money,
medical expertise and an adequate health care infrastructure), political consensus with regard to the relation between individual and social responsibilities and
a long-term perspective. Collective health care inherently nurtures conflicts over
the range of state-intervention, costs and priorities, and political control over
medical professionals and services.

From the background of the crisis of the welfare state since the 1980s, the
foundations of collective health care provisions were and are called into question, in particular because of the rising costs. Costs have continuously gone up
due to improved technological treatment possibilities, increasing numbers of
surviving and chronic patients and the ageing of the population. Ironically, to
a large extent advances in medicine undermined the affordability of socialized
health care and the political consensus on which they were based. The very success of curative medicine, the growing impact of preventive health care and the
promises of biomedical technology provoked rising expectations and growing
demands among the public.[3] Health became a central issue in a whole array of
institutions, agencies, services, commodities and policies addressing insurance,
risk prevention, lifestyle, living conditions, environment and well-being. The
substantive content of health tends to expand continuously and the right to
medical care appears to be infinite. This reflects a more general development
in modern societies: people's increasing reliance on scientific and technological
control has made it more and more difficult for them to accept the contingencies
of human life, including disease and death. Although since the 1960s medicine
has frequently been criticized by social scientists and patients' organizations, at
the same time most people cherish a faith in medical progress and its promise of
prolonging life, minimizing pain and securing a gentle death. At the same time,
tensions between regular and alternative medicine as well as the ascent of new
biomedical technologies have given rise to ethical and political controversies.

From the 1990s on we have seen heated public and political debates about
the organization and financing of collective health care as well as medical ethics.
One of the key questions was to what extent the state can be held responsible
for the health of citizens and the practice of medicine. Critics of the welfare
state argued that it had led to passive and dependent individuals relying on

care from cradle to grave and to an overloaded bureaucratic system that was no longer affordable in a competitive global economy. Praising the benefits of market dynamics, neo-liberals created a strong feeling that the state should withdraw from the social domain. In many countries collective arrangements were being critically reconsidered, reformed or transferred to 'the market'. Rationalization and commercialization brought in managers taking over control from professionals, creating new bureaucracies that to a large extent withdrew from democratic supervision.

Neo-liberalism not only affected the financing and organization of health care, but had other political implications as well. With respect to citizenship, it shifted the emphasis from collective solidarity to individual responsibility, from rights to obligations and from passive entitlement to active involvement. The redefined concept of citizenship, stressing individual autonomy and rational self-interest, suggests that health should be within the control of the individual. The state will be unable to guarantee adequate health care, the neo-liberal argument runs, if citizens do not act responsibly with respect to their own health and that of others. Attempts to curtail direct state intervention in the organization and funding of collective health care, however, have not diminished political interference with public health. The last decades have witnessed a growing involvement of governments in a public health discourse that stresses the danger of health risks and the need to take precautionary measures. There is a broad concern about the health risks of tobacco, alcohol, drugs, 'unsafe' sexual behaviour, overeating, unhealthy foods, lack of exercise, polluted environments, sun-bathing, stress and international migration and tourism. People are being warned of unhealthy lifestyles and admonished to change them. They are urged to have themselves vaccinated for contagious diseases and periodically screened for cancer and other ailments. Public health not only engages the interests of individuals and the state, but also the responsibility of citizens towards each other with regard to the possible unhealthy and polluting effects of their behaviour and consumption. For this reason, for example, smoking has been banned from many public places. One may wonder whether citizens have the democratic right to lead unhealthy lives and the question has been raised whether they are still entitled to the benefits of collective health insurance if they do so.

Recent developments make clear that 'health' and 'citizenship' are elusive categories that are time and again redefined, negotiated and disputed. We believe that they also should be historically analysed, as this volume attempts to do. Current debates about health care as well as about citizenship can be understood against the background of a process that originated in the late eighteenth century, when the contours of modern liberal democracy as well as of scientific medicine emerged. Since then, certain questions about the connection between health and citizenship have surfaced time and again and they are still relevant.

Can health be considered a civil right and what does such a right mean? The right to remain free from state intervention or the right to collective arrangements in the field of health care? Where lies the boundary between medical treatments that should be covered by them and those to be excluded? Given the fact that democratic citizenship not only involves entitlements, but also responsibilities and obligations, can health or the prevention of illness and a healthy lifestyle be imposed on citizens as a civic duty? To what extent is the state allowed to interfere with the (private) lives of its citizens? How should the responsibilities of state, civil society, the medical professions and individual citizens be delineated? How do collective health care arrangements, professionalism and democracy relate to each other? Is health a precondition for the realization of citizenship and to what extent is citizenship a precondition for health? Should the state deal with morally controversial biotechnological developments and related medical treatments? These are the leading questions in this volume.

Our call for a reflection on the changing relationship between health and citizenship does not imply the claim that knowledge of the past leads to clear-cut answers for the present. This volume does not intend to 'solve' current socio-political problems – as products of their age such solutions are always provisional and politically disputed – but rather to analyse the connection between health and citizenship historically and thus put contemporary debates into perspective.[4] We also suggest that health care is entwined with national traditions of state craft and citizenship. With this volume we want to develop not only a historical but also a comparative perspective. By soliciting chapters about five different countries (Great Britain, the Netherlands, Germany, Belgium and France), we hope to throw light on the way in which their health care cultures and systems were influenced by national models of citizenship.

This introduction offers a general outline of the relationship between models of citizenship on the one hand and the definition of health and illness and the practice of health care on the other. We will first explain why the linking of health and citizenship is relevant for medical historiography and how it might offer a new perspective on familiar subjects. Secondly, we will elaborate on the concepts of health and citizenship and demonstrate that they are essentially contested and historically layered concepts. Thirdly, we will offer a historical overview of the changing relation between (public) health and citizenship from the late eighteenth century to the present. We will conclude by returning to recent developments and problems in public health and medical ethics.

Health and Citizenship in Medical Historiography

Whereas studies by historians and political scientists on citizenship are manifold, the concept has hardly been applied explicitly in medical history. Medical historians who have worked on the development of public health and health policies, have not systematically explored the relation between health and citizenship. When they did examine it (usually implicitly), their narratives tend to be one-dimensional as well as teleological. Older, presentist historiography of public medicine suggests that the growing rapport between medicine and the state was both desirable and more or less foreordained, the ultimate outcome being socialized health care in the democratic welfare state.[5]

More recent work in the field is influenced by a Foucaultian perspective, according to which the interlocking of (scientific) knowledge and (professional) power resulted in the disciplining of bodies and minds. Michel Foucault and his followers argue that the modern idea of health was historically constituted when medicine and the human sciences delimited the normal and the abnormal. The medicalization of social relations turned what was considered as deviance into pathology. As exponents of an anonymous 'biopower' and 'governmentality', physicians played a key role in imposing social order and conformity.[6] From a similar angle sociologists such as Eliot Freidson and Irving Zola have focused on the strategies of physicians to expand their field of action by 'medicalizing' individual as well as social problems. Doctors were enabled to dominate the health care system because the state had granted them a large degree of professional autonomy in matters of (public) health.[7]

To a lesser extent, the history of public health has been inspired by Norbert Elias's theory of the civilizing process. The essence of this process is the shifting balance from external social constraint towards internalized self-control and it is brought about by functional specialization, social differentiation, lengthening chains of interdependence between more and more people and changing balances of power between social groups. In this view, the growing preoccupation with health and the introduction of collective arrangements are explained in terms of civilized manners, which the middle class supposedly imposed on the labour class and which were gradually also adopted by the lower orders. While the Foucaultian and professionalization perspective stress the disciplinary power of the medical profession, the Eliasian view emphasizes that the spreading and internalization of health norms was a consequence of changing social relations in society as a whole.[8]

Despite their differences these approaches all focus on the interplay of social coercion and rational (self-)control as the fundamental characteristic of modern liberal-democratic society. Without rejecting this viewpoint altogether, we feel that it is one-sided and incomplete. Medicine indeed became increasingly involved in social issues, but its impact on society was differentiated and diffuse.

By including the development of citizenship, we would like to draw attention to the complications and ambiguities in the changing interaction between medicine, professionalism, state intervention and politics. The expansion and socialization of medicine in the course of the last two centuries should not be interpreted as an inevitable and singularly linear development. Neither was medicine a uniform and overpowering social force that imposed its definitions and practices on society. The health policies of voluntary organizations and the state did not always accord with each other and they might conflict with the ambitions and interests of the medical profession and other social groups.

By focussing on the role of citizenship with respect to health (care), we attempt to shift attention from the social control perspective to an outlook that acknowledges human agency and redresses the balance between repressive and empowering effects. The development of modern medicine and public health was intertwined with the rise and expansion of democratic citizenship and civic participation. Their relation was one of conflict and restraint as well as mutual facilitation. The medicalization of social issues can involve serious infringements on civil rights and the subjection of individual interests to those of the collective or the state, but it can also function as a neutralizing and pacifying strategy to relieve social tensions and protect and advance individual rights. Medical knowledge, which has increasingly multiplied in a large diversity of scientific and popular viewpoints on health and illness, was not only deployed to further the power of the medical profession, insurance companies, pharmaceutical industries, state agencies and welfare bureaucracies. Information about health and illness has also increasingly been used by voluntary associations, social interest groups, patient organizations and individual citizens for their own purposes. As citizens, individuals should not be considered as passive victims of a monolithic and controlling medical juggernaut, with no other choice than to conform to its dictates. Citizens may play an active role in defining health and illness and in utilizing regular or alternative health care services.[9]

Health and Citizenship as Contingent and Contested Concepts

Health and citizenship are ambiguous and multiple-layered concepts. Both are open to a variety of definitions and interpretations. Their meaning as well as the connection between them are historically contingent and embedded in changing socio-political frames of thought, debate and practice, which not only reflect, but also shape their social realities. The contemporary debate about citizenship as well as about health care, for example, is closely linked with neo-liberal and neo-conservative criticism of the welfare state and of the controversial socio-political legacy of the 1960s and 1970s. Health and citizenship are essentially contested concepts: their definition and application are not self-evident, but always open for debate, negotiation and strife. Only a historical survey of the changing connotations of health and citizenship can shed light on their diverse meanings and shifting mutual relationship. Together, they relate to key issues like life and death, collective and individual well-being, independence and dependence, coercion and liberty, social solidarity and individual responsibility, public and private, professionalism and self-help, and humanitarianism and technocracy.

It is difficult to give an unambiguous definition of health, not only because it involves an array of aspects that no single description can fully cover, but also because the term can be used in both a descriptive sense and a normative one. As a concept, health may refer to a particular state of affairs as well as to specific ideals to be pursued. The simplest definitions describe health as the absence of disease or as the unimpeded physiological functioning of a body, enabling life's basic biological functions such as survival and reproduction. Such definitions, however, have been criticized as too limited and biologically reductionist. They have been replaced by broader descriptions that incorporate values concerning people's social functioning, reflecting a shift from preserving towards optimizing health in the sense of, as the World Health Organization has defined it, 'a state of complete physical, mental and social wellbeing'.[10] As such health not only refers to the ability to cope with everyday life without being hindered by some physical or mental malfunctioning, but it may also apply to the individual capacity to carry on in society and realize specific goals in life.

From the eighteenth century onwards, the elastic meaning of health has been expressed in the tendency to interpret more and more aspects of life – such as education, reproduction and sexuality, mental and behavioural disorders, addiction, criminality, labour relations, lifestyle, diet and family life – in medical terms. In the process, health came to be associated with the bourgeois catalogue of virtues, in which such notions as individual independence, self-sufficiency, self-control, responsibility, soberness and moderation, regularity and order, willpower, industriousness, achievement, utility, thrift, investment, cleanliness and moral purity occupied a prominent place. These qualities were geared to a controlled and progress-oriented life. As an essential precondition for optimal productivity, health in particular represented economic value. Partly as replacement of the Christian ideal of salvation, the idea gained currency that health was a good that could be actively pursued, not just by the individual but by society as a whole. Enlightenment thought assumed that advancing scientific knowledge of disease would automatically lead to the control of the human body and behaviour in such degree that overall health would improve. The pursuit of medical knowledge was considered to be an ethical and also political imperative grounded in the rational explanation of nature.

From the eighteenth century onwards, health and hygiene were essential ingredients of the bourgeois ethos and identity. They embodied key values with which the rising middle class distinguished itself from aristocratic idleness, frivolity and decadence, as well as from lower class disorderly conduct and debauchery. Health was associated with cleanliness and moral purity, whereas sickness was linked to dirtiness and depravity. As such, health represented the opposite of the way of life and attitudes of the poor and working class, whose irrational, impulsive, undisciplined and intemperate behaviour could only lead to endemic diseases. Whereas the aristocracy had asserted the exclusive character of its blood and the antiquity of its ancestry in order to maintain its status, members of the bourgeoisie stressed the health and vigour of their body and progeny.[11]

The political-philosophical roots of the middle-class health ideology can be traced back to the ideas of Thomas Hobbes (1588–1679) and John Locke (1632–1704).[12] Hobbes distinguished two bodies: the natural body of the individual and the man-made body politic, the state. By nature a human being, according to Hobbes, is driven by a restless pursuit of lust and the avoidance of discomfort, giving rise to a continuous urge for power and, given the scarcity of means, a struggle of all against all. This 'natural state' was ended because in the interest of their own safety people of their own free will surrendered the right to use violence to a sovereign, thus eliminating the war of all against all. Thus Hobbes formulated the liberal notion of the social contract and of fundamental civil rights. As he argues, the body is owned by the individual self, who possesses the inalienable right to protect it from pain and death, to sustain it and keep it in optimal condition.

Hobbes's notion of possessive individualism has been elaborated by Locke. He conceptualized not only possession of one's body, but also that of material goods as an inalienable individual right. This right to material possession followed from the right to possession of one's own body: what the body produces by means of labour, Locke argued, is the rightful property of the person who owns that body. In his view, individuals not only own their body and the products of their labour, but their thoughts, feelings, acts and experiences as well. Locke was one of the first to formulate the idea of a self-contained and continuous self as the essence of the individual. His *Essay Concerning Human Understanding* (1694) marks the conceptual transition from the Christian soul that is part of a supernatural order to the secular self as a self-reflective monitoring agent who considers his own inner life and outward behaviour.[13] Locke's view of the autonomous and self-responsible person is closely linked to his political doctrines, which hold that society is an aggregate of separate individuals rather than a collective entity. The state, founded on a rational and voluntary contract, is to protect the fundamental property rights of (male) individuals and not interfere in their private lives. Individual autonomy and freedom should be guaranteed, so that citizens can freely develop themselves. Possessive individualism was the core liberal value driving people to improve themselves and fulfil their potential, bringing about social progress in the process. As such, it was the basic principle underpinning liberal thought on citizenship as well as health.

The meanings of citizenship are at least as diverse as those of health and even more contested. Since the 1980s, citizenship has become a fashionable concept all over the political spectrum through which dissatisfaction with specific developments in present society are articulated and certain solutions are put forward. Several social and political issues have been formulated in terms of citizenship: the crisis of the welfare state, ongoing individualization and the presumed loss of social cohesion, growing ethnic and cultural diversity, the declining trust in parliamentary democracy and globalization. Discussions focus on the supposedly disturbed balance between rights and duties. All suggested solutions tend to take the direction of a revitalizing of civic virtues, which are defined in terms of individual autonomy and self-reliance as well as of active involvement and social obligations.

In general, citizenship is about what draws individuals together into a political community and what keeps that allegiance stable and meaningful to its participants. The sociologist Bryan Turner has broadly defined citizenship as 'a set of practices which constitute individuals as competent members of a community' and which 'over time become institutionalized as normative social arrangements'.[14] This overall definition can be specified by pointing to three basic constituents of citizenship, the liberal-democratic ideal in particular. First, citizenship has to do with rights and entitlements granted and guaranteed by the state on the one hand and with responsibilities and obligations towards the state on the other. Secondly, citizenship is about political and civil participation on the basis of a combined sense of individual autonomy and public commitment: it presupposes a capability of self-direction that is irreconcilable with subordination and dependence. Thirdly, citizenship refers to the more or less enduring allegiance between the individual and civil society, the social space of free association that is separate from the state, the market and the private sphere.[15]

The best way to clarify the notion of citizenship is by outlining its various historical forms in the Western world since the Renaissance. Overall, citizenship is a result of a modernizing process that replaced local, fixed and hierarchical patterns of membership in family, feudal and corporate networks with more abstract, flexible and egalitarian conditions of social belonging on a larger scale. The first forms of self-government emerged in autonomous towns, in which the public space of the Greek *polis* as an arena of debate for independent men served as a venerable model. The rise of modern liberal citizenship, which was inspired by the Enlightenment idea of the 'natural rights' of man, was a consequence of the centralization of states and their expanding influence on society. These provoked a growing sense of solidarity among their subjects and the assertion of their common rights vis-à-vis the government. Centralization and democratization went hand in hand: the revolutionary conflicts from the late seventeenth century onwards gradually transferred sovereignty from the body of the monarch (based on divine right and tradition) to the body politic of his subjects (based on a social contract), transforming dynastic states into nation states. The liberties granted by the state and the consensual means of governance following in their wake had to be actively secured by citizens. The implementation and expansion of rights – with respect to the number and range of legal, political and later also social rights as well as to the number and range of people who were entitled to them – was realized through political activism and struggle. The reverse implication of this democratization of citizenship was the growing interference of the state in society.

Ideal Types of Citizenship

The contours of citizenship took shape in the field of tension between freedom and equality, rights and duties, individual autonomy and the common good, uniformity and diversity, state and society, state administration and self-government, inclusion and exclusion and active (civic) and passive (civil) involvement. Passing over different national traditions, roughly five ideal types of citizenship, partly successive, partly overlapping, can be distinguished in Western history since the Middle Ages: (1) classical republican citizenship, defined by self-government and civic virtues; (2) classical liberal citizenship, stressing civil rights against intrusion by the state; (3) liberal-democratic citizenship, centring on political rights, in particular suffrage and political representation; (4) social-liberal and social-democratic citizenship, through which welfare entitlements are granted; and (5) neo-republican citizenship, that emphasizes civic responsibilities and obligations.

Classical republican citizenship, the early-modern interpretation of the Greek ideal of the *polis*, implied that citizens were both governors and governed and it stressed civic virtue, the obligation to serve the state. Republican citizenship was not only defined by administrative and military duties, it presumed undivided loyalty and total patriotic commitment. The republican ideal conflated state and citizenship and it subordinated personal life and economic endeavours to the public cause. It was not a democratic right, but an exclusive, honourable status. Only independent, propertied and reasonable men qualified as full citizens. To the extent that this ideal was realized, the location was the small-scale city-state, in which only privileged males could dedicate themselves to politics. Only during the Jacobin phase of the French Revolution did the republican ideal serve as a model for citizenship on a national scale. Jacobinism prescribed citizenship as the patriotic identity of every adult Frenchman as opposed to alternative identities connected to one's family, estate, region or religion. Efforts to realize this ideal, however, involved coercion, civil war and terror.

Classical liberal citizenship, entailing civil rights on a national scale, emerged in the late eighteenth century as a product of the Enlightenment ideal of natural, inalienable human rights, as proclaimed in the American *Declaration of Independence* and the French *Déclaration des droits de l'homme et du citoyen*.

They established the basic civil rights of individual freedom against unlawful intrusion by the state, such as the integrity of the person, the private sphere and property, equality before the law and freedom of religion, thought, speech, press and assembly. Liberal citizenship is based on the Lockean notion of the free and independent human being, who should be able to create his – not yet her – own destiny. Although it also refers to membership of a particular state, it is first and foremost about individual freedom and equality of opportunity. Liberalism stresses the importance of 'negative freedom': the right of citizens to be protected against improper interference by the state or third parties. Neither the state nor any other institution should be able to impose any particular vision of the good life or collective purpose. As long as individuals did not intrude upon the rights and liberties of other citizens, they should be free to determine their own ends. Whereas republican citizenship was exclusive and stressed active duties, liberal citizenship was inclusive and largely relied on the passive enjoyment of rights. Another difference is that the latter is only a partial state: whereas republican citizenship had absorbed the person in its totality, liberal citizenship only conferred legal status. In liberalism, the state and politics are not goals in and for themselves, but rather the instruments that should safeguard the individual's autonomy and self-development in private life, civil society and on the market.

However, classical liberal citizenship still resembled its republican predecessor to the extent that political rights and participation were still exclusive and elitist. For the better part of the nineteenth century suffrage and eligibility were restricted to the minority of the male population that met certain requirements of property, independence and education. The granting of political rights was geared to the liberal values of possessive individualism and independent contractual exchange. Women were excluded from political citizenship (and to some extent even from full civil citizenship) and the same was true for lower middle-class and working-class men – to say nothing about the poor, colonized peoples or, in the United States, black slaves. Through the gradual extension of suffrage in the late nineteenth and early twentieth century, liberal citizenship was democratized. More and more people acquired full political membership of the national community. Universal suffrage and eligibility established the right of all adult citizens to have access to the parliamentary process and be represented in government. This was the outcome of the struggles of the labour and feminist movements, of the introduction of a comprehensive national system of education, of mass-mobilization during the First World War and, last but not least, of the response of the governing elites to the threat of revolution. They tried to counter massive upheaval by granting political and also, to an increasing extent, social rights, in return for co-operation and national integration.

Social-liberal and social-democratic citizenship originated in the late nineteenth century and, through the workings of the welfare state, matured in the

second half of the twentieth century. This form of citizenship involves entitlements (and obligations) that concern economic and social security, including
income, education, health and welfare. Such entitlements, in particular income-
guarantees in case of sickness, disability, unemployment or retirement, provided
formal rights with a material foundation. Social citizenship was the answer to the
contradiction between liberal ideals (individual autonomy and opportunities) on
the one hand and capitalist realities (social and economic inequality) on the other.
The argument underpinning social citizenship is that civil and political rights can
only materialize when there are no social and economic impediments to their
exercise. Social security, welfare assistance, state-funded education and collective
health care arrangements are put in place in order to mitigate socio-economic inequalities induced by the free market. The main goal of the various emancipation
movements emerging from the late nineteenth century onwards was to remove
obstacles blocking the realization of citizenship for disadvantaged groups: first
the working-class men, followed by women, and later, from the 1960s on, also
youths, ethnic minorities, homosexuals, the handicapped and medical patients.
The 1960s protest movement and other emancipation movements of the 1960s
and 1970s can be seen as a continuation of the development of liberal-democratic
citizenship, embracing now an array of social institutions and also what until then
had been considered as the private sphere. Unequal relations of power in society as
a whole were questioned and politicized. There was a strong belief that the welfare
state would fully realize the egalitarian and integrative potential of democratic
citizenship and thus enable all people to participate in civil society and politics.

The most recent model of citizenship, the neo-republican one, evolved from
mounting neo-liberal and neo-conservative criticism of social citizenship. In
the 1980s and 1990s, debates on citizenship centred on the presumed decline
of civic virtues in Western democracies and they marked the end of the tacit
post-war consensus, which had been articulated most clearly by the British sociologist T. H. Marshall in his *Citizenship and Social Class* (1950).[16] Defining
equality as the core value of democratic citizenship and considering liberalism as
its starting-point, Marshall distinguished three historical phases in its development: civil, political and social citizenship – as discussed above – which were
institutionalized in constitutions and law courts, in parliaments and in welfare
arrangements respectively. According to Marshall, the history of modern citizenship is basically a progressive extension of rights. After the gaining of civil
liberties and universal suffrage, the realization of social rights constituted the
pinnacle of democratic citizenship. The welfare state would guarantee the well-
being and full participation of all citizens in society. Social security, universal
education and comprehensive health care would eventually remove all inequalities that hampered individual emancipation and civil participation.[17] Marshall
postulated a fundamental antagonism between citizenship and capitalism.

Although capitalism had generated individual freedom and high standards of living, full citizenship in the sense of equal opportunity for all could only be realized through the domestication of the market-economy by the state.

Marshall's social-democratic model, which formed an influential paradigm for the post-war welfare state in Western Europe, came under pressure from the early 1980s on. Critics, ranging from neo-liberals and neo-conservatives to feminists, communitarians and political theorists, argued that his model was inadequate, both for understanding the historical development of citizenship in different countries and for meeting the challenges contemporary Western democracies were facing. Marshall's account of the development of citizenship in terms of succeeding phases and linear progression seems to be modelled on the British example and holds true for countries like France, the Netherlands and Belgium as well, but it does not apply to countries like Germany and the former communist world.

In Germany the absence of a successful bourgeois revolution and the incorporation of the middle class and the working class in the nation from above by an authoritarian government, resulted in a superficial realization of political citizenship and a significant implementation of social citizenship. Neither Nazi Germany nor the Soviet Union and other communist countries provided substantive civil and political rights, but social citizenship was developed to a large extent. This suggests that the establishment of social citizenship before the full realization of civil and political rights may obstruct the development of civil society and democracy. Neither does Marshall's model reflect the development of citizenship in the United States. American citizenship, rooted in the classical liberal notion of possessive individualism with its connotations of independence, self-interest and contractual exchange, continued to be centred on civil and political rights and duties. As far as an American conception of social citizenship exists at all, it focuses on obligations to the community rather than welfare entitlements. Welfare and social work are associated, not with civil rights, but with voluntary and private charity implying altruism, unilateral gift-giving and getting something for nothing.[18]

Marshall's story is basically about liberation from oppression and deprivation and the political struggles to obtain, extend and give substance to formal rights. However, as his critics point out, these rights have largely been articulated as passive entitlements while the other side of democratic citizenship, participation in public life and taking on social obligations, has been neglected. Marshall did not address questions about the relation between rights and duties and about the intrinsic quality of citizenship in terms of competence and responsibility.

The crisis of the welfare state prompted the neo-liberal attack on social citizenship, first in the United Kingdom under Margaret Thatcher and in the United States under Ronald Reagan and later in other Western European countries. The economic crisis of the 1970s and early 1980s and the growing volume of beneficiaries undermined the solvency of the welfare state. In the decades that followed it became the object of recurrent political controversy. Critics asserted that the welfare state was dysfunctional, both in its economic and in its welfare effects. It was trapped in a cycle of rising expenditures, taxes and wage costs, an overloaded public sector, decreasing entrepreneurial incentives and economic investments and an increasing exit rate from the labour force because of unemployment, early retirement and the massive distribution of employment disability allowances. Welfare provisions were not liberating, they added, but rather kept beneficiaries tied in dependence and strangled individual initiative. Also, more and more citizens – calculatedly or not – were abusing the welfare system. The sense of civic responsibility necessary to sustain the welfare state appeared to be crumbling. At the same time the welfare state had not removed poverty and social marginalization, but contributed to the rise of a dependent underclass and social disorganization. Such, in neo-liberal eyes, were the perverse effects of the rights-based, 'duty-free' practice of social citizenship that the welfare state had engendered.

The legitimacy of state-guaranteed social rights was also challenged on the basis of classical liberal principles. State intervention in social-economic life, which entailed that governments embraced certain values regarding how people should conduct their lives, was considered to be fundamentally at odds with the formal task of the state as a neutral arbitrator, which should restrict itself to upholding the law and securing civil and political rights. By blurring the boundaries between state, society and the private sphere, the welfare state became an overloaded apparatus for satisfying an endless array of personal demands and transformed responsible citizens into demanding welfare clients. Moreover, welfare from the cradle to the grave involved a state with paternalistic dimensions. Increasing bureaucratic regulation and tutelage by the helping professions threatened basic civil liberties and resulted in dependency and demoralization.

Neo-conservatives and communitarians backed up the neo-liberal rejection of social citizenship. In their view, the extension of welfare benefits in combination with the 1960s liberation movement had bred selfish, irresponsible and consumerist individualism. The result was an erosion of social cohesion, public morality and civil manners, while citizenship had degenerated into passivity: between elections, citizens had become spectators of rather than active participants in the democratic process. Moreover, democracy was undermined by declining political participation, growing voter-apathy, decreasing membership of political parties and social organizations and growing ethnic and religious diversity. Similar concerns, which were increasingly shared by representatives of the political left and advocates of participatory and deliberative democracy, became even more pressing in connection with concern about the continued existence of a marginal 'underclass' which had grown and diversified as a result of mass immigration from the underdeveloped countries. Even in the welfare state many people were suffering from poverty, unemployment, bad health and educational deprivation. Lacking autonomy, self-reliance and the social skills required for full participation in modern society, they could hardly be considered as full citizens. In addition feminists suggested that Marshall's concept of social citizenship still presumed a definition of politics as distinct from the private sphere of the family and a patriarchal approach to women. To a large extent, they argued, social security arrangements were geared to the traditional family: women, in their unpaid caring role of housewife and mother, depended on male wage-earners (or welfare recipients) and were thus designated a position as second-class citizens.

Criticism of Marshall's model was boosted by socio-economic and cultural changes in the Western world from the 1970s. The growing complexity, fragmentation and variability of the social fabric as a consequence of economic liberalization and globalization, the pluralization of individual lifestyles and cultural and ethnic diversity, affected the transparency of society and the belief in social engineering, on which the welfare state was based. The post-war welfare state was built on a more or less socially integrated and culturally homogeneous nation state, which had a large degree of control over a largely nationally organized and industry-based economy. Further, the gender-division of labour between male breadwinners and female caretakers in the family was taken for granted. Economically, the emphasis shifted from the manufacturing industry to high technology, information and services. Socially, alongside the traditional family, a plurality of alternative living arrangements evolved, which together with the ongoing process of individualization and emancipation of women, resulted in stronger claims for economic independence of individuals. Globalization and European integration as well mass immigration and increased ethnic and cultural pluralism affected the autonomy of and the loyalty to the nation and also the homogeneity of its culture. Cultural and religious heterogeneity have shaken the experience of shared citizenship.

In the 1980s and 1990s, a new ideal of citizenship was articulated in public debates by politicians as well as political and social scientists. This neo-republican model came down to a revitalization of liberal-democratic citizenship by infusing it with elements of the older republican ideal of active citizenship. It implies that the resilience of modern democracy depends on the attitudes of citizens, the mutual engagement of the state and its population and the vigour of civil society. Shifting the emphasis from social rights and benefits to duties and responsibilities, the new ideal focuses on the intrinsic quality of the practice of citizenship. Under the banner of 'civic-mindedness' it refers to an ensemble of social abilities and public virtues: independence, self-control, reasonableness, open-mindedness, the capacity to discern and respect the rights and opinions of others, tolerance without being indifferent, social and political participation and 'civil' behaviour in the public sphere.

To these virtues neo-liberal and communitarian merits were added. In the neo-liberal perspective, dominated by economic considerations and a strong belief in the benefits of a free market, citizens should be self-supportive and self-reliant, while the state should limit itself to facilitating private initiative, enterprise, labour force participation and education. Communitarians deny that these neo-liberal tenets are sufficient for realizing good citizenship. Rejecting naked self-interest and fearing social atomization, they hold that individuals are dependent on communities sharing a common basis of togetherness and account-ability. Apart from conservative norms and values such as law and order and the work and family ethic, they stress the significance of community-spirit and mutual assistance and care as civic virtues. Communitarianism is guided by the idea that the democratic public spirit can only be realized by active participation in civil society. While the role of the state is minimal in neo-liberal ideology, it is quite significant in the neo-republican and communitarian approach, making it acceptable to social democrats as well. The state should not just constrain the market and set the basic rules for civil society in order to prevent disproportional inequality and dependency. It should also create the preconditions for the devel-opment of active and competent citizenship, for example through teaching civic virtues and democratic values in schools, mandatory national service for youths, projects aimed at the cultural integration of ethnic minorities and the advance-ment of responsible and healthy lifestyles. At the same time welfare benefits have been trimmed and continue to be trimmed down and social rights are balanced by more duties and obligations than before. The welfare state has embarked on a new course by replacing 'passive' social security rights with more participatory structures. Absorption into employment, the work ethic, flexibility and mobility in the labour market, continuing education and the incentive to develop one's talents and abilities as well as one's health to their fullest extent, are key elements in new welfare regimes and the neo-republican ideal of citizenship. These policies have been accentuated as a consequence of the financial and economic crisis since 2008, which has put the tenability of the welfare state to the test.

The following four sections will discuss the implications of shifting models of citizenship (respectively the classical liberal, liberal-democratic, the social-liberal or social democratic and the neo-republican ideal type) for health and illness from the late eighteenth century to the present.

The Birth of Liberal Citizenship and Public Health

Although the body politic and the natural body had been metaphorically asso-ciated with each other since Antiquity,[19] traditionally medicine was mainly individual and private rather than collective and public as well as curative rather than preventive. There had been some state supervision and intervention in the sphere of medicine since the Middle Ages. In response to recurrent plague epidemics and in order to cope with the sick poor, (city-)governments had taken a variety of incidental measures, such as quarantine and *cordons sanitaires*. Medical practice was often regulated in state-licensed corporate organizations and physicians and surgeons were called upon in times of emergency such as war or, as forensic experts, in the administration of criminal justice. However, for the most part medical practitioners were self-employed and patient–doctor relations generally involved a personal contract or charity on an individual basis.

The private character of medicine continued to a large extent in the nineteenth and twentieth centuries, but from the end of the eighteenth century onwards, health care was also explicitly defined as a public issue and as a part of state policy. The political dimension of health and disease took shape against the background of the growing role of the state in the pursuit of a rational and efficient organization of society, an aspiration that was intensified by the secular optimism of the Enlightenment and the French Revolution. Foucault has characterized this new policy in terms of 'governmentality' and 'biopolitics'.[20] While traditional political regimes legitimized themselves through legal and religious arguments for sovereignty and the aim of rulers was to keep or augment their personal power, modern government consisted of the rational control and calculated management of a country's natural resources, population and economy. In traditional regimes the exercise of power was 'negative' with rulers affirming their sovereignty by taking the possessions and lives of rebellious subjects. The modern employment of power, on the other hand, was 'positive': it set out to control and regulate human life in order to improve the quality of the population in general and the labour force in particular. This implied that the advancement of the health of both individuals and the population as a whole was considered as a precondition for increasing the strength and productivity of a country.

The concept of 'medical police', introduced in some absolutist central-European states and adopted by Russia, Austria, Hungary, Denmark and Italy in the late eighteenth century, represented the first governmental attempt to establish a permanent public health policy. The classic formulation was the six-volume *System einer vollständigen medicinischen Polizey* (1779–1819), published by the physician Johann Peter Frank. He proposed that medical councils made up of civil servants and physicians be charged with the supervision of the health of the population and the prevention of contagious diseases. All this was part of the enlightened despotic project known as cameralism, which aimed at the centralization and rationalization of administration. By surveying all relevant physical and social living-conditions as well as individual habits with the help of systematic registration (statistics), an orderly and healthy society would be promoted in the interest of the state. Since in practice the means for implementation – financial and otherwise – were lacking, medical police was to remain a blueprint rather than a reality. Moreover, the project was conceived as part of a benevolent yet paternalistic instrument in the hands of autocratic rulers without engaging their subjects as active citizens and therefore it lacked backing by relevant groups within society itself.[21]

More long-lasting was the impact of the Enlightenment philosophy of natural rights and popular sovereignty as well as the liberal-capitalist doctrine of possessive individualism, stressing self-help and civic improvement. The Enlightenment belief that science and technology, through the rational control of nature and society, would bring about a better future implied optimism about progress in medicine and health care. The Enlightenment *philosophes* located morality within nature rather than in a Christian spiritual realm. Some compared themselves to physicians: as anatomists and radical diagnosticians of state and society, they would be able to analyse social and political pathologies and indicate a cure. Many were convinced that unspoilt human nature offered the foundation both for moral behaviour of the individual and for harmonious relations between the individual and society. In the context of the emergence of a science of man, physicians began to consider health and disease in terms of the interconnectedness between the individual, his living environment and society as a whole. Such ideas brought a closer rapport between health politics and the emergent bourgeois civil society. In France, Great Britain and the United States, the concern for public health was advanced by democratic impulses as well as by the economic rationality of possessive individualism and utilitarianism.[22]

During the French Revolution health care was discussed as a political issue. The Constituent Assembly committees on poverty and public assistance targeted illness as one major cause of poverty and proclaimed that 'society owes the ailing poor assistance that is "prompt, free, assured and complete".'[23] Rejecting traditional Christian charity and advocating scientific efficiency in the service of patients, in 1791 medical reformers proposed public health programmes and a national network of medical practitioners. Medical benefits would not only entail rights for citizens, but obligations as well: participating in medical interviews and physical examinations; fulfilling doctor's orders; following a healthy regimen and hygiene; undergoing preventive measures such as vaccination; and allowing autopsy of dead bodies in the interest of medical science. The basic idea was that the health of the nation ultimately depended on the responsibility and compliance of 'citizen-patients'. Motivating them to keep and restore their health was part of a wider advocacy of revolutionary civic virtues like self-respect, public commitment, respect for other citizens and national solidarity.[24]

The far-reaching revolutionary plans for public health care, however, came to nothing because of lack of money and expertise, political strife, the exigencies of war and – perhaps surprisingly – because of opposition by physicians. Afraid of becoming (underpaid) civil servants, they insisted on the individual relationship between doctor and patient. They prioritized reform of medical education and the organization of their profession over the creation of a public health system, establishing what has come to be known as 'the Paris school of medicine'. The revolutionary achievements in medicine included the replacement of traditional corporate rights, privileges and monopolies by licensing based on meritocratic principles; the innovation of medical education along clinical lines; and the organization of a new type of hospital in order to advance medical teaching and research along the lines of bed-side observation, systematic scientific analysis, pathological anatomy and the use of new diagnostic techniques. The French Revolution also entailed major reforms in the care for the insane. Replacing the fatalism of moral and religious views of insanity with an ameliorative medical approach, Philippe Pinel was one of the founders of modern psychiatry that sought to cure and rehabilitate the insane in the context of the new therapeutic facility set up to that end, the mental asylum.[25]

Even though the revolutionary ideal of the 'citizen-patient' was not realized, the link that was established between health and citizenship was to become a reference point during the nineteenth century. Reform plans were to a large extent inspired by the so-called *Idéologues*, a group of physicians and philosophers who believed in the possibility to transform both citizens and society through medical knowledge and social hygiene.[26] Assuming that the physical, the mental and 'the moral' were interconnected, they demanded a central role for vitalist physiology and medicine in the development of a comprehensive science of man. The study of man in its totality, synthesizing physiological and medical knowledge of the human body, passions, mind and moral attitudes, should be grounded in the empirical methods of observation and inductive reasoning. The intellectual source of *Idéologie*, which was expressed most systematically in the works of the philosopher Antoine-Louis-Claude Destutt de Tracy (*Eléments d'Idéologie*, 1804) and the physician Pierre Jean Georges Cabanis (*Rapports du physique et du moral de l'homme*, 1815), was sensationalism. This radical form of empiricism held that sensations are the primary sources of human perception, knowledge, understanding, judgement and behaviour.

Starting from the sensualist premise that the body and mind are both an integral part of nature, the *Idéologues* focused on the way human thinking and behaviour were determined by man's inborn dispositions, needs and capabilities as well as by his variable physical and social environment. Similarly, health and well-being were thought to depend on the interplay between individual nature, habit and living conditions. Therefore, they claimed authority for physicians in many dimensions of human life. The organization of society should be based on knowledge of how individuals, as interrelated physical, mental and social beings, functioned. Scientific information about bodily and mental operations would enable people to gear their behaviour to rational principles and improve their lives. Thus the science of man would replace tradition and religion as a moral standard and serve as a guide for good citizenship and the reform of society.

Believing in the perfectibility of man and society, the *Idéologues* embraced the revolutionary principles of individual liberty and equality of rights. They also supported the new republican order because its anti-clericalism encouraged free and unbiased scientific inquiry into the nature of man and society. Many of them were involved in revolutionary politics, but at the same time they feared the dangers of anarchy, ideological discord, uncontrolled collective violence and state terror, which were also part of the French Revolution. In their view the science of man was an important neutral instrument to establish and preserve social stability. The *Idéologues* shared the concern of succeeding republican governments to foster fitness for good citizenship. Their common aim was the moulding of self-conscious and loyal citizens who would adopt the general will as their own and who would subscribe to the rational foundations of social harmony. The ideal citizen was the healthy, balanced and well-tempered individual, who, through responsible and well-adjusted behaviour, contributed to the harmony and the progress of society as a whole.

The ideas of Cabanis and Destutt de Tracy about health as an issue of public policy inspired one of the founding fathers of the United States, Thomas Jefferson and several political thinkers associated with him. They also came to believe that biological, social and mental dimensions of man were interlocked and that their development depended on social, economic and political conditions. The enjoyment of health was considered a precondition for the complete enjoyment of civil liberty, which required a responsible and democratic government. According to Jefferson, despotic regimes bred ill health while democratic government was beneficial for health.[27]

Idéologie, which foreshadowed positivism, was not the only movement to construe a socio-political role for medicine. Inspired by French Enlightenment thought and against the background of the Industrial Revolution in his home country, the influential English philosopher of utilitarianism Jeremy Bentham also nourished far-reaching ideas about social reform in general and a politics of health in particular.[28] Like the *Idéologues*, Bentham was opposed to tradition and religion and he strongly believed in empiricism and the malleability of man and society. Bentham assumed that the principal human drive was hedonistic and egoistic: the avoidance of pain and discomfort and the striving after pleasure and happiness. A rational ordering of society should be based on scientific knowledge of human nature and of the practical ways to regulate behaviour in order to lead it in a social and moral direction. According to Bentham's hedonistic calculus the greatest happiness of the greatest number could be realized by making utility, a rational measure for right and wrong, into the dominant ethical principle and by introducing social engineering along the lines of secular and economic efficiency.

Bentham attributed a prominent role to medicine – in his view the first human science that had successfully adopted the empirical method of natural science – in his utilitarian reform projects. Considering a politics of health as an indispensable element in the advancement of social progress and harmony, he compared medicine to legislation and the administration of justice. Just as the doctor cured the individual body using a scientifically based treatment, which was attuned to the type and seriousness of the disease, the judge healed the social body by his balanced verdict, which should be proportional to the character and seriousness of a conflict or a crime. Both had essentially the same purpose: fighting grief and promoting the greatest happiness for the greatest number. Further, medicine and criminal justice resembled each other because of their potential preventive effects. Impressed by Edward Jenner's claim in 1796 that smallpox could be prevented by vaccination with cowpox, Bentham advocated various public health measures like fighting filth and poverty, providing clean air and water and improving labour conditions. In this context Bentham also pointed to the need of statistical registration of the population: creating transparency in society was a precondition for efficient surveillance and state intervention. As such, it was in line with his design of the Panopticon, the architectural structure he advocated as a model for prisons, poor houses, work houses, factories, mental asylums, hospitals and schools.

Bentham's historical reputation has been coloured to a large extent by Foucault's depiction of him as the architect of the surveillance society. The Panopticon has become infamous as the quintessential machinery for the connection of knowledge to power, resulting in the disciplining of bodies and minds and a chilling economic efficiency.[29] However, selectively focusing on the repressive effects of the Panopticon does not do justice to Bentham's work, which was largely inspired by democratic aspirations. Initially, he had assumed that social reform could be brought about by appealing to the reasonableness and benevolence of established authorities. However, when they disappointed him he grew convinced that the interests of traditional rulers and their subjects were in opposition to each other. Although Bentham was not in favour of revolution and championed gradual change, he opposed the monarchy, the House of Lords and the Anglican Church. He came to believe that freedom of information and debate, a considerable extension of suffrage, representative democracy and active citizenship would pave the way for the greatest happiness for the greatest number. The state should not limit itself to keeping law and order, but should also guarantee a decent subsistence level and equality of opportunity. To Bentham, good health for the greatest number was not just an economic desideratum, but also a democratic achievement. In the mid-nineteenth century his approach made itself felt in the British sanitary movement and it would be echoed in appeals for medical reform on the European Continent. The socio-political involvement of medicine would affect and complicate the relations between health and liberal-democratic citizenship.

The Sanitary Movement and Liberal-Democratic Citizenship

The Industrial Revolution and the emergence of a self-critical bourgeois civil society advanced social concern for the environmental causes of disease. The rise of the sanitary reform movement, first in Britain and France in the 1830s and 1840s and later, from around 1850, in Germany, the Netherlands and Belgium, was prompted by a combination of demographic, epidemiological, socio-economic and political factors. The disruptive effects of a fast growing population, industrialization and urbanization entailed massive poverty, unsanitary living conditions, nutritional deficiencies and new health hazards. Many people suffered from endemic diseases like smallpox, measles, rickets, tuberculosis, malaria, diphtheria, scarlet fever, typhoid, typhus and infantile diarrhoea, while cholera struck Europe in four lethal waves in the 1830s, 1850s, 1860s and the 1890s. The growing fear of social disorder sparked off public and political responses. Governments were facing a growing pressure, not only from physicians, but also from other professional and interest groups (like engineers, lawyers, civil servants and statisticians) and public-minded citizens (philanthropists, moral entrepreneurs, evangelicals and feminists) to take responsibility for health matters. Together, they put public hygiene on the agenda as an urgent problem calling for collective action and state intervention. In the course of the second half of the nineteenth century several infrastructural measures were taken with respect to urban cleansing such as sewerage, drainage, water supply and garbage collection. Public health laws were enacted, establishing national and local medical inspection boards and health councils and introducing (compulsory) vaccination and inspection of dangerous trades, food supplies, public buildings and private dwellings.[30]

Since the French Revolution, France had been the leading nation with respect to public health schemes. During the 1830s and 1840s however, Great Britain, the first industrial nation, set the tone in sanitary reform. Between the 1830s and the 1870s, a set of public health laws was enacted that was more comprehensive than legislation in any other European country and any American state. This is remarkable, given the fact that the liberal philosophy of *laissez-faire* was strongest in the Anglo-Saxon world. In Britain, central government was relatively weak, while individualism and civil society were strong. Sanitary reform was initiated by voluntary private initiative springing from philanthropic impulses and utilitarian considerations about social efficiency and national improvement. The undisputed leader of the British sanitary movement in the 1830s and 1840s was Edwin Chadwick, a lawyer and former secretary to Bentham. Chadwick devised the new Poor Law that was enacted in 1834. Following utilitarian principles, it differentiated between the deserving and undeserving poor, between those being unable and those being able to work. Since deserving poverty appeared to be caused by ill health to a considerable degree, Poor Law medicine expanded in order to increase the numbers of the poor being able to work. A survey of the health of the working classes in England and Wales, published by Chadwick in 1842, suggested that the diseases of the poor were caused by environmental filth that generated putrid vapours, the so-called *miasmata*. Whereas tradition-ally, poverty and ill health were explained in terms of moral failings, Chadwick shifted the emphasis to the environment and the living conditions of the poor. His preventive solution, for which the operative slogan was cleanliness, was not so much medical as social and above all technical. In his view engineering was crucial for sanitary reform: the provision of clean drinking water, effective sewerage and drainage, paving, removal of garbage and filth from the streets, control of industrial effluents and offensive trades, the supervision of dwellings and the establishment of standards of environmental and personal hygiene.

Chadwick's analysis was underpinned by statistical research mapping the dis-tribution of disease and death and correlating such biomedical data with various parameters like geography, class, income, age, sex and occupation. The statisti-cal 'biometer' – developed by the leading French sanitary reformer Louis René Villermé – came to serve as a standard for comparing health situations in vari-ous places. In the 1820s and 1830s Villermé had pioneered this scientific method by producing numerous socio-medical studies. Although his work also indicated that poverty and illness frequently went together, Villermé's solution differed from Chadwick's. It boiled down to the moral regeneration of the lower classes, civiliz-ing and disciplining them out of poverty through philanthropic benevolence and paternalism. Such an approach hardly lent itself for purposive state action. After the bourgeois July Revolution of 1830 leading sanitary reformers embarked on a new course by embracing liberal policies and positivistic social science.[31] Economic modernization, industrialization in particular and administrative reform were con-sidered important for the advancement of public health. During the revolution of 1848 physicians, who were partly inspired by Saint-Simonianism, were involved in attempts at political and social reform, but these were not lasting. French sanitary legislation was far from compelling and the state was slow to translate it into prac-tical policies, despite the French centralist and *étatist* tradition.

In Germany, appeals for sanitary reform were also triggered by social and political tensions. Just before the outbreak of the revolution of 1848, the Berlin physician Rudolf Virchow had been commissioned by the Prussian government to carry out an investigation on a serious typhus epidemic in Upper Silesia. In his report Virchow explained its outbreak in the context of the geography, economy, social relations and culture of the region. His conclusion was that the spread of typhus had been caused largely by poverty, ignorance, backwardness, conservatism, political and religious repression as well as the Prussian govern-ment's reluctance to improve the living conditions of the Polish population in Silesia. Only through removing the obstacles posed by traditional culture, socio-economic modernization and especially, as Virchow wrote, 'full and unlimited democracy' and 'education with its children freedom and well-being', was a structural improvement of the people's health condition feasible.[32] For Virchow, who was supported by other liberal physicians and sanitary reformers, there was no difference between public medicine, science and politics. Medical students should be trained in natural science and physicians should serve as attorneys of the poor. As one of the most outspoken liberal leaders of the democratic left in Berlin he applauded the revolution of 1848. In the journal *Die medicinische Reform* (Medical Reform), which he co-edited in 1848 and 1849 and which advocated 'the great struggle of criticism opposing authority, natural science opposing dogmatism', Virchow argued that endemic diseases and recurrent epidemics were symptoms of social malaise.[33] Only thorough socio-political reform would offer an effective and humane prescription.

As a medical researcher Virchow was associated with an ambitious group of Berlin scientists. They attempted to link physiology and medicine to chemistry and physics and reorganize science radically on a materialist and experimental basis. Their scientific programme was in strong opposition to the Romantic *Naturphilosophie* and implicitly also to autocratic political regimes and dogmatic religion. In their explanation of biological phenomena they rejected the vitalist understanding of life as a hierarchically organized whole and at the same time propagated liberal-individualistic values.[34] Significantly, Virchow, who became famous because of his path-breaking research into cellular pathology, metaphorically associated the cells of the body as the autonomous units of life with the individual citizens in a republic. Cells lived in what Virchow called a 'cellular democracy', while the body could be viewed as a 'republic of the cells'.[35] In the 1860s and 1870s Virchow was one of the leaders of the Progressive Party (*Fortschrittspartei*) and as a long-time member of the liberal opposition in the Prussian Chamber of Deputies he criticized Bismarck's authoritarian government in the Prussian *Obrigkeitsstaat*. He also devoted his energies to the reorganization of Berlin's sanitary and public health facilities. Virchow and his associates clearly claimed that medicine involved politics and that a healthful existence should be a constitutional right of citizenship.

In the Netherlands and Belgium, hygienics, which evolved from the 1840s, was also rooted in liberal political ideology. Using statistical evidence, some leading physicians established that there was a causal relationship between the spread of epidemic diseases on the one hand and living conditions and social and political influences on the other. Hygienists argued that science-based and state-supported preventive public health care could provide a major contribution to social progress, national regeneration, economic prosperity and social harmony. People should not resign themselves to disease or premature death, but should take destiny into their own hands: active intervention in social conditions was urgently called for. The Dutch and Belgian hygienists were guided by the liberal ideal of citizenship, pertaining to free individual development and productive virtue. At the same time they viewed society as an organism, arguing that the whole was more than the sum of its parts and that harmonious collaboration constituted the foundation of social order and the improvement of the quality of life. Citizens owed it to themselves as well as to their community to lead industrious and virtuous lives, but many people fell ill through no fault of their own. Since all citizens should have the right to keep and improve their health, government should take the appropriate preventive measures with the help of the medical profession.[36]

In many countries ambitious plans for sanitary reform were proposed, but their implementation was controversial: they were entangled with delicate issues like individual versus collective rights and responsibilities, the legitimate sphere of influence of central government and the sanctity of local autonomy, private property and enterprise. Public health schemes were often inspired by liberal-democratic impulses, but at the same time staunch defenders of liberal principles opposed them. One of the legacies of the French Revolution with respect to democratic citizenship was the dilemma of civil liberties and individual freedom against solidarity and the common good. Conceptualizing politics as distinct from the private as well as the economic sphere, classical liberalism emphasized the principle of minimizing state interference in society. The programme of sanitary reform, on the other hand, was based on the recognition that some sort of intervention was necessary to secure a more or less harmonious functioning of society in accordance with public interest. Liberalism vacillated between *laissez-faire* philosophy (allowing individuals to pursue their own interests) and utilitarianism (seeking the greatest good for the greatest number).

Many liberals – and conservatives tended to support them – rejected public health measures and legislation because they believed that such compulsion would undermine personal freedom, the operation of the free market and local autonomy. Since civil rights and liberties were highly cherished and a sense of urgency for sanitary reform often seemed to be lacking, its implementation frequently met with opposition or indifference. Compulsory health regulations might provoke popular resistance, which was difficult to ignore for political leaders who, with the extension of suffrage in the last decades of the nineteenth century, had to take the expanding electorate into consideration. Controversies about compulsory smallpox vaccination, the compulsory treatment of tuberculosis by isolating patients and the medical regulation of prostitution in order to combat sexually transmitted diseases were cases in point. In Britain for example, the country that was at the forefront of sanitary reform, the laws and regulations concerned were repealed or watered down.[37]

Implementation of public health measures was also hampered by the ambiguous attitude of the medical profession. There was no monolithic block of physicians pressing forcefully for the incorporation of medicine within the state administration. Apart from social reformers, like Bentham and Chadwick and members of the urban medical elite, the majority of physicians did not take much interest in public health schemes. While the elite committed itself to science and social progress, the rank and file of the profession was pursuing narrower professional interests relating to income, working conditions and social position. For most of the nineteenth century, the large majority of physicians worked in private practice and constituted a group of minor entrepreneurs of rather low prestige. The public image of doctors was one of intra-professional squabbling and weakness. They were dependent on the approval, trust and fee-for-service payment of their (upper and middle class) patients and competition between practitioners, including non-licensed healers, could be fierce. Traditional patronage and corporate organization had been replaced by meritocratic ideals. Physicians operated largely on the free market, which might be lucrative, but which for many of them was also insecure.[38]

Although employment in public health positions represented professional opportunities for physicians, as a group they remained rather ambiguous and divided about the role of the state in health care. Apart from national differences between the Anglo-Saxon world, where physicians generally operated on the market as a free profession and continental countries like Germany and France, where the medical profession was more closely associated with the state, in general the professionalization of medicine was double-edged. On the one hand physicians were striving for autonomy and self-organization in order to be able to shape the conditions of their occupation themselves. Large segments of the medical profession, which were attached to economic liberalism and the concomitant bourgeois values of individual initiative and independence, feared being subordinated by the state. On the other hand, they were keen on safeguarding some degree of state regulation to protect their professional status and licensing procedures and to reinforce their control of the medical market. As soon as such occupational objectives had been realized more or less, professional medical organizations tended to retreat into defending their privileged interests. Cherished professional values, such as exclusive scientific knowledge, expert authority and compliance of the patient were largely at odds with public health schemes, in particular if these implied a more democratic and egalitarian vision of medicine. At the same time, physicians who were involved in sanitary reform and public health, tended to shift their focus from a liberal-democratic programme of social progress to a more narrow scientific and technocratic approach.[39]

When, in the last decades of the nineteenth century, liberals were confronted with the advent of mass democracy and the social question, they began to recognize that they had to abandon the principle of *laissez-faire* in its pure form. In order to cater to the needs of an expanded electorate, the state had to shoulder greater social responsibilities. In order to create more equal social and economic preconditions for materializing the ideal of democratic citizenship, social liberalism paved the way for increasing state intervention in society. As a consequence, more and more sanitary goals were realized, and at the same time the character of public health changed. In the 1830s and 1840s the sanitary project had started as a broad movement aiming for social reform. Connecting disease to poverty and the detrimental effects of urban, industrial society and tending to consider health as a right of citizenship, a broad coalition of public-spirited social reformers, advocated public health aims on socio-economic, humanitarian and political grounds. The miasmatic theory of disease, offering an atmospheric explanation of disease causation, underpinned an environmentalist programme of disease control. In the last decades of the nineteenth century, however, medical expertise increased its hold on public health, replacing the idealistic involvement of voluntary groups. From the 1880s and 1890s onwards, bacteriology and epidemiology toned down the relevance of the larger social environment while reinforcing a biomedical and technocratic approach. Whereas bacteriology was looking for disease-causing organisms in the laboratory, epidemiology set out to understand the spread of diseases through statistics and identify individuals and social groups who harboured injurious germs. Both were geared to the contagion theory of disease and implied that public health was to be based on specialist scientific knowledge and expert authority and that the role of lay social reformers should be limited.[40]

The growing role of medical professionalism in public health can be explained against the background of the tension between the increasingly felt need to respond to social problems and disturbances in a democratizing mass society on the one hand and the liberal reluctance to state-intervention on the other. Since liberal democracy was based on the principle that the government should respect and guarantee civil liberties, the liberal art of social policy was often not based on direct state interference. It rather took the form of 'governing at a distance' or indirectly with the help of professional expertise outside the state apparatus. By delegating the execution of social policies to more or less independent, state-regulated – but not state-controlled – helping professions and their administrative networks, such interventionist strategies were removed from the disputed terrain of democratic politics and ideological controversy. Professionals applied putatively neutral scientific knowledge about what is normal, virtuous, healthy and efficient. By using various methods – education, persuasion, disciplining, inducement, management, incitement, motivation and encouragement – socio-political concerns about poverty, social unrest and disorder, criminality, depravity, abnormality and disease could be translated into expert language and dealt with by technical means. The lack of democracy associated with professionalism was compensated by the professional ethos, which presupposed personal integrity, scientific competence, technocratic efficiency and disinterested dedication to the public good.[41]

Professionalism became a crucial feature of the liberal-democratic order, but at the same time they were at odds with each other. Next to the positive or inclusive link between professionalism and democratic citizenship, which we will discuss in the next section in the context of social citizenship, there were also negative, exclusive ones. The first relates to the development and growing popularity, from the late nineteenth century onwards, of alternative forms of healing, such as homeopathy and counter-cultures of health, like in the German *Lebensreform* movement. These movements doubted the liberal belief in progress through science and technology and they also resisted state-supported professionalism. Alternative and 'natural' healing practices involved disputes about the exclusive right of professional physicians to medical treatment and the legitimization of such a monopoly by the state versus the right of citizens to decide for themselves and to withdraw from professional regimes.

Another negative relation concerns the fundamental ambiguity of the liberal order. While in principle committed to equal rights and opportunities, in practice it often subordinated democratic values to what was considered the collective good, national interest and economic efficiency. Under the cloak of professional regimes, the liberal threshold of individual rights and liberties might be crossed or even violated. A case in point is the turning away from environmental and social reform approaches to biological ones in public health, social hygiene and psychiatry. This shift manifested itself not only in the rise of bacteriology, but also in the growing impact of degeneration theory, Social Darwinism, criminal anthropology and eugenics in the late nineteenth and early twentieth century.

Two years before Charles Darwin published his *Origin of Species*, the French psychiatrist Benedict Augustin Morel, in his *Traité des dégénérescences physiques, intellectuelles et morales de l'espèce humaine* (1857), had devised a theory of retrograde evolution. According to Morel, pathological phenomena were caused by the combined effect of environmental and hereditary influences. Adapting the Lamarckian idea of the inheritance of acquired characteristics, Morel explained how a pathogenic environment and the extraordinary demands of modern civilization affected the behaviour and constitution of individuals, who consequently passed on the damage to their offspring. Following their inevitable biological course, inherited physical and mental disorders deteriorated over the generations and would ultimately result in racial decline. The spectre of degeneration presented a dismal counter-current to the predominantly optimistic outlook that the Darwinian emphasis on natural selection seemed to propagate.

In the second half of the nineteenth century the theory of degeneration found widespread acceptance, especially in France, Belgium and Germany.[42] Projecting the stigmata of deviance onto the lower stages in the evolution of mankind, the idea of degeneracy suggested a causal relationship between normality and progress and between abnormality and decay. Physical disorders, mental retardation, insanity, nervous disorders, sexual perversion, alcoholism, prostitution, suicide, crime, the declining birth rate and sometimes even political agitation and women's emancipation were all treated as the effects of widespread biological decline. Concern about degeneration signalled a crisis in the optimism that had characterized both liberalism and positivist science. The broad social acceptance of hereditary thinking signified a turn away from environmentalism and optimistic notions of social reform. It undermined Enlightenment faith in benevolent nature and the hope that through the scientific discovery of its rational laws, individual and social diseases could be cured. Degeneration theory was grounded in determinism: forces outside of and predating the lives of individuals were believed to shape them in ways beyond their control. Thus, disease and other abnormalities were considered to be the result of natural destiny.

The theory of hereditary degeneracy as well as Social Darwinism interpreted social and political issues in biomedical terms. The Enlightenment concept of human nature, stressing the fundamental similarities shared by all men and forming the basic assumption of democratic equality, was superseded by an increasing emphasis on inborn differences and 'natural' inequalities between (groups of) men: those of race, gender and class as well as of the contrast between rationality and insanity. Society was no longer viewed as the sum of its individual citizens freely interacting and associating, but rather as an organism in which the hierarchical interdependence between its parts was a guarantee for its stability and harmony. Society was compared with a living body that could suffer from illness and its supposed decay was discussed as a natural fact. Thus, the concept of degeneration and other biological theories not only naturalized existing social and political relationships, but also provided a rationale for medicalizing a wide variety of social problems. This biomedical perspective reflected deeply felt conservative and liberal fears of the 'dangerous' classes in cities and other social groups regarded as public nuisances, of recurring revolution and class struggle and of mass democracy, socialism and the emancipation of women. An increasing amount of 'non-social' and 'unreasonable' behaviour in mass society as well as growing demands for further democratization were believed to undermine the bourgeois ideal of controlled freedom. Discussion of the danger of degeneration expressed a more general fear among the middle classes of 'the primitive', which was supposed to be embodied in the residuum among the poor, the insane, criminals, alcoholics, prostitutes and sexual perverts. Labelling them as atavistic misfits in an evolving world, physicians and social theorists conferred the stigma of mental and social inferiority to such people. Stressing the naturally determined inequality between individuals and groups, degeneration theory and social Darwinism made it possible to distinguish between various levels of social integration within modern society. Thus, the biomedical sciences implicitly set a standard for citizenship and offered an instrument to legitimize the exclusion of several social groups from political rights.

The more liberalism allied itself with nationalism and its concomitant values of moral integration and national vitality, the more the right of the state and professional experts to set the standards for collective survival overrode the claims of private interests. Against this background, segments of the medical profession allied themselves to purity movements, stressing the need to promote morality and to outlaw obscenity, indecency and depravation. They garnered much support in predominantly protestant countries like Great Britain, Germany and the Netherlands. By the late nineteenth century, the concern over depopulation and biological decline became something of an obsession affecting many nations, France in particular, but also Great Britain and Germany. National rivalries, for example between France and Germany, were framed in Darwinian terms of demographic battles for the survival of the fittest. In Great Britain the experiences of the Boer War in South Africa led to concerns about the physical deterioration of the nation as a whole and efforts to strengthen 'national efficiency'. The ability of the nation to defend its vitality against internal weak spots became the criterion for its external security. Embracing a social-hygienic role, physicians expanded their professional domain by claiming expertise in what they framed as social pathologies, such as alcoholism, crime, sexual perversion, mental disorders and educational deprivation.[43]

Around the turn of the century, the precepts of eugenics seemed to promise a rational mastery of the laws of evolution. Such trends occurred in many countries, albeit in different degrees and with more or less serious consequences as far as civil rights were concerned. Several American states and Scandinavian countries, for example, enacted eugenic laws enforcing measures like institutional segregation and mandatory sterilization of those regarded as 'unfit'.[44] In Germany in particular eugenics gained an increasing following among the medical profession in the first decades of the twentieth century.[45] Under the Nazi regime, physicians endorsed nationalist and racist policies. In the Third Reich social issues like poverty, crime, 'asocial behaviour', sexual deviance, ethnicity and the Jewish 'question' were largely defined and dealt with as biomedical problems. Employing the rhetoric of medical emergency, many leading Nazis considered their politics as applied biology. In their world view, the German people suffered from deadly diseases. Their 'cure' was racial purification, moving from coercive sterilization, euthanasia and segregation for 'hygienic reasons' to direct medical killing and genocide. Nazi racial hygiene dictated a 'total cure' of the nation through its purification from Jews, gypsies, ethnic minorities, psychiatric patients, mentally retarded and hereditary sick people and homosexuals. Physicians played an active role in large-scale, mandatory sterilization and euthanasia programmes as well as enforced medical experiments on humans in concentration camps. The Nazi regime did not corrupt a supposedly neutral biomedical science: its radical policies built on the strong affinity of the German medical profession with biomedical reductionism, its absolute trust in scientific expertise and its lack of democratic values. In fact medicine had been politicized early on and, conversely, it lent Nazism a specifically scientific and technocratic character.[46]

Collective Health Care and Social Citizenship

The Nazi regime, which has been characterized as a 'biocracy', can be considered as an extreme example of the undemocratic, coercive and excluding effects of medicine's linkage with state policies. However, beginning in the nineteenth century and intensifying in the twentieth century, more democratic and inclusive liaisons between medicine and the state developed, and they were more enduring.

The sanitary movement of the nineteenth century, both in its earlier social-environmentalist and its professional biomedical form, was not just a medical project targeting disease and unhealthy living conditions. Sanitary reformers also addressed questions of social order and integration of the working class and poor into the industrializing, urbanizing and democratizing mass society. Public health was one of the first social projects in which professional groups – not only physicians, but engineers, lawyers and civil servants as well – used their expertise to make themselves advocates of the public interest and civil virtues. Crossing the boundaries between the private and the public and wavering between the voluntary and the coercive, 'the social' emerged as a domain for professional intervention in the lives of the dispossessed.[47] Sanitary reforms included the missionary zeal to civilize the lower strata of society and educate them into middle-class values, at the same time making life for the middle classes less dangerous and more pleasant. The miserable health conditions of the lower orders, especially the possible spreading of contagious diseases like cholera, also endangered the health of the middle class. And out of well-understood self-interest, the middle classes became prepared to pay for collective arrangements in the field of public health and to allow for a certain degree of state-regulated professional intervention.[48] Although it implied paternalism and disciplinary strategies, sanitary reform simultaneously, through articulating what was healthy and clean as well as normal and virtuous, was also geared to making responsible citizens out of the working class and the poor. Professional regimes not only put constraints upon people: as democracy advanced they also operated by co-opting them and by encouraging and guiding their self-control, self-direction and self-development. Targeting individuals and groups who supposedly did not behave in their own self-interest or who seemed to be indifferent to their own advancement, professionals like physicians were involved in the constitution of citizens who would be capable of regulating themselves and bearing a kind of controlled freedom.

The late nineteenth and early twentieth century not only witnessed the realization of various sanitary reform plans, but also the introduction of the first social insurance schemes for workers covering sickness and disability. The state would increasingly assume responsibility for the accessibility of health care provisions for all of its citizens. Older practices of subsidized health care as an aspect of charity and poor relief were increasingly replaced by collective insurance schemes and state guaranteed entitlements. All of these reflected the growing political emancipation and enfranchisement of the working class and the poor. Health care benefits – and obligations – were an important ingredient of social citizenship.

In several industrial nations the health risks of industrial workers – not only sickness, but also injuries caused by accidents on the work-floor – were taken into account as a result of the pressure of the socialist movement, trade unions, social reformers, enlightened capitalists and medical professionals. Sickness, disablement and life-insurance funds, developed by voluntary associations, mutual aid societies, trade unions and political parties, contributed to the collective identity and political mobilization of the working class. Sooner or later such endeavours were taken up and extended by the emerging welfare state and they would also include unemployment, widowhood and retirement. In Germany the first social insurance legislation laws for workers covering sickness, disability and accidents were introduced in 1884 by Bismarck's government. They were part of the strategy to counteract the spread of socialism and to bind the working class to the state. In other countries, like Great Britain, France, the Netherlands and Belgium, social liberals, seeking to balance individual freedom and some basic social security through collective arrangements, laid the foundations of the welfare state. Both the authoritarian German government and the more liberal-democratic governments of other Western European countries increasingly followed a middle way between liberal *laissez-faire* and socialist collectivization. Social security arrangements offered themselves as exemplary solutions to the social question, reconciling labour and capital in the interests of social stability and turning potential revolutionaries into loyal citizens, who were expected to internalize middle-class values. Collective insurance would foster a rational, methodical and responsible conduct of life and would bind claimants and beneficiaries into a system of solidarity and mutual obligations.[49]

When epidemic diseases had successfully been overcome, other public health issues began to assume prominence: poor nutrition, infant mortality, vaccination, child-raising, domestic hygiene, alcoholism, venereal diseases, tuberculosis and other endemic chronic illnesses. New forms of public health care and social hygiene, originating from voluntary associations as well as initiated by local and national governments, concentrated less on the social environment and more on individuals and their behaviour. New methods and institutions, such as health-education, social work, house visits, maternity allowances, material assistance, out-patient clinics and social hygienic welfare centres, were based on a mixture of support, encouragement, regulation, surveillance and compulsion and they especially addressed women. Specialized sanatoria, public and private, for tuberculosis and nervous and other disorders, involving segregation in rural areas, a medical regime, pedagogical instruction and various degrees of coercion and discipline, multiplied rapidly in the late nineteenth and early twentieth century.

The new model of social citizenship that social insurance and collective health care arrangements forged, came to be considered in terms of rights instead of a mere favour. They fostered in the lower classes a sense of entitlement that might further politicize them, the more so because tensions arose over provision and payment of benefits as well as over the coercion that new public health policies entailed. On the other hand, many public health activities depended on the more or less active co-operation of the targeted populations, which they might be willing or not willing to give, depending on whether such interventions accorded with their self-interest and enhanced their living conditions.[50]

Although social and medical insurance and the expansion of public health activities entailed an extension of the professional domain of physicians, which they generally embraced, many physicians were ambivalent about social medicine in as far as it might lead to a loss of professional autonomy. Their growing involvement as advisors and medical examiners in collective insurance schemes implied the control of medical practice by welfare bureaucracies and insurance companies. Social politics in the field of health care often provoked resentment and more or less successful resistance from the medical profession, distrustful as many physicians used to be of any threat to the liberal model of a 'free' profession and of any tendency to transform them into state functionaries.[51]

Despite objections by the medical profession, the provision of collective health insurance for all citizens in order to make medical services broadly accessible, became an issue after the First World War in many countries – at the same time as universal suffrage – at least for men – was introduced all over the Western world. The 'Great War', which took a heavy toll of the life and health of so many male citizens, was the final confirmation that health was a national concern and belonged to the responsibilities of government. After Germany had set the example for social legislation and the communist regime in the Soviet Union for socialized medicine, national health insurance schemes were discussed and partly implemented in Britain and France between the two world wars. The economic depression of the 1930s and the post-Second World War reconstruction prompted states in the Western world to become far more active in social planning. In the Netherlands a national sickness fund for lower income groups was introduced by the German occupying force during the Second World War. After the war the United Kingdom, as part of the construction of the welfare state, took the lead with the introduction of a National Health Service for all citizens in 1948. Other countries, like New Zealand, Canada and Sweden, also took the path of national-ized health care provision. In the Federal German Republic, the Netherlands and Belgium, gearing their welfare systems to social market economies, a combina-tion of private insurance and socialized sickness funds continued to prevail. The French state, relying on corporate planning, gradually realized a comprehensive national health insurance system for all citizens between 1945 and 2000.

The collectivization of health care essentially occurred in one of two forms. Great Britain, some Scandinavian countries and the former communist countries, among others, opted for nationalized, publicly funded and govern-ment-organized health care, in which physicians lost much of their professional autonomy. Most other European countries opted for a budgetary funding system, with government, in consultation with the medical profession, setting the rules and conditions and citizens having the obligation to purchase health insurance, either from a private insurance company or, for those in the lower income range, through public health funds. Although in these countries the organization of health care was largely in the hands of social and (semi-)private organizations, it was monitored and supervised by the government, while the medical profes-sion still managed to secure considerable autonomy. In the United States there was – and still is – strong resistance to any notion of socialized medicine. Here a stronger emphasis on the market as provider of medical services has prevailed, including the need to have private health insurance to pay for them. Medicaid and Medicare, introduced in the mid-1960s, were essentially government-subsi-dized medical insurance for social security recipients and the elderly.[52]

As a result of broad coverage and open-ended fee-for-service, in many coun-tries collective health insurance schemes and care systems have forced up costs much higher than expected.[53] In the welfare state the thing modern citizen-patients value most in life, is their health. The rising demand for health care follows from the increased treatment and prevention options, growing life expec-tancy and the increasing frequency of controllable chronic diseases, the higher expectations regarding health and the development of advanced medical tech-nologies. Also, the domain of medicine expanded, moving from treatment and prevention of disease towards the preservation and improvement of health and well-being, including the realization of personal wishes regarding, for example, appearance, parenthood and euthanasia. New biomedical technologies – such as in vitro fertilization, surrogate motherhood, psychotropic (designer) drugs, embryonic stem cell research and genetic engineering – are (or will probably be) no longer used as a cure for ill-health only. The line between therapy for patholo-gies and the enhancement of body and mind tends to be blurred. Furthermore, a host of social issues, for example, abuse of women and children within the nuclear family, traumas and victimhood, sexuality, diet, addiction, disability and work-related problems and conflicts, sports and lifestyle, have partly been put under a medical regime. From the 1960s and 1970s onwards, the health care system in the welfare state more and more became a domain without limits. The boundaries of health and normalcy were stretched according to the expanding supply of health care services as well as the insatiable needs of the citizen-patient. The view of health as an inalienable right of social citizens entailed continuously rising costs. At the end of the twentieth century, this budgetary problem of the welfare state was crucial in bringing about a neo-liberal re-orientation with respect to health care as well as citizenship.

The New Public Health and Neo-Republican Citizenship

The growing impact of neo-liberalism since the 1980s, emphasizing the benefits of the market and a new, neo-republican ideal of citizenship in terms of freedom and autonomy, has entailed major shifts in health care. The endeavour to curb costs and to push back state regulated welfare schemes involved the introduction of economic considerations and market mechanisms in the organization and delivery of care. A more or less free market of health products and services and the dynamics of competition were expected to bring about a balanced mediation of supply and demand as well as transparency to all parties involved. In reaction to the soaring costs of high-tech medicine and the rising demand it excited, managers were set to work alongside physicians to align medical expertise with budgetary discipline and economic efficiency. Thereby new forms of administrative and bureaucratic regulation emerged, which were withdrawn from democratic control.[54]

At the same time medicine continued to broaden its scope to the protection of the still healthy from sickness by means of the detection and prognosis of possible illnesses in the more or less distant future. The predictive and preventive approach, fostered by the growth of epidemiological surveys and new techniques of medical surveillance, screening and monitoring, is based on a view of health and illness as a continuum, a statistical style of reasoning and the notion of risk. The so-called new public health is part of a wider emphasis on anticipating and preventing dangers and undesirable events like illness, abnormality and deviant behaviour. Sociologists such as Ulrich Beck, Anthony Giddens and Robert Castel have pointed to the rise of risk calculation and management as ways of dealing with growing uncertainties and contingencies in technologically advanced and deregulated liberal societies. Considering everybody at any moment as a potential patient, predictive and preventive medicine focuses on health risk profiles in relation to factors such as age, social class, occupation, gender, living-environment, lifestyle and consumption. Interventions take diverse forms such as genetic testing, periodic check-ups, screening and monitoring of groups at risk for specific illnesses, supervision over the health of children, public education about 'risky' lifestyles, products or environments, community and personal skills development and health promotion.[55]

The new public health is all about providing individuals with information about their health status and possible health risks in the near or more distant future, so that they can act to reduce those risks and preserve or even improve their health. At the same time the risk discourse, although embracing the neo-liberal slogan of transparency, does not provide ultimate certainty, but, on the contrary, generates its own discord about what constitutes a risk, its implication and how to respond. Scientific and expert knowledge on health risks is intrinsically provisional and time and again gives cause for disagreement, not only among experts, but also between expert and popular views. Medical information is increasingly located in the free market, where competition and various players with different interests are involved: physicians, medical researchers, public-health experts, epidemiologists, the manufacturers of foods and medical instruments, the pharmaceutical and fitness industries, health magazines and patients and their support organizations.

Conflicting and changing knowledge about sources and levels of risk, brought on by the ever-expanding range of information, services and products, has moved public health policy and expert systems towards identifying the individual as ultimately responsible for the assessment and avoidance of risk and danger. Patients as well as healthy individuals are framed as active and self-conscious 'health consumers', who are or should be well-informed about their health-status and who supposedly can take responsibility for their own health and well-being. The rise of 'healthism' implies that people are expected to be active in keeping and optimizing their health by adapting a healthy lifestyle including a balanced diet, regular exercise, stress-management, curbing smoking and drinking and avoiding unsafe sex. Such demands fit in with the neo-republican ideal of citizenship stressing a reflexive, competent and entrepreneurial self. Healthism requires the replacement of passive 'welfare dependency' rights by active citizenship, shifting the emphasis from entitlements to duties and responsibilities. Individuals whose behaviour is deemed contrary to the pursuit of curbing risk and advancing health, are likely to be considered as lacking self-control, rationality and responsibility. As such they appear not to be fulfilling their duties as citizens and the question has already been raised whether or to what extent they should still be entitled to collectively funded health care.

Both the neo-liberal emphasis on the free market and transparency and the consideration of health in terms of risk management assume individual autonomy, responsibility, free choice, knowledge, competence and motivation. This neo-republican ideal of citizenship has also put its stamp on debates about ethical issues that have resulted from the increasing medical possibilities to subject the beginning, course and end of human life to manipulation and control. This broadening of medicine's role entails new relationships between doctor and (future) patient and between medicine and other social institutions such as government and insurance companies. Autonomy is the key concept in medical ethics as well as contemporary notions of citizenship. According to this principle, which from the 1970s on also has been advocated by the patient movement, adults have the right – and to a large extent also the duty – to self-determination and self-organization of their lives. In the Netherlands, for example, autonomy serves as the basic principle of patient's rights in medical practice. The Dutch Constitution of 1983 guarantees the right to the inviolability of the human body, while a law enacted in 1995 stipulates that medical treatment should be based on informed consent by the patient.

However, autonomy is not without problems. Not only is it far from self-evident that this high-flown ideal and the related neo-republican civic virtues are achievable for everyone, they are also contradictory to the experience of (chronic) illness and the practice of care. Being ill, implying suffering, pain, dependency, anxiety and confusion, often entails an infringement on or a lack of self-determination. In this sense illness is the opposite of the liberal-capitalist ideal of possessive individualism, on which the modern ideal of autonomy is based. Does not the experience of being ill and the certainty that we will all die make us aware that our ability to own and control our bodies is extremely limited and that in fact the body owns and controls us instead of the other way around? In addition, the emphasis on autonomy tends to privilege cure over care and thus reflects the traditional gender division of labour in health care. In opposition to the intellectual, rational, scientific work of (predominantly male) doctors, aiming at cure and thus restoring autonomy, nursing, associated with menial tasks as well as emotional support and nurture, has been conceptualized as a natural female activity. Care, which presupposes dependency of patients, in particular those that suffer from chronic illnesses, was and is often considered of a lower status compared to the progress made by medical science in the field of curative treatment.[56]

Also the neo-liberal conceptualization of the patient as a freely choosing consumer is problematic. Patients do not always have the proper information at their disposal to be *able* to choose – full transparency is more often a promise than a reality – and it is questionable whether they always *want* to have a choice. Moreover, the conditions in which patients typically find themselves differ from those of consumers on the free market. Despite commercialization and privatization, the largely monopolistic offerings of collectively funded health care and the conditions imposed by health insurers limit patients' freedom of choice. The neo-liberal promotion of customer-friendliness by gearing the supply of medical services to the demand of health consumers, is at odds with the increasing standardization, scaling-up and bureaucratization of health care and the growing influence of intricate and specialist scientific knowledge and medical technology.

The principle of autonomy also seems to be inadequate to solve the ethical problems and political controversies that arise in the context of the practices of predictive and preventive medicine as well of biotechnology. Apart from the question what might be the implications of biomedical technology for the definition of what will count as a human subject and citizen, human and civil rights are at stake.[57] Let us point to three sets of questions and problems as far as the present relationship between health and democratic citizenship is concerned.

First, the suggestion that health and illness depend on individual choice and responsibility not only plays down the differences between individual bodily constitutions, but also underestimates the extent to which ill health is still being determined by social-economic and cultural factors. There is a real danger that the new preventive interventions will benefit the healthier part of the population instead of those with fewer opportunities due to deprivation, lack of education, unemployment or ethnic and religious background. Predictive and preventive medicine may give rise to a dynamic of health standards being forced up. The consequence might be that those who cannot meet them – for example the chronically ill, the elderly, the physically and mentally disabled and psychiatric patients – are downgraded and marginalized as second-class citizens, despite their formal rights.

Secondly, in some ways predictive and preventive medicine may even undermine the very principle of autonomy. By providing knowledge about the chance of becoming ill later in life, they call into question the open future, which the principle of autonomy presupposes. Such predictions not only have an impact on personal life and further feelings of uncertainty, but may also entail serious social consequences such as refusal by insurance companies, banks, mortgage lenders or employers to consider those diagnosed with potential future ill health. Predicting health risks may result in discrimination and social exclusion and thus undermine the democratic principles of freedom, equality and solidarity, which are the foundation of civil and social rights. This raises the question whether governments have a task to safeguard civil rights vis-à-vis the practices and consequences of predictive medicine. As information on individual health profiles and risks is increasingly stored in data banks, the accessibility and the control of such information touches on the civil right of privacy and the inviolability of the body.

The third set of problems concerns the professional power of medicine to define what constitutes a health risk, who is at risk, what the consequences of such risks are and which measures should be taken. Informed consent, which is now an important principle in medical ethics and which has confirmed the patient as a citizen-patient, is difficult to realize in predictive medicine. For a variety of reasons, people may feel compelled to undergo its interventions: anticipation of regret about non-participation and feeling responsible for the health of next-of-kin, while at the same time not being able to assess either the value of its knowledge claims or the practical consequences of its predictions.

On the other hand there are indications that professional medical expertise, which legitimates itself by stressing scientific rationality and control, is increasingly disputed by critical citizens. Whereas in the past the medical profession was often accused of being authoritarian and paternalistic, now trust in public health programmes seems to be declining because their rational and technocratic approach is far removed from the daily experiences and lay meanings of health and illness. Further, increased access to a wide range of health information and to popular opinions about health and illness have undermined the credibility of experts and government agencies responsible for the top–down implementation of health policies. In the Netherlands for example, large-scale vaccination programmes to prevent epidemics of Mexican flu and cervical cancer met with widespread distrust and even resistance, thus undermining the effectiveness of such measures. The same holds good for campaigns to prevent heart and vascular diseases and other ailments though the promotion of healthy lifestyles. Health experts and government officials who urge citizens to be autonomous, expect them to take responsibility for their health according to rational insight. However, in practice autonomy may also imply that citizens choose not to be rational in this sense, that they have their own ideas about what is healthy or desirable and that they establish other priorities in their lives. Growing distrust among citizens seems also to be triggered by the fear of increasing government surveillance and control, which endanger the security of the private sphere. At the same time government is criticized for not adequately tackling public health problems. In the Netherlands the unhealthy consequences of environmental pollution and factory farming – such as antibiotics in meat-products and an outbreak of Q-fever – are cases in point.[58]

All of this raises the question of whether people should follow professional and governmental definitions of health risks or whether the lay public should be democratically enabled to form and express their own opinions about the merits, results and consequences of preventive and predictive medicine and biotechnology, as well as the ethical issues that are involved. Perhaps governments are tasked with initiating public debates in order to advance active, well-informed citizenship in the domain of health and illness, clearing the way for a range of viewpoints, whether or not experts consider these views to be rational. Also, more participatory structures of public health, in which citizens' own perspectives and experiences are taken into consideration, could be developed.[59] In this way citizens could be enabled to discriminate between good and bad uses of these medical practices on the basis of democratic empowerment and fundamental human and civil rights.

This volume is organized in three parts, each of which is devoted to a specific type of citizenship. Because developments differed across Europe and because there was always a time lag between the introduction of political ideals and their implementation, it is impossible to suggest a clean periodization with clear caesuras. The types of citizenship are ideal types; therefore, the periods partly overlap. Each of the parts is preceded by a short introduction, which will also introduce the chapters.

PART I: LIBERAL CITIZENSHIP AND PUBLIC HEALTH

After the French Revolution had proclaimed the principles of liberty, equality and fraternity, it was up to post-revolutionary generations to take a stance towards them. This section is concerned with the dilemmas of liberal citizenship, in relation to developments in (public) health care during the nineteenth and early twentieth century. All four chapters are about the relationship between citizens and the state in a period in which Europe was going through profound social (industrialization) and political (democratization) changes. Over the course of the nineteenth century, liberal democracy gradually took shape and the first contours of public health in industrial society appeared. Inherent tensions between liberal-democratic principles troubled the relation between health and citizenship. Each of the chapters discusses the contradictions within liberalism with respect to state intervention, the role of medicine in society and the protection of individual rights. Their common focus is the problem of reconciling freedom and distributive justice.

Matthew Ramsey outlines the tension between the promises of the French Revolution with respect to public health care and the liberal aversion to direct intervention by the state in society. Among other things, the constitution of 1791 had promised a broad system of public assistance, but the liberal respect for individual autonomy, private property and free enterprise hampered the enactment of compulsory legislation. Two major projects – one on poor relief and the other on medicine – sought to make medical assistance available to the poor. The authors of both projects, however, expressed distrust of a state apparatus exercising uniform control over poor relief and the provision of health care. As the project for poor relief evolved, it increasingly diminished the role of the state, emphasizing the contributions of voluntary philanthropy. In fact neither project was ever implemented. Indeed, again and again, arrangements for medical assistance to the poor reaffirmed liberal misgivings about state-intervention. In public assistance, commonly seen as a duty of society rather than as a right of the citizen, the state merely advanced private philanthropy and mutual aid – a policy that continued to dominate until the 1930s. To a large extent, public health measures depended on the good will and resources of local authorities. Over the course of the nineteenth century, a series of piecemeal measures extended the reach of medical assistance programmes at the level of the municipality and the *département*. In 1893, a medical assistance act made the provision of health care for the indigent an obligation for the municipality, the *département* and the state. The programme was highly decentralized, and many individuals who were too poor to pay for private insurance or membership in a mutual aid society, were not poor enough to qualify for government assistance. In the end, the French Revolution fell short of its high expectations. It had dismantled the network of local charitable institutions of the *Ancien Régime*, but it did not succeed in putting a new national system of public assistance in its place. Ramsey concludes that despite the high flown ideals of the Revolution, French citizens have never shared a common right to health care, and do not fully do so today.

The implementation of public health policies never went uncontested, especially when commercial interests were involved, especially in a liberal political context. By exploring the case of the British shellfish trade – an economically important yet unregulated industry – Anne Hardy shows that the state could not simply impose civic responsibility on society on the basis of unequivocal scientific evidence on the risks of the shellfish trade. In a way, entrepreneurship implied a one-sided interpretation of liberal citizenship in terms of freedom at the cost of the public interest. The suggestion that typhoid and gastro-enteritis might be transmitted to humans by eating sewage-contaminated shellfish caused a major food scare in Great Britain around 1900. After the connection was suggested by epidemiologists, the different interest groups quickly co-opted bacteriology in an attempt to either confirm or refute the claim made by epidemiologists. Since bacteriology was still in its infancy, its claims were contested. Its uncertainties were exploited by the liberal interests of free enterprise, which sought to reject moves by the state to impose hygienic controls on the shellfish industry. Thus, the decade around 1900 witnessed a collision between economic group interests and collective health interests. The issue raised questions of scientific authority, of the pros and cons of state intervention, and of the social responsibility of the food trade towards consumers. Hardy explores the clash of interests over shellfish borne typhoid, and the ways in which scientific knowledge was used by the different parties to argue their case. Initially, the fish trade had been determined not to give in to the regulatory demands made by science and the state. It had sought to destabilize bacteriological knowledge and ignored political calls to take responsibility for its products. However, under the pressure of loss of public trust (and hence market share), the trade had to give in and move towards self-regulation. One could argue that this is a case of citizenship and civic responsibility forced on entrepreneurs by the market – rather than by science or the state. Negotiated in the years between 1895 and 1905, the outcome of this crisis is suggestive of a preference for self-regulation and minimalist state intervention that may still be observed in British attitudes towards food safety.

Frank Huisman moves the focus from the domain of public health to individual health care. By looking at the debate on Dutch medical legislation that was current in the 1910s, he explores the strained relations between patient autonomy and professional medical authority. The debate is a perfect illustration of the democratic paradox. Liberal democracy was based on the principle that the state guarantees civil liberties. To liberals, social policies should not be based on direct state intervention but rather be delegated to professionals outside the realm of the state. By delegating policies to putatively neutral outsiders, their intervention was separated from political controversy. Over the course of the nineteenth century, this method of depoliticizing social issues had come to be accepted for the domain of public health. In individual health care, however, classical liberal principles were still very much alive. This became clear when in 1913, three Dutch lawyers submitted a petition to the Dutch parliament requesting the abolition of the monopoly of treatment for physicians. Because of all the inherent tensions mentioned above, the petition was taken very seriously. The social liberal ministers of the Dutch government were challenged by classical liberals to 'repair' earlier legislation. The three lawyers questioned the expertise of the medical profession and disputed the exclusive right of physicians to give medical treatment. Medicine should be in the service of the patient instead of the physician, they argued, and patients – being free citizens – should have the right to consult the healer of their choice. The petition caused much social and political commotion. As many as 7,700 people expressed their approval by signing it. While the petition was under consideration, many articles, brochures and pamphlets – pro and contra – were published. At stake was the authority of medicine vis-à-vis the rights of patients as free citizens. Huisman's chapter addresses the fundamental question also raised by the petition: how should the paradoxical relationship between patient autonomy and professional expertise be organized? He discusses this debate against the background of tensions between classical liberal principles and social liberal ideals. After a landslide victory in the general elections of 1917, however, the new government of Christian-democrats decided to leave things as they were.

In their chapter on *Lebensreform* movements in Belgium, Evert Peeters and Kaat Wils also look at disputes over the exclusive right of professional physicians to give medical treatment. Although Belgium is reputed to have been the most liberal country in nineteenth-century continental Europe, liberal physicians were in favour of state intervention in the field of health care in order to secure public health on the basis of scientific insights *and* their own professional interests. Nonetheless, although Belgium developed rather progressive initiatives in health care during the 1840s, the momentum of reform had been lost by the late nineteenth century. The liberal hygienist movement was hampered by the strong Catholic hold on government as well as by divisions within the Belgian medical profession. In the 1890s, a 'political counterculture of health' took shape, claiming the right of citizens to withdraw from professional regimes. They doubted the liberal belief in progress through science, and they resisted state-supported professionalism. For them, health was a personal affair in which the state had no right to intrude. Inspired by the anti-modernist German *Lebensreform* movement, they embraced alternative cultures of health. Peeters and Wils observe that the communitarian utopia of naturopaths and the social engineering of hygienists were alternative expressions of the same ambition. Both similarly diagnosed society, considering it as an organism on the verge of degeneration. However, naturopaths did not believe in the need for state-supported collective action. The cures which they proposed were neither collective nor disciplinary in nature. Contrary to the proposals of hygienists, the movement of natural healers advocated a strictly individual reform of lifestyle which the modern autonomous and self-responsible citizen had to perform on his own initiative, without external pressure. Alternative healers in Belgium contrived a project of health care in which citizens and their individual experience of illness and health played a central role. Opposing the dominant hygienist discourse with its patriotic and even nationalistic emphasis on the health of the nation, natural healers construed an alternative, more or less politicized ideal of a self-sufficient community.

As Ramsey remarks, the French Revolution had opened a new space for innovation and contestation in many fields, including health care. A debate on liberties and benefits should always begin with a debate on the nature and limits of liberty itself. As the chapters of this first part abundantly make clear, the outcome of these debates was by no means self-evident or straightforward; rather, it was highly dependent on national contexts, the interpretation of political principles and the financial possibilities of the moment.

1 BEFORE *L'ÉTAT-PROVIDENCE*: HEALTH AND LIBERAL CITIZENSHIP IN REVOLUTIONARY AND POST-REVOLUTIONARY FRANCE

Matthew Ramsey

In France, all citizens and, indeed, all regular residents are now guaranteed access to health care through the law on la Couverture Maladie Universelle, or CMU, passed in 1999 and implemented in 2000. The CMU, however, is not simply an act enforcing a fundamental right of the sort enunciated in 1948 in the Universal Declaration of Human Rights. The declaration proclaimed that

> everyone has the right to a standard of living adequate for the *health* and well-being of himself and of his family, including food, clothing, housing and *medical care* and necessary social services and the right to security in the event of unemployment, *sickness*, disability, widowhood, old age or other lack of livelihood in circumstances beyond his control.[1]

The language of the French text is less robust:

> A *couverture maladie universelle* is created for residents of metropolitan France and the overseas *départements* which guarantees to everyone health care coverage through a medical insurance policy [*une prise en charge des soins par un régime d'assurance maladie*] and, to those persons with the lowest incomes, the right to supplementary insurance protection and exemption from the requirement to pay charges up front [and then apply for reimbursement].[2]

Although *la prise en charge des soins* might suggest that the state assumes broad responsibility for health care, the expression here has the narrower technical sense of coverage by an insurance policy. Everyone is guaranteed health insurance, but the terms of the coverage remain undefined.

In 2000, shortly after adoption of the CMU, the European Union promulgated a Charter of Fundamental Rights. One article recognized an 'entitlement to social security benefits and social services providing protection in cases such as maternity, illness, industrial accidents, dependency or old age'. Another proclaimed a 'right' of access to health care, but stopped short of imposing new standards on member states and to some commentators seemed more the statement of a general principle than a basic right:

> Everyone has the right of access to preventive health care and the right to benefit
> from medical treatment under the conditions established by national laws and prac-
> tices. A high level of human health protection shall be ensured in the definition and
> implementation of all Union policies and activities.[3]

France remained committed to its own model for linking citizenship, rights and
health.[4]

Health Insurance and the French Welfare State

The CMU, like all the components of the French welfare system that emerged
in the aftermath of the Second World War, was the culmination of a long historical process. In the case of health care, the first national insurance law, passed
in 1928 and modified in 1930, applied to wage-earning workers with incomes
below a certain level and covered about 25 per cent of the population.[5] The
post-war social security system initially provided compulsory health insurance
for industrial and commercial wage earners, with the exception of some already
covered by a special scheme. Over time, new plans and occupational groups were
added. By the time the CMU was enacted, less than 1 per cent of the population remained uncovered. The end result is a remarkably complex system run by
quasi-public insurance funds supported by payroll and income taxes and supplemented by private insurance. Patients have free choice of physician; most obtain
coverage through their employers.[6]

The French welfare state is often called *l'État-providence*, an expression that
gained currency in the 1860s, primarily among critics, who warned of a dangerous tendency of the state to substitute itself for individuals. The term had
roughly the same force as 'nanny state' in English a century later, though over
time it came to be used in a more neutral sense. *L'État-providence* is arguably a
misnomer, in the absence of uniform state-run programmes funded entirely by
tax revenues. The substance is very similar, however, to what is usually understood as a welfare state and the basic framework is established in constitutional
law. The underlying principles were stated in the preamble to the constitution
of the Fourth Republic (1946), which started with the rights enunciated in the
Declaration of the Rights of Man and the Citizen of 1789 but added a set of
social and economic rights.[7] A long-standing critique from the Left had held that
the formal individual rights proclaimed in the Declaration meant nothing to the
dispossessed. The sociologist Dominique Schnapper argues that these new rights
made it possible 'to pass from formal citizenship to real citizenship, to assure that
individual citizens really exercise their rights', as the French revolutionary tradition of the sovereignty of the citizen required.[8] According to the preamble, 'The
Nation assures the individual and the family the necessary conditions for their
development' and also 'guarantees to everyone, notably the child, the mother

and old workers, the protection of health, material security, rest and leisure'. All those unable to work because of 'age, physical or mental condition, [or] economic situation' enjoy the 'right to obtain appropriate means of existence from the collectivity'.[9] The constitution of the Fifth Republic (1958) subsequently incorporated both the declaration of 1789 and the preamble of 1946.

Although the word 'right' appeared only once in the preamble, the text as a whole seemed to embody what was often called a second generation of rights, supplementing already established civil and political rights. They include, according to some jurists, a 'right to health', though that specific phrase appears in neither the constitution nor statutory law. It could refer to the provision of health care but also to protection against harmful products like tobacco or environmental hazards like asbestos.[10] Some recent commentators write about a third generation, including, for example, 'the right to live in an environment that is balanced and respectful of health', proclaimed in France's Environmental Charter of 2004. The charter was incorporated into the French Constitution the following year.[11] The concept of generations fits easily into a Whig narrative of progress, perhaps best exemplified in a lecture on 'Citizenship and Social Class' delivered by the English sociologist Thomas Humphrey Marshall in 1949. For Marshall, the steady growth of rights – civil in the eighteenth century, political in the nineteenth and social in the twentieth – had gradually reduced class inequalities, though it would never eliminate them. These rights affirmed that there is 'a kind of basic human equality associated with the concept of full membership of a community – or, as I should say, of citizenship'.[12]

The new body of rights, however, was not homogeneous and the preamble of 1946 was marked by tensions.[13] That fundamental rights might conflict had been clear since the French Revolution, which struggled to reconcile equality and liberty. But the 'second generation' of rights created a disjuncture between two different kinds of rights, often called individual and collective. Some writers distinguish between 'rights of' (free speech, for example) and 'rights to' (health care or shelter, for example). The terminology most widely used now by French scholars opposes *droits-libertés* to *droits-créances*. The former allow individuals to act freely without government interference so long as they do not infringe on the rights of others. *Une créance* is a claim, literally a debt due as opposed to a debt owed. The citizen is the creditor and the nation is the debtor, although as critics like to point out, there is no precise accounting that would allow one to specify the amount of the debt. The authors of a standard treatise on public liberties write that *droits-créances* 'confer on their holder not a power of free expression and free action but a claim [*créance*] on society, which, in order to satisfy it, is obliged to provide positive benefits which involve the creation of public services'.[14] They call, in other words, for governmental action rather than restraint.

A question hotly debated among French jurists is the extent to which the government is compelled to act in particular cases. Can a citizen turn to the courts to have a *droit-créance* enforced, or is the right rather an obligation of the nation as a whole that is not comparable to a subjective right enjoyed by an individual?[15] There is general agreement, however, that *droits-créances* can become concrete only through legislation that creates specific entitlements and that the government has the authority to set limits required by budgetary constraints or particular policies.[16] Such debates are, of course, part of a larger ongoing discussion on entitlements in a welfare state. Marshall, for example, writes that

> benefits in the form of a service have this further characteristic that the rights of the citizen cannot be precisely defined ... It may be possible for every citizen who wishes it to be registered with a doctor. It is much harder to ensure that his ailments will be properly cared for.[17]

This debate on liberties and benefits overlaps another debate on the nature of liberty itself. It begins with a distinction between negative and positive liberty, memorably developed by Isaiah Berlin in a lecture delivered in 1958.[18] He was not the first to use the terms. The radical philosopher Thomas Hill Green, who greatly influenced British 'New Liberalism' in the late nineteenth and early twentieth centuries, distinguished between 'negative liberty' and 'positive freedom, which consists in an open field for all men to make the best for themselves'.[19] The basic concept is older still. Negative liberty consists in freedom from constraint or interference, within certain limits. Positive liberty is something both broader and vaguer, the ability to realize one's fundamental purposes and become fully oneself. It aims for 'human development in its richest diversity', to quote the line from Wilhelm von Humboldt that John Stuart Mill took as the epigraph for *On Liberty* (1859).[20] The next step and the central question in the debate, is to ask to what degree positive liberty depends on assistance and intervention, requiring society and the state to do more than leave individuals alone. Education, whether private or public, is one commonly cited area of intervention. One could also argue that health is a precondition for self-development and that maintaining it may require external assistance as well as the individual's own efforts. This aspect of positive liberty may give rise to *droits-créances*. The final issue is to what extent upholding positive freedom may require some limits on negative liberty. Green, for example, emphasized the ways in which unlimited economic freedom for the most advantaged individuals had led to poverty, injustice and loss of freedom for the majority.

Rights and Assistance in the French Revolution

Like the debates on the rights of citizens, French programmes for delivering services have deep historical roots. The French social insurance legislation of 1928 and 1930 owed a good deal to the model established in Germany by Bismarck in the 1880s. The German government implemented it in the region of Alsace-Lorraine, which France had ceded to Germany in 1871 after the Franco-Prussian War. When France recovered its lost territory in 1919, the insurance programme remained in place and strongly influenced subsequent proposals. The legislation owed something as well to French traditions reaching back nearly a century before Bismarck. As the historian Paul Dutton has argued, the French health care system, together with its American counterpart, 'reflects the various interpretations of their eighteenth-century revolutions'. At the heart of these interpretations lay a central question involving far more than health care: 'whether individual liberty should be sacrificed for the sake of collective equality and the common good'.[21] Dutton cites Patrice Higonnet's comparative study of the American and French revolutions.[22] The same tension is also central to two major works by Higonnet on the French Revolution.[23]

Higonnet attributes the instability of the French Revolution to a failure to develop a successful synthesis of communitarianism and individualism. He characterizes the society of the *Ancien Régime* as fundamentally corporatist in its values and not particularly open to the ideology of possessive individualism, though corporate institutions had decayed. The Revolution opened a new space for innovation and contestation. In the period 1789–91, French legislators 'followed the principle of individualism more closely than had ever been done in any society'. A counter-reaction followed after the fall of the old monarchy in 1792. Different social groups embraced divergent values, with a 'basically individualist-minded possessing elite' confronting 'the deep-seated communitarian longing of French working people for a more regulated economic and social life'. For tactical reasons, the Jacobins (radical democrats) struck a bargain with the people, employing 'an increasingly meaningless communitarian rhetoric' while making a few practical concessions such as the price controls. They did not, however, change their profound individualist convictions and in the longer run individualism and property rights prevailed.[24]

In places, Higonnet uses the terms 'universalism' and 'communitarianism' interchangeably; he characterizes universalism as 'the communitarian legacy of tradition and civic humanism'.[25] For present purposes, it would be helpful to distinguish universalism (contrasted with particularism), on the one hand, from communitarianism (contrasted with individualism), on the other. The principle of universalism holds that the same rights apply to all humans in all times and places – *les droits de l'homme*. Within any society, all citizens have the same

rights and obligations, a point heavily emphasized by abbé Sieyès in his cele-
brated pamphlet *What is the Third Estate?*[26] Particular groups are not entitled to
privileges. The principle of communitarianism affirms the rights – or better the
claims – of the collectivity as opposed to the individual. The state, in addition
to enforcing individual rights may in some ways limit them for the larger good.

In the French Revolution, the universalist ban on privileges and the affir-
mation of equality before the law were generally unproblematic. The tension
between communitarianism and individualism raised more difficult issues, as
Higonnet shows. The case of the guilds and other corporations proved particularly complex. With respect to non-members they were holders of special
privileges, such as a monopoly on a trade in a guild town. Such privileges violated
the universalist principle of freedom of occupation and were finally swept away
in 1791. With respect to their members, they constituted a community which
both imposed restrictions, such as setting prices and standards for products, and
provided benefits, such as assistance to the sick, the unemployed and widows.
The power to regulate work and markets violated the principle of economic
freedom. The provision of assistance, however commendable in itself, rewarded
membership in a particular community rather than citizenship.[27]

The case of health care is still more complex. Where medical practice was
concerned, the public interest trumped freedom of occupation. Although the
abolition of the old corporations temporarily produced what some physicians
dubbed 'medical anarchy', this was not the legislator's intent. As Michel Foucault
has written, 'In fact, no one, not even the most liberal of the Girondists, dreamed
of freeing medical practice entirely and opening it up to a free regime of uncontrolled competition'.[28] As part of the post-revolutionary settlement, French
medicine wound up in 1803 with one of the strictest professional monopolies
in the world, enjoyed by state-certified individuals rather than members of privileged corporations, as under the *Ancien Régime*. Although regularly defied by
unlicensed practitioners, it persisted as a legal principle, despite challenges from
radicals like François-Vincent Raspail, whose annual handbooks of health were
designed to allow laypersons to dispense with the services of physicians and pharmacists in all but the most serious cases.[29] In public hygiene, however, despite the
common image of France as the land of the strong state, private property rights
generally trumped the public interest. Throughout most of the nineteenth century the French public health system was weak and decentralized.[30]

The revolutionaries' projects for the public provision of drugs and medical
services raised another set of questions, because they applied only to the needy.
Like public assistance more generally, medical assistance involved the transfer
of resources from some individuals to others, albeit less directly than in traditional charity. Although the nation might benefit from having healthier citizens,
the primary beneficiary was the recipient of aid. Universalist principles did not
apply as they would in a national health insurance plan or health service, except
in the sense that every citizen might someday be both sick and poor.

In a widely cited article on 'man's right to health', Dora Weiner argues that the early phase of the Revolution (1789–91) produced a new vision of social medicine but failed to realize it because of political divisions and lack of resources.[31] It is unlikely that anyone proclaimed a right to health in so many words, but this period saw a proliferation of proposals for reforming health care and providing medical assistance to the poor. One prominent contribution, submitted by the Société Royale de Médecine, called for district physicians, one of whose principal tasks would be to provide free services to the poor, as well as a system for distributing medicines to needy patients in the countryside.[32]

Weiner presents such proposals for programmes of medical assistance as part of a novel eighteenth-century conception of social welfare as a right. Reaching back to Enlightenment debates over the problem of poverty and mendicancy, she quotes Turgot's dictum in his article 'foundations' in the *Encyclopédie*: 'The poor person has indisputable claims [*droits* – the term can also be translated as 'rights'] on the wealth of the rich'. She fails to note, however, that he goes on to invoke the classic liberal argument that charitable institutions actually promote idleness and poverty.[33] She also quotes Francois-Alexandre de La Rochefoucauld, duc de Liancourt, a member of the National Constitutent Assembly (1789–91), who wrote in 1790 that '*la bienfaisance publique* … owes the indigent sick person prompt, free, certain and complete assistance'.[34] Liancourt's use of the term *la bienfaisance* is worth underscoring. Coined from the adjective *bienfaisant* – beneficent, doing good – it was free of the religious associations of 'charity' or 'alms'.[35] *La bienfaisance* is an obligation as well as a virtue. Both *la bienfaisance publique* and society 'owe' assistance to the poor.

Weiner's article focuses on two rival bodies in the Constituent Assembly, the Poverty Committee (formally the Comité pour l'extinction de la mendicité, or committee for the elimination of begging) and the upstart Health Committee (Comité de salubrité), which encroached on some of the other committee's jurisdiction.[36] The former, chaired by Liancourt, was primarily concerned with public assistance for the deserving poor and the latter, chaired by Dr Guillotin, with medical education and practice; but both produced a plan calling for district physicians to treat indigent patients. Neither proposal was adopted.

In 1993, Weiner published a major book entitled *The Citizen-Patient in Revolutionary and Imperial Paris*. In addition to giving a useful account of the new health-related institutions established in the French capital between 1789 and 1815, it returns to the broader question of access to medical services. Weiner once again invokes the idea of a right to health or, in some places, 'health care'. In this version the citizen-patient has duties as well as rights. They include promoting public and personal health, cooperating with care providers and showing consideration for other patients.

Weiner's emphasis, however, is on individual rights rather than duties and on the collective responsibility to uphold them. She again cites the duc de Liancourt, writing that 'he defined a social obligation that stems from the ancient

moral principle that man is his brother's keeper and from the philosophic doctrine of the natural rights of man'. In the debates on the remaking of French
politics and society, she argues, health care became a 'constitutional right'. In
this 'democratic vision of citizen-patients with equal access to equally good care',
the government was obligated to make the principle a reality by subsidizing care
for the poor. In the end, what Weiner characterizes as 'an ambitious attempt to
spell out nationwide health care for the poor' becomes something much larger.
In her view, even though reformers from the late Enlightenment through the
Consulate lacked the means to put their plans into action, their work 'laid the
foundation for health care in a democracy'.[37]

This strong interpretation of the Revolution's projects as an anticipation
of modern health care systems has been widely influential, as has the broader
view of the schemes for public assistance as forerunners of the welfare state.[38]
Although there is clearly a family resemblance between modern *droits-créances*
and the revolutionary proposals for a national system of assistance, there are
some problems with this interpretation. For one thing, the proposals on national
medical reform focused on assistance to the poor; it is hard to see how they
adumbrated a national health care system. Indeed, much of the discussion that
follows in this chapter deals with the central issue of poor relief, since there was
no question until the second half of the twentieth century of providing health
care for the population as a whole.

Then there is the question of the 'right' to health care. It is not hard to find
expressions of a right to assistance for those who were truly unable to provide for
themselves. Sieyès, who insisted on the equality of rights while accepting social
and economic inequalities, argued that such citizens had 'just claims [*droits*] on
the assistance of their fellow citizens'. His proposed declaration of rights, published in 1789, recognized a 'right to assistance'.[39] Despite Sieyès's considerable
influence in the Constituent Assembly, however, it did not include such a right
in the declaration it formally adopted one month later.

Liancourt affirmed a similar principle in the reports he drafted for the Comité
de Mendicité. His 'plan of work' for the committee stated that 'every man has
a right to subsistence'. This 'fundamental truth of every society, which urgently
demands a place in the Declaration of the Rights of Man', was the key to eliminating mendicancy. Given this right, assistance was not a kindness (*bienfait*) but
a duty for more fortunate citizens and the 'inviolable and sacred debt of society'.[40] He reiterated this theme in the committee's first report, on the general
principles that would guide its work, invoking justice, liberty, the rights of man
and natural law. France, he wrote, would be the first state to provide for the poor
in its constitution. Up to now it had been a question of giving charity to the poor
'but never to assert the claims (*droits*) of the poor man on society and those of
society on him'. The nation, however, would provide only for those unable to

provide for themselves. 'If one who exists [an allusion to a fundamental right of existence] has the right to say to society: *Make me live*, society has the equal right to respond: *Give me your work*'.[41]

The committee's third report invoked 'the right of the poor person' as a reason for rejecting the terms 'charity' and 'alms' in favor of 'assistance' (*secours*) but reaffirmed that 'men capable of work will have the right to assistance only in sickness and old age'. An early version of the committee's proposed decree, which called for compiling rolls of eligible recipients, stated that inclusion on the roll would give the 'right to free assistance in times of sickness, infirmity and old age'.[42] The fourth report addressed the tension between 'the rights of poverty' and the property rights of taxpayers. Protecting property was 'the sacred duty of the laws', but devotion to humanity was 'more sacred still'. Indeed, 'wherever there exists a class of men who lack subsistence, there exists a violation of the rights of humanity'.[43] The committee's work, however, did not result in legislation.

The Committee on Public Assistance of the Legislative Assembly (1791–2) continued the work of the Comité de Mendicité, though with no more practical success. In a report presented to the Assembly on the committee's behalf two months before the fall of the monarchy in August 1792, Bernard d'Airy stated as its first principle – 'which is missing from the declaration of the rights of man [but is] worthy to be placed at the beginning of the code of humanity' – that 'every man has the right to subsistence, through work if he is able-bodied, [or] through free assistance if he is unable to work'. While recognizing the 'sacred right of property', he defended public assistance in terms that suggest what we might think of as a form of social insurance based on participants' contributions as much as a fundamental right. Children deserve assistance because of the work they will contribute to society in the future, the sick or temporarily disabled because of their past and future work and the elderly because of their past contributions – though d'Airy made room for the permanently disabled as well.[44]

This rather narrow conception of a right to subsistence was neither radical nor new at the end of the eighteenth century. It offered a bare minimum of sustenance to those who could not support themselves and called for punishing those who could work but avoided doing so. Conceding that minimum was the widely accepted limit to possessive individualism. In John Locke's version of natural rights, the principle that 'no one ought to harm another in his Life, Health, Liberty or Possessions' and its corollary, that each individual has the right 'to preserve his Property, that is, his Life, Liberty and Estate, against the injuries and attempts of other men', might seem to reduce the right to life to the right not to be murdered. But Locke was at pains to insist that property rights did not give the proprietor the right to make others starve and force them to choose between death and slavery. An individual who lacks sustenance is not secure in the enjoyment of either life or liberty. Although the claim is more implied than clearly stated, it would follow that sustenance is itself a kind of right.[45]

Nevertheless, the Constituent and Legislative Assemblies chose not to recognize a right to work for the able-bodied or a right to assistance for those unable to work. The Declaration of the Rights of Man and the Citizen of 1789 was based on a negative conception of freedom and its limits: 'Liberty consists in being able to do everything that does not harm others; thus the exercise of the natural rights of each man has only those limits that ensure the enjoyment of these same rights by the other members of society'.[46]

Under the radical Republic (1792–4), Maximilien de Robespierre went further but stopped short of explicitly proclaiming a right to assistance. In a speech of 2 December 1792 on *les subsistances*, he argued, in terms reminiscent of Liancourt's observations on property rights and the claims of the poor, that the first of all imprescriptible rights was the right to exist. Property rights, highlighted in the Declaration of Rights of 1789, had to be subordinated to it.[47] The same theme reappeared in Robespierre's draft declaration of rights the following April: 'The principal rights of man are those which preserve his life (*existence*) and liberty' and 'the right of property is limited, like all the rest, by the obligation to respect the rights of others'. Two articles of the proposed declaration developed the practical implications. First, 'society is obligated to provide for the subsistence of all its members, either by providing them with work, or by ensuring the means of existence for those who are unfit to work'. Secondly, 'the indispensable assistance for someone who lacks bare necessities is a debt for someone who possesses non-essentials'.[48] Robespierre's draft recalls the proposals of the Comité de Mendicité, but it is striking that it characterizes assistance as an obligation of society and of the rich, but not as a right.

Similar language appears in the provisions for welfare and education that were famously included in the Declaration of Rights of 1793 and less famously in the Constitution of 1791. Article 21 of the declaration, whose phrasing is very close to Robespierre's, reads: 'Public assistance is a sacred debt. Society owes the means of support (*la subsistance*) to indigent citizens, either by finding work for them or by assuring the means of existence to those who are unfit to work'. Article 22 states: 'Everyone needs education. Society must promote the progress of public reason with all its power and make education accessible to all citizens'. Education appears here as a universal need rather than a universal right. The Constitution of 1791 ordained the creation of new institutions: 'A general establishment for public assistance will be created and organized to bring up abandoned children, relieve the disabled poor and provide work to the able-bodied poor who have not been able to find it'. And 'A [system of] public education will be created and organized, common for all citizens, [and] free for those parts of education that are indispensable for all men'. It did not proclaim a right to assistance or schooling, even though these clauses appear in a section entitled 'Fundamental provisions guaranteed by the Constitution', which opens by stating that 'the Constitution guarantees certain *droits naturels et civils*' – that is, the rights of man and the citizen.[49]

What emerges from these texts is a view of public assistance, including medical assistance, as an obligation of the community and the government but not a right of the individual. It is not what we would call an entitlement. In some ways this stance recalls the traditional conception of charity, which was not a right of the recipient but a moral obligation for the donor. This particular relationship between community and individual places the locus of control with the former, a critical consideration in the distribution of goods such as food, shelter, health care and education. There are some limits on the right to free speech, but within those limits you can exercise it as often and as much as you wish. Not so with a putative right to health care. It was difficult even to specify a necessary minimum, as was typically done for sustenance – enough not just to sustain life but also to allow the beneficiary to work. Was every citizen, no matter how sick, entitled to any medical intervention needed to sustain life, no matter the cost?

In practice, the Revolution dismantled the network of old regime charitable institutions – the old nursing orders, for example, were dissolved on 18 August 1792 – without establishing a national system of public assistance of the sort envisaged by the Comité de Mendicité.[50] At the local level, some Jacobin clubs took a keen interest in improving health as well as voluntary assistance to the needy.[51] In Paris, district assistance committees, initially supported by voluntary contributions, provided support for the deserving poor. Among other services, they maintained dispensaries or distributed medicines.[52] Legislation at the national level was the work of the National Convention in 1793–4. A law of 19 March 1793 on the organization of public assistance established a plan for distributing funds according to local needs. It also called for medical practitioners to serve poor individuals who were recipients of outdoor relief, abandoned children and other children registered on the poor rolls.[53] New legislation passed on 28 June 1793, shortly after the Jacobins assumed control of the Convention, aroused great hopes by promising funding for the elderly, the disabled and the working parents of large families who did not earn enough to support their children. The first instalment, however, was not approved until seven months later, on 1 February 1793, or 13 Pluviôse Year II in the revolutionary calendar adopted in October 1793, and it proved to be the last. The most radical measure that would have benefited the poor, the 'Ventôse' decrees, adopted on the 8th and 13th of that month in Year II (26 February and 3 March 1794), called for confiscating the property of émigrés and turning it over to poor citizens who were good patriots. Implementation, however, fell far short of the expectations the legislation had aroused.

Finally, an ambitious law of 22 Floréal II (11 May 1794), intended to relieve poverty in rural areas, established a Grand Livre (literally, 'great book') de la Bienfaisance Nationale to register the deserving poor. The emphasis was on rewarding those who had contributed to the nation through their labour rather than simply aiding the indigent. In addition to pensions, the measure provided for three salaried medical practitioners in each district as well as medicine, food and temporary financial support for the impoverished sick.[54] In this case, the Convention began to implement the new legislation without delay, but funds ran short and the uniform network of district health officers did not materialize. Two months later, on 23 Messidor Year II (11 July 1794), shortly before the fall of Robespierre and the Jacobins, the Convention nationalized the charitable endowments that had funded assistance to the needy, without adequately replacing the lost income.

The conservative turn that followed the fall of Robespierre, together with the economic disruptions cause by hyperinflation in 1795–6, undid the schemes of the National Convention. Its welfare legislation was formally abolished in October 1795. The Directory regime (1795–9) developed a new model of *la bienfaisance publique* as opposed to *nationale*, which built on the unrealized projects of the Constituent Assembly but repudiated the ambitions of the National Convention and diminished the role of the state. Poor relief would be local and mainly voluntary, administered by boards of private citizens and subsidized only to a limited extent by the national government.[55] Many towns assigned medical practitioners to the *bureaux de bienfaisance*, the institutions for outdoor relief established in 1796.

After the Revolutionary Decade

Similar principles, based on a liberal conception of citizenship, were to apply for most of the nineteenth century.[56] Everyone would enjoy negative civil liberties and the benefits of constitutional government and representative institutions, elected initially by a propertied elite and then, after 1848, by universal manhood suffrage. But there was no social guarantee. Assistance would be a moral obligation for the donor but not an individual entitlement. The state had no legal obligation to meet the needs of the poor, though it could play a useful role by coordinating and providing limited subsidies for measures taken at lower levels of government and by encouraging voluntary efforts. One increasingly common utilitarian argument, reflecting the dislocations associated with industrialism and rapid urban growth, held that public assistance was not merely a moral obligation but also a social necessity, a bulwark against crime, class conflict and revolution. That did not, however, make it a right.

Early-nineteenth-century liberals, like their Enlightenment predecessors, feared that public assistance might do more harm than good. Adam Smith's French disciple Jean-Baptiste Say rejected the notion that the poor had a claim on the state or on private individuals. Would-be recipients had to show that

> their misfortunes are a necessary consequence of the established social order [as opposed, for example, to their own laziness, improvidence, or other inadequacies] and, at the same time, that this social order itself would not offer them any resource for escaping their troubles.

In any case, it was not possible to relieve all misfortunes, even those that were undeserved. Such generosity would only cause the poor to multiply and depress their general condition, through what we would now call moral hazard. A Malthusian streak ran through liberal arguments against the dream of a world without poverty.[57]

At mid-century, the liberal politician and writer Adolphe Thiers, a fierce defender of property rights, adopted what he saw as an intermediate position between the proponents of purely private philanthropy and those who preferred to entrust assistance entirely to the state. He recognized the need for public *bienfaisance*, since the efforts of individuals and religious charities would not suffice. He insisted, however, that it must be voluntary and unconstrained like its private counterparts, with this difference, that the state had to exercise greater prudence in spending public funds. The victim of misfortune could appeal to our sympathies; 'he does not, however, have the right to force us to help him'. That would transform him from a 'sacred object' into a 'criminal'.[58]

Although still attached to traditions of private Christian charity, many Catholics accepted a version of *la bienfaisance publique*. Under the Restoration and July Monarchy the most prominent advocate of such a programme from a Catholic perspective was Joseph Marie, baron de Gérando, member of the Paris hospital council and author of two widely read texts on public assistance.[59] Inequality was part of a providential design, in which pity and charity serve to restore lost harmony.[60] In more practical terms, *la bienfaisance* would forestall a 'war of the poor against the rich'. Indigence, like great wealth, was the product of economic freedom in modern societies. The beneficiaries had a collective moral obligation to the less fortunate. Society could not simply wash its hands of them, as radical Malthusians suggested. Yet this obligation did not justify 'legal charity [the mocking oxymoron was borrowed from Malthus] equating this right with a sort of political or civil right'. A state guarantee of welfare would do more harm than good and the government in any case could not fully replace private charity, *la prévoyance* (savings and other provisions for future contingencies) and self-help. In the case of medical assistance, however, Gérando did not rely in the first instance on the charity of individual practitioners but called for district physicians as found in Italy and elsewhere and for ambulatory clinics on the German model.[61]

The strongest challenge to the limits of *la bienfaisance publique* came from the small but vocal socialist minority, who identified with the communitarian legacy of the Revolution. They believed that post-revolutionary France had failed to meet the social and economic challenges of the new industrial world, even though it had maintained and developed some of the political reforms introduced by the Revolution. This perspective entailed a new view of both the Revolution and citizenship. In the social realm, the work of the revolutionaries had been almost entirely negative, destroying the *Ancien Régime* but putting nothing in its place. Citizenship involved association with others in communities, not just the pursuit of individual interests. Although they differed on what a just society would look like, notably the status of private property, the early socialists agreed that a new form of social organization was required. This vision had important implications for health and health care. A properly organized society in which no one lacked adequate food and shelter would have a lower incidence of disease. Medical knowledge would be disseminated as widely as possible and preventive medicine based on public and private hygiene would have a much larger place than curative medicine. Physicians would still play a role, but they would no longer constitute a privileged elite exploiting the sick as capitalists exploited the workers.

Three examples will illustrate the range of socialist views on social reorganization, citizenship and health. Victor Prosper Considerant, the leading disciple of the utopian socialist Charles Fourier, called for 'true Liberalism, new Liberalism, social Liberalism', which would promote peaceful progress and the 'evolution' of society. Both progressive and conservative, this programme would recognize the rights of property and labour alike, rejecting both revolutionary communism and 'blind reaction'.[62] As for health care, in the Phalanstery or Fourierist ideal community, physicians would promote health through hygiene. In lieu of fees they would receive a 'dividend' at the end of the year, like all other members of the community, which in their case would be inversely proportional to the number of sick people.[63]

Étienne Cabet, the leader of the Icarian movement, may have been the first writer to use the word 'communism' and was among Considerant's targets. He described his ideal society in his *Travels in Icaria* (1848), whose title page proclaimed the basic Icarian principles: 'All for each. Solidarity, equality-liberty. First right: to live. To each according to his needs. First duty: to work. From each according to his abilities. The happiness of all'. The term 'solidarity', which appeared throughout the century in critiques of liberal individualism, had replaced the third element in the revolutionary triad liberty–equality–fraternity. Cabet's ideal society would have neither money nor private property; citizens would work for the Republic and the Republic would provide for their needs. Health care would rely on self-help, supplemented when necessary by public institutions and practitioners. Rather than serving primarily an indigent clientele, the public hospices would accommodate 'all the citizens without exception, when they have serious illnesses'. Each head of household would receive training in hygiene and the rudiments of medicine and would be provided with a 'domestic pharmacy'. Students in medical schools would be supported by the Republic and after passing examinations would qualify as national physicians or surgeons.[64]

François-Vincent Raspail denounced physicians and pharmacists as 'licensed health merchants'. The poor were protected from their misdeeds simply by being unable to pay the price. To restore the credibility and dignity of the health professions, Raspail proposed to diffuse medical knowledge as widely as possible as a counterweight to the obscurantism of the faculties and to open the teaching of medicine to all physicians. The professionals would remain, but removed from the marketplace. The medical profession would become a 'permanent magistracy', organized hierarchically according to merit and seniority. A practitioner would be guilty of misappropriation of public funds if he required or accepted direct payment from any citizen.[65]

In practice, post-revolutionary France made little progress towards a national system of medical assistance for the poor, in the face of inadequate funding, resistance to centralized state control and limited support within the medical profession.[66] The revolutionary idea of a network of district physicians continued to attract support but was initially implemented in only a few *départements*.[67] The only nationally coordinated system of medical services, required by a decree of 1805, was a network of epidemic doctors and supplies of remedies, a revival of an institution of the *Ancien Régime*.[68]

In 1845, a national medical congress composed of nearly 700 physicians, pharmacists and veterinarians met in Paris to discuss medical reform. It considered but rejected a proposal for district physicians. A minority of physicians saw appointments in government service as a career opportunity, but the majority could not accept the idea of becoming public functionaries and feared that they would lose fee-paying patients to salaried rivals. The concept reappeared in a major bill on medical education and practice proposed in 1847 by the Comte de Salvandy, the minister of public instruction. It met with opposition from the medical profession as well as from Catholics who resented the State's monopoly of medical education and expected challenges to religious orders that provided charitable care. Salvandy was working on a revised version when the Revolution of 1848 intervened.[69]

The February Revolution awakened hopes for a 'social-democratic' republic, which would not only establish universal manhood suffrage but also address the 'social question' of poverty and unemployment. The provisional government included the socialist Louis Blanc. As in 1789, the moment seemed ripe for medical reform. The orthopaedist Jules Guérin, editor of the *Gazette médicale de Paris*, saw 'a true social revolution' in the events of that year. He did much to popularize the term 'social medicine', which he defined as including all the relations between medicine and society. He was careful, however, to distinguish between social medicine and 'socialist medicine', which he characterized as 'medicine considered ... from the point of view of the doctrine of socialism'.[70]

The Second Republic, which lasted until Louis-Napoleon Bonaparte was proclaimed emperor Napoleon III in 1852, turned increasingly conservative after the heady February days. The constitution completed in November 1848 promised work or assistance to the needy, but the legislative committees failed to produce the necessary laws.[71] The government did not create a national system for assistance along the lines imagined by the revolutionaries of 1789. Nor did it reform health care, despite the presence of a significant number of physician legislators – fifty-two out of 900 representatives in the Constituent Assembly and forty-two out of 750 in the Legislative Assembly elected in 1849, a little over 5½ per cent in each case.[72]

The Second Empire (1852–70) made modest contributions to expanding medical assistance. In the mid-1850s, the government encouraged but did not require the *départements* to create systems of free medical care for the rural poor. Baron Haussmann, the prefect of the Seine, established a municipal system in Paris to provide comprehensive medical care for the needy, which some other major urban centres took as a model.[73] The imperial government also encouraged mutual aid societies, which often provided health care as well as subsidies to compensate for wages lost because of illness.

New Visions under the Third Republic

It was the Third Republic (1870–1940) that finally revived the Revolution's vision of welfare and medical assistance at the national level.[74] A stable regime developed in the 1870s from a compromise between moderate monarchists, who were willing to accept a republic so long as it was conservative, and republicans willing to accept a conservative regime so long as it was a republic. The beginnings of *l'État-providence* subsequently emerged from the growth of republican factions that rejected the original compromise and the convergence of new forms of liberalism and reformist socialism.

The new liberalism was more solicitous of the least advantaged citizens than classical liberalism had been, more willing to compromise on property rights and laissez-faire policies and more tolerant of government intervention. Liberals had gradually adapted to and accepted democracy, which an earlier generation had feared would give power to the uneducated and un-propertied masses. Now they accepted at least as much social intervention as was needed to alleviate the worst effects of poverty, disease and the loss of earning power due to injury, illness or old age. The result was a modified conception of liberal citizenship, which stopped short of proclaiming a right to well-being but revived and reinforced the Revolution's conception of an individual and collective obligation to the least fortunate members of society.

The proponents of this approach thought that they had found a middle way between liberalism and socialism that would respect the rights and duties of both the individual and society. They rejected, on the one hand, the untrammelled laissez-faire philosophy of the 'economists' and, on the other, attacks on property. They would respond to the Left's critique of the inequalities generated by industrial capitalism, while protecting individual rights against state power. Government intervention could be justified only insofar as it promoted personal liberty. The collectivity was not a higher interest in itself, to which individuals were subordinated.

The various expressions of this position were labelled both 'social liberalism' and 'liberal socialism', the term preferred by the philosopher Charles Renouvier. The terminology itself was not new; we have seen that the socialist Victor Considerant called for both a new liberalism and social liberalism. There are some parallels with earlier efforts by liberals like Thiers to steer a middle course between those who insisted that philanthropy should be entirely private and those who believed that assistance should be exclusively in the hands of the state. What was new at the end of the nineteenth century and the beginning of the twentieth was the prominence and political influence of an ideology opposed to both radical individualism and radical collectivism, which shaped legislation and policy in France as in Britain in the years before the First World War.

The contribution of the New Liberals to building the welfare state in Britain, culminating in Lloyd George's National Insurance Act of 1911, is well-known. Developments in France are less familiar in the Anglophone world and were more complex. France had no analogue to the Liberal Party or, indeed, any large national party until 1901. The Republican, Radical and Radical-Socialist Party, founded in that year, was to be the largest single party until 1936 and although some of its left-leaning members were sympathetic to social liberalism, it lacked a coherent unifying programme. The great cleavages in the first decades of the Third Republic opposed convinced republicans first to monarchism and then to the Catholic Church. During this time, however, a variety of thinkers developed loosely related social and political theories that emphasized the need for social cohesion and a concept of citizenship that called for a strong sense of community as well as individual rights. They included, among many others, the economist Charles Gide, proponent of 'cooperatism' and a strong critic of Manchester-style free market economics; the sociologist Émile Durkheim, who linked individual autonomy to social solidarity; and the philosopher Alfred Fouillée, who developed a social ideal that would maximize both the individuality and autonomy of each citizen and the solidarity of all.[75]

The key elements of the French version of the new liberalism came together as an intellectual synthesis and political force in 'solidarism', which was to constitute the quasi-official ideology of progressive reform of the pre-1914 Republic.[76] Its leading exponent, Léon Bourgeois, had been chairman of the committee on social insurance in the Chamber of Deputies before serving as prime minister for six months in 1895–6.

Solidarism began with a rereading of the heritage of the French Revolution, emphasizing the duties as well as the rights of the citizen. This basic principle recalled the Directory constitution of 1795. The constitutions of 1791 and 1793 were based on a 'Declaration of the Rights of Man and the Citizen'. The constitution of 1795 proclaimed duties as well as rights, a reaction against the perceived excesses of the radical Revolution in 1793–4. Duties to society included respecting the law and its agents and serving and defending the country. Duties to fellow citizens included a version of the Golden Rule: 'Do not do to others that which you would not have them do to you'. 'Do continually for others the good that you would wish to receive from them'. Property, which already appeared twice in the list of rights, reappeared in the list of duties. Citizens were obligated to respect it, because 'the maintenance of properties' was the foundation of 'the entire social order'. Moreover, the section on rights dropped the articles of the declaration of 1793 on education and public assistance as a sacred debt of society.[77]

While still respecting the principle of private property, solidarism modified it in ways that, unlike the Declaration of 1795, moved the entire framework in a progressive direction. It began with a broader conception of duty, an expanded version of the idea of social debt articulated in an earlier phase of the Revolution. Liancourt had described a 'debt' owed by society to the indigent and Robespierre a debt owed to the poor by society in general and more specifically the rich. For Bourgeois, every person owed such a debt to society and fellow citizens in general, since individuals do not exist in isolation from society and cannot survive and flourish without it. The relationship between individual and society implied what Bourgeois, borrowing from Fouillée, called a 'quasi-contract', which modified natural rights and was the foundation for the social debt. Charity towards the less fortunate had been a moral duty, whereas solidarism was mandatory and the social duty it entailed was an enforceable obligation. In return, society owed certain things to its citizens. The right to existence trumped the right to freedom and each citizen possessed an equal right to self-development.[78]

In concrete terms, society should provide, among other things, education, labour legislation and, where appropriate, assistance. Some solidarists reached the conclusion that these social obligations meant that individual citizens enjoyed an entitlement and legally enforceable right.[79] Meeting these obligations, however, was not primarily the responsibility of the state, as it was for most socialists. Although open to a role for government, solidarists remained distrustful of *l'État-providence*. They preferred voluntarist and local solutions and were drawn to the model developed in Belgium in 1899, which relied on state subventions to mutual aid societies and avoided the German model of compulsory social insurance.[80]

This form of social liberalism, then, could be called both individualist and collectivist. On the one hand, it treated private property as the foundation of liberty, accepted that inequalities would arise as the result of different levels of talent and sought to avoid placing limits on individual accomplishment. On the other hand, it insisted that society should not exacerbate inequalities by, for example, failing to provide adequate education for all. The more advantaged citizens should contribute more in the form of higher taxes. Society would protect all citizens from life's misfortunes by insuring them against risks such as sickness, accidents and unemployment.

The influence of solidarism can be seen in changes at the national level that occurred at the end of the nineteenth century. A national welfare office, the Conseil Supérieur d'Assistance Publique (CSAP) was established in 1888; its director, Henri Monod, became head of the Conseil Consultatif d'Hygiène Publique the following year, creating a critical link between health and welfare policies. This connection and the extraordinary number of medical practitioners who served on the CSAP and in the Chamber of Deputies, help explain why the first important new law on public assistance, adopted in July 1893, provided medical services to the poor, rather than food, shelter, or money.[81] The legislation made medical assistance an obligation for the *commune*, the *département* and the state – in that order, following the principle of subsidiarity. Although it did not employ the language of rights, it made a commitment to each eligible individual: 'Every sick Frenchman who is without resources receives, free of charge ... medical assistance at home, or if it is impossible to provide effective care at home, in a hospital'.[82] The new provisions mainly affected rural areas, since municipalities with an existing medical service could opt out. The law did not provide state funding or prescribe a particular model, leaving the design of the programme to lower levels of government.[83] Nor did the legislation make access to health care anything even remotely resembling a constitutional guarantee for all citizens. In the long-established tradition of medical assistance, it was aimed at the needy rather than the population at large.

In addition to solidarism, the beginnings of *l'État-providence* owed something to the ideological transformations of socialism and its emergence as a significant political force at the end of the nineteenth century. In the first decades of the Third Republic, French socialism was highly factionalized.[84] Nor did socialists enjoy the electoral success of the Social Democrats in neighbouring Germany. At their pre-war zenith, in the elections of 1914 – a landslide victory for the left – they won 17 per cent of the seats in the Chamber of Deputies. They contributed directly to passing only one major piece of social legislation before World War I, the old age insurance law of 1910.

Even before that legislative victory, however, socialists played a key role in debates over public provisions for the well-being of the population, including health care. They emphasized class rather than citizenship, starting from the premise that not all citizens were in fact equal, even if all enjoyed certain civil and political rights. They differed among themselves, however, on the means of redress. Revolutionary and Marxist socialists rejected 'bourgeois' social laws, which they saw as palliative measures designed to protect the status quo. This was the position of the Workers Party (later the French Workers Party), founded in 1882 by Jules Guesde and Paul Lafargue, Marx's son-in-law. It became the largest single socialist party in late-nineteenth-century France. Guesde objected to insurance schemes funded by payroll taxes, though he came to support insurance paid for in other ways. Some socialists accepted that an insurance plan could be 'revolutionary' if workers alone ran it.[85]

Guesde's critics, many of them influenced by the libertarian socialist tradition of Pierre-Joseph Proudhon, rejected Guesde's authoritarianism and doctrinal purism, as well as the goal of seizing control of the state through revolution. They called for a non-violent approach, using social democracy to improve the lot of workers. Starting at the local level, the movement would gradually replace capitalism with socialism. One key exponent of this position was a physician, Paul Brousse. He was uninterested in doctrine and focused instead on practical improvements that could be achieved through municipal socialism. His emphasis on doing what was possible led Guesde to denounce him as a 'possibilist'; he happily accepted the label and contrasted his position with his adversary's 'impossibilism'.[86]

The most prominent reformist socialist at the end of the century, Jean Jaurès, emphasized political rather than class struggle, practical goals and ideological flexibility.[87] In 1902 he joined with the possibilists and other reformist groups and independents to form the French Socialist Party, under his leadership. A merger between Guesde's French Workers Party and another revolutionary socialist group created the Socialist Party of France. The two parties participated in elections but disagreed on whether a socialist should participate in a 'bourgeois' government. Guesde's negative response was a condition for the union of the parties in 1905 as the French Section of the Workers International. The Guesde faction rapidly declined, however, and Jaurès's view predominated on many key issues, including social insurance on the German model, which he hoped eventually to extend beyond workers to all citizens. Jaurès laid out his vision during his campaign for the legislative elections of 1906, a year after parliament had passed a law guaranteeing assistance to the indigent elderly, disabled and chronically ill. With the legislation of 1905, Jaurès declared, 'we have proclaimed the right to life'. What was needed now, however, was an alternative to the old model of assistance to the needy. 'Thus the Republic, stimulated by socialism, pressed by the working class, is beginning to set up social insurance applicable to all risks, sickness as well as old age, unemployment and death as well as accidents'.[88] Albert Thomas, a socialist who was close to Jaurès, emphasized the significance of a worker's contributions to insurance plans. The income he received in old age would no longer seem like charity and 'his retirement would assume in the eyes of all the character of a new right'.[89]

In practice, the first major step away from the tradition that associated health care programmes with poor relief came with the social insurance legislation of 1928 and 1930, which emerged from a project first proposed in 1921 and was finally enacted, with significant changes, only after protracted parliamentary debates and negotiations. It fell far short of creating a truly national system of health insurance. Coverage was limited to, as well as required of, workers with incomes below a certain level. Moreover, public assistance – as opposed to insurance – continued to play a large role in providing French citizens with access to health care. The medical assistance act of 1893 remained in effect until 1953, when la Sécurité sociale finally supplanted it. It is also worth noting that the 1930 programme was governed by private law and was independent of the state bureaucracy. As we have seen, even the post-1945 social security system does not fully fit the model that the term *l'État-providence* might suggest: the state directly guaranteeing the well-being for all citizens.[90]

The contemporary French model of universal – though not entirely equal – access to medical care, in the form of health insurance, reflects its historical origins. Although the health care system far exceeds in size, complexity and cost what the planners of two centuries ago could have envisaged, the mixture of private and public funding, local and national control, freedom of choice and state guidance, bears the marks of the model of liberal citizenship that emerged from the French Revolution. It continues to reflect the enduring tension among the revolutionary principles of liberty, equality and fraternity.

2 AN OYSTER ODYSSEY: SCIENCE, STATE AND COMMERCE IN ENGLAND, 1895–1905

Anne Hardy

The recognition of physical health as a right, but also as a responsibility, of citizens of a modernizing state shaped public health activity in England, as elsewhere in Europe, in the nineteenth century.[1] Nonetheless, the implementation of public health policies did not go uncontested and the ways in which tensions between the desires of the state and the views of citizens were negotiated often proved influential in determining long-term state policies, as the case of anti-vaccinationism clearly demonstrates. Difficult enough in direct confrontation between state and citizen, such negotiations became yet more complex where commercial interests were involved. These problems were especially notable in relation to the food industries, where questions of state regulation, commercial responsibility and the health interests of the community were variously negotiated by individual industries over many decades from the late nineteenth century. One early example comes from the shellfish trades, which in the mid-1890s found themselves increasingly held responsible for the dissemination of typhoid in Britain.[2] For a short time at the turn of the nineteenth century, classic liberal values of individual rights and freedom of economic interest clashed with state and medical concerns over public health, disease transmission and the welfare of the wider community. This case study shows that health policy and market interests were shaped not just by top-down government and political philosophy but also by events and actors on the ground, especially in a liberal political and economic context, such as existed in late nineteenth-century England.

Between 1895 and 1903, a sharp contest developed between concerned medical men and public health officials on the one hand and the fish trades on the other, over the sanitary regulation and monitoring of shellfish supplies and the extent to which shellfish could be blamed for causing typhoid in the community. It was a contest eventually settled, effectively, by a clear-sighted representative of the fishing interests, which implemented internal regulation in co-operation with the new science of bacteriology. The contest itself reflects the tensions inherent in nineteenth-century liberalism: individual rights versus the state intervention and group interests against the collective interest. The principal actors involved were the fish trades, the medical men and the fish-eating public. The role of the state in supporting the efforts of state public health officials to effect state control over the fish trades was minimal. English government and the governing class were still too much in sympathy with individual economic interests and with the tradition of free trade, to intervene where powerful financial interests were at stake. Yet the position of the fish trades shifted over time, under pressures of market loss and public trust, towards self-regulation. In this process, we can see the reshaping of English citizenship within a liberal political context. Throughout this confrontation, the young and as yet contested, science of bacteriology and its practitioners played a prominent role.

Typhoid and the Oyster: Winter 1895

The story began in January 1895, when the *British Medical Journal* reported that an unusual prevalence of typhoid among the wealthier sections of London society over the Christmas period had been attributed to oysters, which were a standard seasonal celebratory fare.[3] The same issue carried a note by Sir William Broadbent, Physician-in-Ordinary to the Prince of Wales and famous for his successful management of Prince George's illness from typhoid four years earlier. Broadbent recorded that he had from time to time seen cases of typhoid apparently attributable to oysters and he had now become convinced of the connection. 'The contamination of oysters by typhoid can only be accidental', he noted, 'and is therefore probably preventable'. He went on to describe the 'six separate incidents' that had convinced him. First, a young man convalescent from influenza, who developed bronchial catarrh and was confined to his room for three weeks: he had consumed oysters freely during that time and was the only member of a large household with 'faultless' sanitary arrangements, to be stricken. The second case was of two young men living in the same house, who had enjoyed an oyster supper after visiting the theatre together ten days previously. The third, a clergyman and his twelve-year-old daughter at Daventry, the only members of the household to have eaten oysters sent down from London. And finally, several cases among City gentlemen who had eaten oysters at lunch and were similarly the only members of their households to suffer.[4] Broadbent's cases represent a wonderful window on the oyster-eating habits of the English middle class; but, given his popular profile and standing as Physician-in-Ordinary to the Prince of Wales, they were also highly damaging to public confidence in the safety of English oysters.

Barely had Broadbent pronounced, when news of an outbreak of typhoid at Wesleyan University, Connecticut, USA, in October/November 1894 was published in the medical press.[5] There had been twenty-five cases, thirteen very severe, with four deaths. None of the fifty women students at the college had suffered; it turned out that the damage had been done at a series of fraternity suppers held on the occasion of freshman initiations on 12 October. This was the first major outbreak of oyster-borne typhoid recorded. In the words of the biology professor H. W. Conn, who investigated the outbreak for the State Board of Health, it was

> especially interesting in the history of epidemics. A more typical example of an out-
> break of typhoid due to a single source of infection has hardly been found in the
> history of medicine and the example furnishes a demonstration of a new source of
> danger for this disease.[6]

Conn's conclusion was stark: 'One thing is sure. The public health is placed in jeopardy when oyster dealers, for the sake of producing plumpness, place oysters in the mouths of freshwater creeks in close proximity to sewers'.[7] In both Britain and the United States, it was a common belief among oyster cognoscenti not only that sewage was rendered harmless by sea water, but also that it was ben-eficial in fattening and enhancing the flavour of shellfish destined for the table.[8]

The *British Medical Journal* report on the Wesleyan University poisonings was published on 12 January 1895. At the end of the month followed publi-cation of the Chief Medical Officer's report into the distribution of cholera in England in 1893, which also implicated sewage-contaminated shellfish as the cause of infection.[9] The accumulated effect of these revelations, all published in the medical press during January 1895, was an immediate and thorough-going food-scare. Already on 12 January the *Fish Trades Gazette* was lamenting of the medical journals:

> Will they ever have done with scaring the public? ... The *B.M.J.* ... will make our grey
> hair go down in sorrow to the grave. And all on account of oysters ... Are the public
> to forego oysters at the bidding of medical alarmists at the end of the nineteenth
> century? Why the very idea is absurd.[10]

By mid-February, however, the tone was less ebullient. Time was, the writer declared, when the medical profession 'gave us a lift'. Now, it had laid down a law that 'every bi-valve is a bacillus in ambush, consequently the public won't buy the bi-valve any more'. The impact of the scare was later confirmed by the Cen-tral Medical Department's investigator (the Central Medical Department was the predecessor of the Ministry of Health). The English oyster trade had been temporarily paralysed with such severe financial loss to the oyster merchants and their staff that representations had been made to the Board of Trade. Not only was public health at stake as a result of the oyster merchants' practices and the recent medical revelations, but also the future of that large national industry.[11]

The Medical Department's response to this crisis – although stated to be the result of the 1893 cholera inquiry – was to undertake an inquiry into conditions in the English coastal oyster industry, supplemented by a bacteriological investigation of the various known pathogenic 'sewage' organisms in relation to oysters. This was notably more comprehensive than the Department's response to meat-poisoning and contaminated milk: it involved both the traditional epidemiological survey, the coastal inquiry, and utilization of the new bacteriology in exploring the economy of potential pathogenic organisms in nature. It seems likely that the human dimension of the problem facilitated this broader investigative approach: here was a direct connection to existing problems of sewage management and disposal. It had, indeed, already been noted in this connection that, 'man had only himself to blame ... the mollusc was only the unwilling vehicle of infection'.[12] Whereas the possible environmental sources of salmonella and tubercular infections in animals potentially led medical epidemiologists into the uncertainties of veterinary epidemiology (a subject then virtually non-existent) and of professional entanglement with veterinarians and the powerful agricultural industry, in addressing problems created by human excreta they were on home ground.

The Medical Department's inquiry into the oyster layings was undertaken by one of its star investigators, H. Timbrell Bulstrode. Published in November 1896, it offered a thorough survey of the English oyster industry, as well as a detailed account of the local conditions existing in oyster beds located around the coasts of England and Wales.[13] Bulstrode investigated fifty-four layings with exemplary thoroughness, but his conclusions were not entirely unequivocal: it was difficult to demonstrate any substantial risk of sewage pollution in most of the layings examined, but only a few of them could be held to be free of the possibility of chance infection. In the event, Bulstrode condemned fourteen layings and approved eight, finding twenty-two to be associated with various degrees of risk. The report was commended for its 'unbiased character' by both the *Lancet* and the *British Medical Journal*. Both journals hoped that it would serve to draw public and official attention to the issue of contaminated oysters and their role in causing typhoid. The *British Medical Journal* was, however, concerned lest the accompanying report by the bacteriologist Edward Klein, which appeared to minimize the risks of direct sewage contamination, should detract from the power of Bulstrode's deductions.[14] Bulstrode's report was a miracle of scrupulous, almost loving, attention to the detail of the coastal environment and the condition of the shellfish in the layings investigated, but the responses from the fish trades would confirm the associated report to be a mixed blessing.

Klein's inquiry was focused on the bacteriology of oyster-borne disease. Unlike Bulstrode's pioneering investigation, this was not a new area of inquiry. The first investigations into the survival of cholera and typhoid bacilli in sea-water had been published in 1889, when it was reported that both kinds survived three to four weeks in sterilized sea-water, but rapidly disappeared in the natural medium – a result attributed to an unsuccessful evolutionary struggle with other water organisms and which appeared to endorse the traditional belief in the purifying qualities of the sea.[15] By the mid-1890s, further confirmatory and contradictory researches had been published and the problematic nature of available bacteriological techniques in securing dependable results recognized.[16] As Christopher Hamlin has so well documented, bacteriology remained a contested science at the turn of the nineteenth century.[17] Yet the question of the viability of these organisms in sea water remained and was recognized to be important because, as the *British Medical Journal*'s investigator phrased it: 'those interested in denying the possibility of infection through oysters have made use of these results in support of their statements'.[18] It was in this context that Klein's investigation was of special significance. His results furnished ammunition for the defenders of the status quo in the oyster industry. Although he was able to add judicious weight to existing research indicating that shellfish could carry the infections of typhoid, cholera and gastro-enteritis, Klein was only able to detect the typhoid bacillus itself once in a number of oysters placed in contaminated water.[19] It was a result which the Chief Medical Officer, Richard Thorne Thorne [*sic*], confessed to finding disappointing. The bacteriologist, Thorne concluded, 'can ... tell us of impurity and hazard – often indeed, of the precise nature of specific hazard – but not of purity and safety'.[20] This was a question that lay at the heart of the contest between the public health service and the fish trades.

The Fish Trades and the Experts: Bacteriology in the Community

As the Medical Department was well aware, the shellfish trades were an important industry, estimated to be worth £2,500,000 a year.[21] As an unregulated industry, the trades were combative and enterprising in their own defence. For example, one of the layings condemned by Bulstrode was the one at Southend-on-Sea, an important supplier to the London market, but also a popular holiday destination for East-Enders, for whom shellfish were a traditional celebratory dish. A newspaper's attempt in December 1896 to discover whether Southend oysters had been withdrawn from the market as a result of Bulstrode's 'damaging document' ended in failure. It was ascertained that four thousand Southend oysters were dispatched to London every day, but where in London they went remained a mystery: 'they seemed to disappear somehow en route'. It was implied that their place of origin was disguised in the shops.[22] At London Bridge, meanwhile, one dealer was found advertising his stock as 'non-typhoidal oysters' and another in Little Queen Street had submitted his to the public analyst and received a certificate of 'absolute purity', which he displayed in his window.[23] The *Fish Trades Gazette*, meanwhile, was much dismayed by Bulstrode's condemnations: his reputation was such that his negative opinion was likely to be very damaging to the trade. It suggested that the whole question should be referred to the scientists at the Marine Biological Laboratory at Plymouth, or to the Scottish Fisheries Board, or indeed to 'The Right Honourable Thomas Huxley', who at the time of another scare had pronounced there to be no connection between cholera and the consumption of mackerel.[24]

Beleaguered as they were, the shellfish trades were perfectly ready to exploit scientific uncertainties and to wield denigration as a weapon against the medical profession in general. The *British Medical Journal*'s fears that Klein's bacteriological report would 'put back' the issue of sewage pollution, for example, were amply justified by subsequent events. Of Thorne's disappointment at Klein's inconclusive results, the *Fish Trades Gazette* noted: 'What would the man have? Would evidence that might have ruined an industry been more pleasing to him?' It was more generous to Klein: 'on the whole, Dr Klein has played the part of Balaam and his report may be used as a counterblast to Dr Bulstrode's alarming indictment'. Bulstrode's remarks did not carry the weight they would have done had Klein's researches backed them up.[25] And finally and specifically, the *Fish Trades Gazette* noted the *British Medical Journal*'s interpretation of the Medical Department report: it suggested that germs were so diluted by sea-water that there was little chance of them being absorbed by the oyster: 'We thank thee ... for teaching us these words'.[26]

The Medical Department's oyster investigations made an immediate issue of polluted shellfish and how they were to be judged. Medical journals attacked the trade and bacteriologists disputed bacteriological standards of purity and impurity. The *Lancet* promptly suggested the registration of all oyster layings, fattening beds and storage ponds.[27] The *British Medical Journal* called for the Local Government Board to be empowered to close dangerous oyster beds.[28] The *Fish Trades Gazette* expressed a preference for regulation by the Board of Trade – 'which according to the *Lancet* has no expert sanitary advice at its disposal'.[29] The *Gazette*'s jibe at the *Lancet* was suggestive: the interests of the Board of Trade lay with industry, not with public health improvement. The battle lines were clearly drawn between the sanitarians on the one hand and the fish trades on the other. Bacteriology, however, lay in between – its uncertainty of expertise laid it open to competitive exploitation by both sides.

Despite a low opinion of doctors and scientists and of medical officers of health in particular (discussed further below) the *Fish Trades Gazette* was perfectly willing to use science to fight its corner, exploiting the uncertainties of the new bacteriology and divisions and disagreements among its practitioners. During the 1890s, the journal repeatedly drew attention to the issues surrounding bacteriological analysis, the methods by which shellfish (especially oysters) were judged to be safe or hazardous and techniques for ensuring their purity.

A favourite authority was William Abbott Herdman, professor of natural history at Liverpool University and an energetic advocate of co-operation between scientific research and the fishing industry. Herdman had founded the Liverpool Marine Biological Committee in 1885, which in 1887 had opened its own research laboratory, initially at Puffin Island, Anglesey, later at Port Erin, Isle of Man. In 1891, Herdman was brought into yet closer connection with the fishing industry, when he was invited by the newly established Lancashire Sea Fisheries Committee to organize their marine research laboratory at Liverpool and became their chief scientific adviser.[30]

Following the oyster scare of January 1895, Herdman joined with the bacteriologist Rubert Boyce to research into the effects of pollution on oysters. Their initial results were published in the Lancashire Sea Fisheries Committee's annual report and emphasized that oysters could be cleaned by natural methods: their occasional transmission of disease germs to humans was an insufficient reason for the public to avoid 'an important and highly-esteemed food matter'.[31] According to Herdman and Boyce, the typhoid bacillus could not flourish in clean sea water and their experiments 'seemed to show' that it decreased in numbers in its passage along the oyster's alimentary canal. Their preferred cleaning method was the French 'degorgeoir': tanks of clean water in which oysters were placed for a short while before dispatch to the consumer.[32] In 1897, as befitted a friend of the industry, Herdman again urged 'the exercise of common-sense by the public and of moderation by some sanitary reformers ... do not insist on conditions which will make it impossible to rear any oysters at all'.[33]

Herdman was clearly identified with fish trade interest and from 1898 was working with the newly formed British Oyster Industries Association to ensure improved conditions within the trade. Nonetheless, he sought to maintain the authority of science. 'The oyster, like the woman, is better not to have had a damaged past', he declared in 1898, continuing that a 'more or less damaged character' necessitated that it 'come into court – the scientific laboratories – and request the fullest possible investigation'.[34] In the wider food industries too, Herdman's position was seen as a rational counterbalance to sanitary over-enthusiasm. The journal *Food and Sanitation*, for example, commented on the Herdman/Boyce claim never to have found naturally-occurring typhoid bacilli in any oyster, whether obtained from markets or the sea: 'they give the whole case against oysters away'.[35] Yet the Fisheries Committee report also indicated Herdman's political position. As the *British Medical Journal* noted, its conclusions rested on negative results and negative results had their own problems: 'the fallacies involved in implicitly accepting negative results must be borne in mind'. Nor did the journal agree with the Herdman/Boyce recommendation that the sanitary inspection of oyster layings be vested in the Sea Fisheries Committees: this was a public health matter and should be within the remit of the central or local public health authorities.[36] In other words, the *British Medical Journal* saw the Committees as guardians of trade interests and the government authorities as better guardians of the public interest.

The question of the laboratory findings and of sanitary 'over-enthusiasm' was especially pertinent at the end of the 1890s in regard to the imminent introduction of legislation to regulate the oyster industry. In May 1899, the Local Government Board formulated its Oyster Bill, which provided for the inspection of layings, a ban on removing oysters from insanitary grounds and the regulation of oyster imports from abroad, measures which were to be the responsibility of the county and borough sanitary authorities.[37] These authorities already had responsibility for the disposal of sewage. As the fish trades pointed out, it was unlikely that they would require themselves to undertake the expensive removal or re-location of sewer outfalls. The Bill appeared to take it for granted that the oysters must give way before the sewers and that the outfalls must not be interfered with; there was no suggestion of any possibility of compromise, or of compensation to oyster growers for loss of business.[38] And who was to decide when the risk of pollution was serious, or not worth troubling about? The local fish trades clearly did not trust their medical officers of health to act impartially.[39] Both the British Oyster Fisheries Association and the National Sea Fisheries Protection Association objected.[40] In July the Bill was referred to a Select Committee (parliamentary inquiry) and in August withdrawn: the Committee had substituted the local Sea Fisheries Committees for the Local Government Board as supervisory authority – a measure which the Board of Trade considered impractical.[41]

Quite what passed within the Select Committee is unclear: the loss of the bill meant that neither its text nor (apparently) the proceedings of the Committee reached publication. According to the *British Medical Journal*, the witnesses were essentially representatives of the oyster industry and the Local Government Board – the Chief Medical Officer, Richard Thorne, Mr Provis, the Permanent Secretary and Timbrell Bulstrode. The Committee was chaired by Lord Harris, a well-known cricketer, former civil servant and former Governor of Bombay, who outraged the medical press by expressing the opinion that the bill was concerned with the health of oysters rather than with the health of human beings. Indeed, the Committee had stated explicitly that it wished to hear no evidence regarding injury to humans as a result of eating polluted oysters.[42] Since the bill had been formulated by the central Medical Department and was sponsored by the Local Government Board, this was a substantial misreading of its intent. In the event, the Committee's amendment, substituting the Sea Fisheries Committees (who would safeguard trade interests) for the local authorities as supervisory bodies, ensured that many of the most important coastal oyster layings would go uncontrolled because they lay outside the Fisheries Committee districts. The Local Government Board's decision to abandon the bill was recognition that a stalemate had been reached. The motives of the Select Committee remain obscure, but that they were favourable to the fish trades and to the freedom of industry from sanitary supervision seems indisputable. The Local Government Board and its medical experts had no automatic leverage with the legislature.

Meanwhile there were signs that the industry was beginning to take remedial action against the local authorities: in Kent and Essex, the Sea Fisheries Committee was standardly opposing new sewerage schemes that were likely to contaminate oyster beds and a number of independent oyster bedders also took action; and the British Oyster Trades Association was reported to have begun to flex muscle.[43] Launching an offensive, the *Fish Trades Gazette* declared in February 1901 that nearly all oyster beds in England had been purified.[44] By September 1901, the trade was beginning to feel more secure. Firstly, it had been established that the Sea Fisheries Committees had the power to prohibit the deposit of crude sewage in areas under their jurisdiction; secondly, the judgement for Lord Gifford in a court case against the City of Chichester for polluting his fishing grounds with sewage had determined that sanitary authorities could be deemed responsible for damaging sewer discharge and made to pay compensation; and thirdly, the Board of Trade had declared that all new sewage schemes were liable to be disapproved unless they satisfied the requirements of the Board and of the Fisheries Committees as to the purity of the effluent.[45]

At the same time, the trades responded to the perceived threat from the new bacteriology. Since science might be used to combat science, the trade felt the need to educate its members in scientific language and methods the better to meet the challenge. Early in 1901, the *Fish Trades Gazette* began to instruct its readers in the language of bacteriology: 'a subject but little known to oyster dealers, but one which, in their business, is continually cropping up'.[46] The frequent conjunction of oysters and microbes in press reports, the journal noted, made it important that the trade should be familiar with the action of bacteria and of typhoid bacteria in particular. A series of five 'discussions' followed, dealing with bacteria generally, typhoid bacilli, the work of scientists demonstrating that 'typhoid bacilli do not flourish in sea water' and the virtual absence of bacteria in general in fresh oysters, the distribution of typhoid bacteria in nature and the action of septic tanks in rendering sewage harmless. How effective this educational effort proved remains uncertain, but in 1904, in the midst of yet another oyster crisis, one of the *Gazette*'s correspondents noted how the enforced idleness of the oyster merchants had driven them to the occupation of informing themselves on bacteriological subjects:

> The readiness with which the crack-jawed names of different bacteria are bandied about ... and the depth of knowledge and the subtlety of argument displayed, raise an apprehension as to whether oyster merchants will not all take to bacteriology as a profession.[47]

For the oyster trade at least, joining the bacteriologists had become an alternative to beating them.

The Fish Trades and Public Opinion

The importance of learning the language of bacteriology was underscored by the oyster traders' experience through the 1890s, which amply demonstrated that both press and public were highly sensitive to the risk of typhoid and that the influential public health lobby listened to the pronouncements of bacteriologists. Initially, the *Fish Trades Gazette* took up a combative attitude towards critics of the shellfish trades, which it kept up for much of the 1890s. It was, for example, adept at picking up and republishing the opinions of other contemporary newspapers and journals. Thus it quoted the *Star*, which had summed up the Medical Department Report 'in one Anglo-Saxon word – Rot!' In the *Star*'s opinion: 'We are not a bit awed at the learned twaddle of these well-meaning bacteriologists, who would find microbes in heaven and would have issued a report condemning manna if they had been employed by Moses to report upon its collection and storage'.[48] The *Star* clearly had a low opinion of bacteriologists (as well as a respect for Moses), for months later it was poking fun at 'medical oysteria', declaring that 'if Dr Klein had been a contemporary of Moses he would have found bacilli in the water that gushed from the rock'.[49] On accumulated evidence, including the opinions of other newspapers, the *Fish Trades Gazette* had decided, by December 1896, that the Medical Department was 'ignorant and short-sighted'.[50]

Beyond the bacteriologists and the Medical Department, the *Fish Trades Gazette* writers took a particularly dim view of medical officers of health. Dr Laing of Cowpen, Northumberland, was 'any irresponsible person' for attributing typhoid to mussels from the river Blyth.[51] In December 1896, medical officers were accused of trying to increase the oyster scare: 'Who on earth is Dr A. Wynter Blyth, Medical Officer of Health for Marylebone, that we should accept him as an authority?'[52] The paper became increasingly truculent about 'medical alarmists' – a view that stayed with it for many years. In 1900, for example, it reprimanded the Medical Officer for Folkstone for blaming typhoid on oysters from Whitstable: although a bacillus 'common to sewage' had been found, the typhoid bacillus had not: 'there is no reliable evidence whatsoever that the disease was so caused'.[53] This was in line with the current debates and uncertainties on the precise relations between sewage contamination, specific disease organisms and proof of dangerous contamination of food and water and the *Gazette* made of it a vehicle for a more generalized attack on the public health administration and on the medical profession as a whole:

> This was another illustration of the haphazard way in which many medical officers accept unhesitatingly and repeat, statements which, to a critical mind, would not be accepted for a moment without verification. The cause of this ready belief is probably because medicine is not a science. Medicine is based on empiricism and not on rationalism and men trained to believe what they are told by authority, without rea-

sons being adduced to support statements they are asked to believe, are liable to carry this uncritical and unsceptical mental receptivity with them in all the questions with which they are called upon to deal.[54]

The trade line on the general public and the influence of the press on popular opinion was no more flattering than its opinions of the medical profession. Thus P. Quant declared that it 'takes very little to frighten the public. A couple of paragraphs in the medical papers extensively copied into other journals throughout the country are quite sufficient to ruin a good industry'. He argued that the medical press 'can only live by working up sensations of some kind or another'. And if the medical press were self-interested promoters of damaging allegations, the public was sadly gullible: 'People nowadays do not think for themselves – they allow the newspapers to do all their thinking for them'; 'We are a nervously over-excitable people'.[55] Publicity in the lay press, whether in newspapers or other journals, was clearly thought important in shaping public opinion and the fortunes of trade. In 1900, for example, the *Gazette* welcomed an item in the *Daily Express*, headed 'Oysters Acquitted', which summarized the report of the British Oyster Industries Association and indicated that conditions of oyster culture had significantly improved: 'More of this kind of publicity is required'. As the *Gazette* specifically noted: 'Now that the trade is practically, if not absolutely purified, the public certainly ought to be informed, both for their own benefit and for the benefit of the trade'.[56]

The Oyster Industries Association, founded to safeguard the interests of the trade, came in for repeated criticism for not doing enough to publicize improvements. In particular the journal felt that action should be taken at the beginning of the oyster season in August – which happened to coincide with the British Medical Association's annual meeting. Inevitably, papers on typhoid were read at the latter, 'in all of which reference is made to oysters', which the daily press then seized on, resulting in the annual renewal of the oyster scare.[57] As the trade remained depressed through 1901 and 1902, the calls became more urgent:

> Improving the trade depends upon *publicity*. It was by the public condemnation of oysters that the trade was reduced ... if public condemnation took five or six years to reduce the trade to its present level it will take forty years to restore it to its previous level if the fact that oysters are clean remains unpublished.[58]

There were signs of recovery with the opening of the 1902 season and a degree of equilibrium appeared to have been reached.[59] The *Fish Trades Gazette* responded sharply to the publication of Klein's latest researches into typhoid in cockles and mussels, demonstrating a grasp of contemporary bacteriological understanding: Klein's research was conducted in the laboratory, 'which in no way imitates the conditions found in nature', where sunlight and harmless bacteria combined to destroy potential pathogens; the great majority of mussel beds must be free from

pollution.[60] Yet, despite the vigorous claims of the *Fish Trades Gazette* and stir-
rings to action among oyster bedders and the Oyster Association, 'practically, if
not absolutely purified' proved to be insufficient. A seminal crisis broke over the
English oyster industry in December 1902.

Crisis 1903

Mayoral banquets were an integral part of the annual tradition of local government in provincial England and they commonly took place in the late autumn,
in the last week of November. Within weeks of the banquets held at Southampton and Winchester in November 1902, typhoid had broken out among
the guests who had assembled at the different feasts. After the Winchester feast
sixty-three people fell ill and four died; at Southampton fifty-five fell ill; at Ports-
mouth at the same time, twenty-two people fell ill after eating oysters from the
same source as those supplied to the banquets, although guests at the town's
mayoral feast went unscathed: their oysters had come from Whitstable and not
from Emsworth near Chichester.[61] By mid-December, the *Daily Mail* was said to
be 'working up' a campaign against Emsworth oysters and oyster sales had again
plummeted, although it was later admitted that damage to the Christmas trade
had not been as great as expected.[62]

In light of this fresh disaster, the Worshipful Company of Fishmongers
finally took decisive action. One of the old City of London livery companies,
the Fishmongers regulated the trade of London's Billingsgate fish market – the
central entrepôt for the English fish trades – with a view to maintaining standards and consumer confidence in this fragile product. The Company's inspectors
were instructed to stop the sale of shellfish coming from any known contaminated source; in late December, therefore, cockles which had been deposited in
Lea Creek prior to boiling were banned: bacteriological examination had shown
them to be dangerously infected and unfit for human consumption.[63] Although
this prohibition applied only to the London markets, it was important to the
shellfish industry generally, as a great many provincial centres were supplied
through Billingsgate. The Company was nothing if not thorough. In the months
that followed, it instituted a programme of sampling and testing oysters from
beds supplying the London market, having them analysed and closing those
reported as likely to endanger public health.[64] By September 1903, even the *Fish
Trades Gazette* had come round to the idea that all polluted oyster beds must be
closed.[65] And finally, the Company appointed Edward Klein as its official bacteriologist, responsible for the testing and monitoring of layings, for devising
bacteriological tests of purity for shellfish and methods of ensuring that they
reached market in a safe and saleable condition.

The bacteriological wrangles were not yet over, however, for the question of just what constituted the measure of safety remained. Over Christmas 1903/4, the well-established oyster merchants Messrs Gann were prosecuted for selling polluted 'Princess' oysters unfit for human consumption. The case of 'Gann's Princesses' became something of a *cause célèbre* in the trade: it turned on Klein's judgement that the 'B.coli communis' found in considerable numbers in eight of twelve oysters sampled made them 'decidedly sewage polluted and ... not fit for human consumption'.[66] On a previous occasion, however, Klein had allowed that the presence of 'small quantities' of the bacterium did not mean the oysters were not 'pure': where was the dividing line? Was it a purely arbitrary one drawn by Klein himself? If Klein was an eminent bacteriologist, noted the *Gazette*, so was A. A. Kanthack, who in 1896 had declared to the British Association for the Advancement of Science that b.coli existed everywhere in nature and that it was 'absurd to assume' that its presence in the digestive tract signalled direct faecal contamination.[67] In his recently published report on the mayoral banquet fiasco, moreover, none other than Timbrell Bulstrode had noted:

> Negative bacteriological evidence may be highly misleading, and as regards positive evidence, it is desirable that there should be some agreement among bacteriologists as to the precise significance, both as regards presence and number, of B.Coli Communis and B.Enteritidis Sporogenes before a bacterial standard can be applied either with safety to the consumer or justice to the oyster industry.[68]

A week later, the *Gazette* saw its stand on the Klein's 'extraordinary ruling' triumphantly justified, when the interim report of the Royal Commission on Sewage Disposal declared itself 'dead against the bacteriological test, seeing no grounds for condemning oysters for the mere presence of b.coli or the like'.[69] Kanthack's opinions were again invoked in direct contradiction to Klein and his status as a scientist proclaimed: he had been Klein's predecessor at St Bartholomew's Hospital, but also professor of pathology at Cambridge; 'When he died, in 1897, he was described in *Nature*, which is the leading scientific journal, as the ablest and most brilliant exponent of bacteriology we possessed'.[70] There was no suggestion that bacteriological understanding might have moved on in the intervening five years – indeed, the evidence did not suggest that it had. A further cynical note on bacteriologists was added by 'a correspondent':

> The competition in the profession does not appear to be keen, for illogical reports seem to pass unchallenged and the fees appear to be remunerative. Moreover, a little tact and a few contradictory reports enable a bacteriologist employed in any branch of the investigation to keep the ball rolling indefinitely.[71]

When further reading of the Royal Commission report threw up a divergence of opinion between Klein and Alexander Houston, the Commission's chosen bacteriological expert, the *Gazette* reported with glee. Klein had told the Commission that his standard was based on the view that the normal oyster did not contain *B. coli communis*; Houston, however, had examined over one thousand oysters and found that nearly every one contained 'what Dr Klein said the normal oyster did not harbour' – *B. coli communis* and allied bacteria.[72]

The Royal Commission on Sewage Disposal had been appointed in 1898 to inquire into the methods of treating and disposing of sewage pollution. Its fourth report, however, diverged into the issue of the impact of sewage pollution on shellfish. Its membership included a number of eminent scientists and public health experts: Sir Michael Foster MP, founder of the Cambridge School of Physiology; William Power, the then Chief Medical Officer; Sir William Ramsay, professor of chemistry at University College London; and Dr James Burn Russell, for many years Medical Officer of Health for Glasgow City and latterly a member of the Scottish Local Government Board. That a Commission with such a membership should come out against Klein's bacteriological standard for oysters and assent to the proposition that *B. coli communis* was not significant in public health terms was little short of astonishing. But Alexander Houston's investigations on behalf of the Commission into the ecology of *B. coli* had demonstrated that the organism was widely distributed in nature and in areas far removed from sources of faecal pollution. Although in general oysters stored in pure water contained very many fewer *B. coli* than those stored in polluted waters, it did happen that the occasional mollusc from these pure waters contained as many as if it had been stored in sewage. The 'mere presence' of *B. coli* and related bacteria, the Commissioners concluded, was no justification for the wholesale condemnation of shellfish. And, they warned further, 'It is clear ... that a single examination of chance samples of oysters might be most misleading as to the bacterial flora of the whole oyster contents of a laying or pond'.[73]

This was not welcome news to the medical community. The *Lancet*, for example, reflected the medical community's general dismay when observing that the report was remarkable from the purely scientific standpoint: for the first time in the history of bacteriology, 'a check has been administered to that young and vigorous pursuit'. The journal prophesied that the result would be improvements in techniques and more careful interpretations in the 'unfolding of nature's story' by the bacteriological community.[74]

Towards a Resolution

Yet if the Royal Commission report was seen as a setback for bacteriology, there was little evidence on the ground, in the ongoing polluted shellfish drama, that this was so. The Fishmongers' Company showed no sign of having their faith in Klein undermined and retained his services until his retirement in 1920. The trades themselves had cause to be grateful to Klein's researches. In 1905, at the Company's instigation, Klein published the results of experiments undertaken to assess the vitality of typhoid bacilli in oysters, cockles and mussels.[75] He was able to demonstrate that the numbers of typhoid bacilli in oysters were greatly reduced after four days in water changed every day and disappeared after six days. Similar experiments on cockles and mussels were, however, much less satisfactory. As regards oysters, the trade found this result 'welcome and reassuring' – but it was still not enthusiastic about bacteriologists: 'What we really want is that bacteriologists should be tried by a jury of their peers'.[76] Klein's researches indicated, however, that there was no reason to restrict the sale of oysters from any area, however polluted, provided that they had first been placed in clean sea water, changed frequently, 'for a given period to be decided on'.[77] On balance, the *Gazette* concluded, the trade 'cannot fail to be grateful to the Fishmongers' Company'.[78]

Klein's name remained closely associated with the bacteriology of shellfish for several decades. The Fishmongers' Company was anxious to develop bacteriological controls for shellfish that would both protect the consumer and be flexible enough to meet the needs of the trade in assessing hygienic quality both of layings and of supplies for the retail market. Two different tests were adopted, which remained in use into the 1930s.[79] The first was Klein's 'Short Method', suitable for the assessment of shellfish in the market, because results could be obtained within twenty-four hours or so. Using *B. coli* as the index of cleanliness (despite all previous reservations!), the proportion of contaminated oysters in a sample of ten provided the guideline for cleanliness. Any sample containing 30 per cent or fewer clean fish was rejected; those at 40–50 per cent clean were subjected to further analysis and then if required a review of the topography of the layings from which they came; samples rating 60 per cent and above clean were 'safe' for market. For the evaluation of conditions in shellfish layings, Alexander Houston's 'Long Method' was favoured. Technically far more complex than Klein's, results were only obtained after seven to ten to fourteen days.[80]

If the conclusions of the Royal Commission revealed divisions between bacteriologists and sharpened the search for bacteriological standards for evaluating sewage pollution in shellfish, it was less successful in moving the administrative authorities towards reforming techniques of sewage disposal, or in developing an administrative framework for the environmental protection of shellfish layings. The Commission proposed the establishment of a separate River Board under a central administrative and executive authority to administer and enforce the Rivers Pollution Prevention Act 1876 and to police the condition of shellfish layings.[81] This proposal remained 'in the air'.[82] Various minor attempts to deal with the situation were made by the legislature. The Public Health (Regulations as to Food) Act of 1907 enabled the local authorities to make regulations, but it was not until 1915 that the Local Government Board produced the Public Health (Shellfish) Regulations which forbade the sale of shellfish likely to endanger public health. The regulations offered no guidance to medical officers of health on how they were to decide whether shellfish in the market were clean or sewage-polluted and to a large extent remained a dead letter. The safeguarding of British shellfish supplies against sewage pollution and contamination with pathogenic bacteria remained, essentially, in the hands of the trade itself and of the Fishmongers' Company.[83]

Conclusion

This case study demonstrates the complexities of the political arena within which the English public health initiative operated at the turn of the nineteenth century. While the pronouncements of medical men carried weight with the general public and affected the behaviour of many consumers, the observational and bacteriological evidence on which medical opinion rested remained open to question by interested parties. The growing power of science was, however, demonstrated by the way in which the fish trades, which at first denigrated medical authority, began to co-opt appropriate bacteriological opinion in their own defence. It was an implicit admission that in areas of activity associated, for better or worse, with matters of health, medical support was essential if the wider society was to be convinced that the fish trades were behaving in a socially responsible fashion. The state, however, represented at this point by the legislature, clearly remained unconvinced of the necessity of intervening in trade questions even where the issue at stake was public health. The question of sanitary standards in the shellfish trades was resolved internally, but at the highest level and only after attempted intervention by a government department and a number of local trade initiatives had conspicuously failed. This was an ad hoc process rather than one involving a particular strategy of government. Nor did consumers as citizens play any apparent role in the process, except in so far as they withdrew their confidence from the product in question.

The key actors in this drama were the representatives of the fishing trades, concerned public health personnel and the bacteriologists whose investigations, together with the disease outbreaks, kept the issues alive. As citizens, these two groups, the fish trades and the public health doctors, stood for the two sides of the liberal dilemma: for the rights of the individual and economic interests on the one hand, as opposed to the collective interests of the larger community and state intervention on the other. The outcome of the drama was influenced by several factors which helped to modify the classical liberal stance of the fish trades: economic pressure as markets reacted to adverse publicity; the gradual recognition that bacteriology was an adversary to be reckoned with; and, finally, recognition by the industry's most powerful body that internal regulation was essential if the trades were to retain their economic viability. The drive to reform practices in the shellfish trades came from within medicine, partially backed by the state, to be taken up under pressure of negative consumer input by a reluctant industry which showed a sense of civic responsibility essentially in its own defence. Entrepreneurship and citizenship thus existed side by side in London at the turn of the nineteenth century.[84] In this case, consumer confidence in the product and self-regulation by the industry were at stake, impelling the industry's own supervisory authority to take action.

3 MONOPOLY OR FREEDOM OF HEALING? THE ROLE OF MEDICINE IN A MODERNIZING SOCIETY

Frank Huisman

In 1913, three Dutch lawyers presented a petition to the Dutch parliament. In their request, they argued for the abolition of the monopoly of treatment by physicians, as was formally provided for in legislation dating from 1865.[1] The lawyers disputed the physicians' exclusive right to perform medical interventions because they had serious doubts about their therapeutic competence. And because the lawyers questioned the state's right to intervene in the health matters of individual citizens, they felt that the state should stop favouring academic physicians above other kinds of healers. They argued that medicine should serve the patient rather than the physician, and that the state should be impartial. The petition caused much political and social commotion. As many as 7,700 people expressed their approval of its contents by signing the petition, while the Dutch government was prompted to ask the Central Health Council (the highest advisory body in the field of health care) and two State Committees for formal advice on the issue.[2] During the five years in which the petition was under discussion many articles, brochures and pamphlets were written, both in favour and opposing it. At stake was no less than the cultural authority of medicine.

The controversy on the petition took place in the 1910s, or – in terms of the periodization suggested in the introduction to this volume – in the transitional era between liberal and social citizenship. While nineteenth-century liberalism had been Janus-faced (moving between *laissez-faire* and utilitarian social intervention), something similar applied to the medical profession. On the one hand, physicians strove for professional autonomy while on the other, they were eager to safeguard some degree of state protection against non-academic competitors. In 1865, the Dutch medical profession had succeeded in obtaining this. In the early twentieth century, however, this regulation was put into question. As argued in the introduction, professionalism had become a crucial feature of the liberal-democratic order, while at the same time, the two forces were at odds with each other. The three petition-presenting lawyers had a fine sense of this tension. They decided to address it by forcing a political and public debate on the matter.

A Petition of Three Lawyers

In September 1913, Samuel van Houten (a former Minister of the Interior), Joost van Hamel (professor of criminal law at the University of Amsterdam) and Rudolph van Holthe tot Echten (councillor of the court of justice in The Hague) submitted a petition to the Dutch parliament, in which they requested a liberalization of the 1865 laws on medical practice.[3] Although the issue at stake was very complex, the three lawyers decided to focus on its legal dimensions, which were both criminal and constitutional. Thus, they established the fact that the law of 1865 was violated on a daily basis, which they considered an infraction of justice. At the time, it had been the intention of Minister Johan Rudolph Thorbecke, who had been responsible for getting the law passed by Parliament in the 1860s, to put an end to the confusing patchwork of medical schools and qualifications in medicine. After 1865, only those who had studied medicine at a university were allowed to practice. The three argued that during the past five decades, this goal had not been accomplished. Quite the contrary: the High Council of Justice (*Hoge Raad*) had had to step in quite often to issue jurisprudence in interpretation of the law.[4] As a result, a situation of 'total legal insecurity' had come into being. The three proposed to end this situation by adapting legislation to daily practice. Secondly, they claimed that the law of 1865 violated the right of citizens to make their own decisions in health matters. They wondered what vital state interests were served by punishing irregular healers and they called for legal guarantees to ensure the patient's freedom of choice in case of illness.[5]

Over and above these requirements, the three lawyers argued that it was impossible to maintain the physician monopoly of treatment as long as it had not been proven that health matters were better dealt with by physicians than by others, that freedom of treatment would cause damage to public health and that legislation could be an effective weapon in the battle against the practice of medicine by irregular healers. They called for amendment of the 1865 legislation to allow patients to seek treatment from the healer of their choice. The state should limit itself to regulation of the training and examination of medical students. Further, the state should take legal action against conscious deceit of the public and against any speculation on its ignorance. Finally, the petitioners wanted *all* malpractice to be prosecuted, regardless of whether it had been committed by physicians or irregular healers. What they called for, in short, was a fair political balance between narrow professional interests and the general interest of all citizens.

During the parliamentary debates of 26 and 27 January 1914, feelings were mixed.[6] Some MPs felt that the petition was moving things in a dangerous direction, pointing to the evils done by quacks. Others argued that there was no proof that the (supposedly) good health condition of the Dutch population was due to the work of academic physicians. As a matter of principle, they argued, the state did not have the right to restrict the freedom of citizens in a matter as personal as individual health. The respected MP A. F. de Savornin Lohman, who thought that laws should be in accordance with the 'people's sense of justice',[7] stepped forward as spokesman for those who supported freedom of healing.[8] The government, on the other hand, withheld its point of view for the time being. To Prime Minister P. W. A. Cort van der Linden, a lawyer and a liberal, the issue was fundamental. A decision was called for that would do justice to both the general health interest and the principle of individual freedom of choice. Although he granted that the state should not act as guardian vis-à-vis its citizens, he thought it unacceptable when a liberalization of the law would endanger public health. Cort van der Linden acknowledged that it was not just a simple matter of choosing between autonomy and paternalism. He therefore forwarded the petition to the Central Health Council, the government's supreme advisory council in health matters.

In its report, published in 1916, the Health Council admitted that illegal medical practice was indeed thriving.[9] There was no denying that the major objective of the law had not been achieved. Indeed, the 1865 law was 'nearly a dead letter' according to the Health Council. The number of irregular healers was 'certainly very substantial' and it was not to be expected that the objective of the 1865 law would be realized in the near future. The Health Council was facing a thorny problem: helping fellow human beings in distress should not be liable to punishment, while at the same time there was ample evidence of irregular healers causing damage to individual health. The Health Council therefore advised the government to organize an impartial investigation of healing systems hitherto unexplained by science. Should it turn out that inexplicable forces or faculties existed, the government should seriously consider taking steps to alleviate human suffering. In that case, many legislative changes would be called for: not only would the Law on Higher Education have to be amended, but Criminal Law and the Law on Medical Practice as well.

In line with the advice of the Health Council, two State Committees were established on 31 July 1917. They were asked to look into the legal and the medical dimensions of the issue. The Legal State Committee was made up of six lawyers, including 'the three H's', as they had come to be called, with Van Houten as chair.[10] Very soon, the committee presented its advice, in the form of a proposal for an amendment of the law.[11] The Van Houten Committee encouraged the embracement of the principle of 'limited exclusive competence'. The proposed law wanted everyone offering medical help or counsel to register with their district health inspector. Healers were expected to specify the specific nature of their treatment and training. In addition, the committee defined a number of 'restricted interventions' in which only regular practitioners should be permitted to engage, notably surgery, obstetrics, the prescription of strong medication and the treatment of venereal disease. Finally, all practitioners would henceforth be held legally liable for the effects of a treatment, while none could any longer claim ignorance of the law. According to the committee, the proposed law would be more in line with people's overall sense of justice. Also, it would honour – within certain limitations – the principle of patient autonomy and self-determination; and, finally, it would encourage irregular healers to use their gifts in the interests of public health.

Response of the Medical Profession

For some time an unfavourable wind had been blowing in the Netherlands. From the medical profession's viewpoint, people from the higher echelons of society were peddling concepts and propositions that harkened back to the Middle Ages.

Thus J. F. Selhorst, a physician from The Hague, in a series of articles published in the journal *Vox Medicorum* argued against the three H's and the 'petition movement' they had started.[12] Initially, Selhorst had hardly taken the H's initiative seriously and the same went for most of his colleagues.[13] However, when it turned out that the prime minister was prepared to give their petition serious consideration, even asking the Central Health Council for advice, the medical profession was alarmed and felt the need for a clear collective response. The editorial board of the Dutch journal of medicine, *Nederlandsch Tijdschrift voor Geneeskunde*, the journal of the Dutch Society for the Advancement of Medicine (Nederlandsche Maatschappij tot bevordering der Geneeskunst, NMG), decided to devote a special issue to the matter.[14] This issue, entitled 'Medical Monopoly and Freedom of Healing' (*Artsenmonopolie en geneesvrijheid*), contained twenty-six contributions written by twenty-three authors. Together, they argued for the superiority of science over intuition, claiming that healing practice should always be rooted in science.

Two Amsterdam lawyers had been invited to write an extensive legal defence. The argument of J. Slingenberg came in two parts.[15] First, he used an international comparison of medical legislation – to argue that the introduction of freedom of healing would lead to a deterioration of public health. He presented the United Kingdom and Germany as examples to be avoided. While the UK had always been the classical example of freedom of trade, Germany had embraced *Kurirfreiheit* in 1869. 'Quackery' had been thriving ever since, he argued, and had even 'grown into an important power within the state'.[16] In the second part of his essay Slingenberg defended the principle that 'the good must suffer under the bad'. Just as the carrying of arms in a 'well-ordered society' was forbidden to all in an attempt to prevent anyone from causing damage to a fellow-citizen, so irregular medical practice should be prohibited. In most cases, quacks could not be accused of deceit, because they were consulted by the patient themselves.

Slingenberg argued that it was difficult to collect evidence against irregular healers: not only because witnesses often sympathized with the accused, but mainly because health, illness and healing are difficult categories to define.

Physicians contributing to the special issue argued for 'science' as a demarcation criterion between regular and irregular healers. Although this seemed like an unambiguous criterion, it hardly solved the issue. After all, why should it be assumed that a 'scientific' discipline would lead to a superior profession, deserving state protection? Moreover, if academic medical knowledge was clearly superior, then why was it in need of state protection? These questions were just as essential as they were difficult to answer. From the outside, the medical profession may have looked like a unified whole, but behind the façade of scientific and legal unity, there was an enormous diversity of professional standards.[17] In his introduction to the special issue, Gerard van Rijnberk – professor of physiology and editor-in-chief of the *Dutch Journal of Medicine* – wrestled to define what made medicine a science. Medicine, he argued, included 'all knowledge, tested by experience and experiment, of the material structure, the workings and the defects of the human body, as it is gathered through the ages and taught at university'.[18]

Several essays looked into the basic characteristics of science. While some emphasized the open character of medicine, others felt that its system and method were the discipline's defining characteristics, making it superior to lay knowledge. Thus Willem Nolen, professor of practical medicine, felt that the very openness of the discipline would lead it to progress. Only receptiveness to new and unexpected facts derived from experience could improve medicine, following the path of trial and error. 'Modesty suits physicians well', he argued.[19] By contrast, Cornelis Pekelharing, professor of pathology and chair of the Medical State Committee, was very much devoted to strict scientific methodology. For generations, mankind had used speculation, *a priori* reasoning and mysticism. The nineteenth century had witnessed the final breakthrough of science, in particular in physics and chemistry. According to Pekelharing, pioneers like Bichat, Laënnec, Müller, Dubois Reymond, Helmholtz, Virchow and Henle had supplied medicine with rigorous scientific foundations, causing a fundamental break with the past.

The views of Nolen and Pekelharing point to a contradiction between the clinical and the analytical gaze. The clinician has an eye for the multiplicity of his object and the unruliness of practice. Convinced that health and disease are complex phenomena in which not only physical factors play a role but mental and environmental ones as well, the clinician puts all his trust in his experience, which over time has been shaped and coloured by an array of 'clinical images'. The analyst, however, is looking for unity in diversity. By tracking down patterns, he seeks to reduce the complexity of the real world. Of course we are dealing with two extreme positions here, but it is clear how this contradiction complicated the fixing of scientific and professional standards. Knowing that this was a weakness in their argument, a number of authors introduced the distinction between 'genees*kunde*' and 'genees*kunst*', or science (*scientia*) and practice (*ars*). Medicine as *ars* referred to medical interventions informed by experi-ence – that might, in turn, benefit medical science. Only thus was it possible to distinguish between systematic, scientific knowledge and random, useless knowledge.[20]

The ophthalmologist Pieter Muntendam illustrated this distinction in a dis-cussion of self-help books written by lay people. If the medical monopoly were abolished, he worried, the market would be flooded by such writings. In France and Germany, huge numbers of booklets like *Le médecin des pauvres* and *Das neue Naturheilverfahren* were printed. Muntendam deemed popularization of medical knowledge useful for countering ignorance and superstition, but only if it was supplied by 'sensible, level-headed and skilled physicians', rather than by 'non-experts, who were often quacks of the worst kind'.[21] Writing on medi-cation, professor of pharmacology Evert Cornelis van Leersum argued that the notion of 'old' was wrongly associated with 'well-tried'.[22] According to Van Leersum, good medication was the end product of a slow and lengthy process of critical experimenting and logical thinking against the backdrop of an estab-lished, systematic scientific world view. In his opinion there was no place for accidental findings or medications that were discovered in unsystematic ways and administered without a proper understanding of pharmacodynamic princi-ples. If modern medicine was systematic, rational and consistent, old or popular medicine was incoherent, erratic and merely based on experience.

In addition to the special issue of the *Dutch Journal of Medicine* there was another major response to the petition coming from medical circles: the report from the Medical State Committee (which consisted of medical professionals).[23] This Pekelharing Committee had been assigned to study the value of unorthodox healing methods. It had published an announcement in a number of newspapers in which all 'who believe they qualify' were invited to allow the committee to assess their healing method. Several healers had contacted the committee, taking along one or more patients. Furthermore, three organizations had committed themselves to participate in the study: the Society for Mental Research and Applied Magnetism, the Society *Vis Naturae Medicatrix* and the Committee for Amending the Law on Medical Practice. Based on a study of the treatment of a total of ninety-six patients, the State Committee concluded that healers made poor if not wrong diagnoses, that many phenomena and methods they worked with were already known to physicists and physiologists (and could thus not be attributed to unknown, mysterious forces) and that the results of their treatment were quite limited and in some cases even negative. Having studied the merits of magnetism, Christian Science, somnambulism, herbal medicine, homeopathy and naturopathy, the Committee concluded that there was no evidence of healing methods that resulted in new or surprising cures. Although the committee declared that the healers it had studied were no frauds, it flatly rejected their claims to special healing powers. Potentially favourable results were attributed to (auto)suggestion. Its final conclusion was that the results 'in no way substantiate the view of those who feel that it is in the interest of mankind to recommend the practice of medicine without scientific training'.[24] It was thought dangerous to proclaim freedom of healing, because unqualified healers posed a risk for their patients and even (in the case of contagious disease) for society at large. The Committee's advice to keep the law of 1865 in force was warmly welcomed by the medical establishment.[25]

The Incommensurability of Legal and Medical Arguments

Van Holthe tot Echten responded in *Future Life* (*Het toekomstig leven*), a journal devoted to the study of spiritualism.[26] In response to lawyer Slingenberg he argued that 'quackery' flourished as much in countries with a medical monopoly as in countries with freedom of healing. A more fundamental objection against Slingenberg, however, concerned his assertion that the 'good must suffer under the bad'. Van Holthe tot Echten considered this a reprehensible view that undermined the basis of morality and criminal law.

Van Holthe tot Echten briefly summarized the reasoning of physicians thus: 'having knowledge is better than having no knowledge at all and we are the ones who own medical knowledge'.[27] He countered that precisely in the domain of medi-cine (scientific) knowledge alone is not enough: 'What if there were knowledge that "physicians" do not own, knowledge of how our inner personality construes and maintains the body ... then what?'[28] He was not just thinking of the fluidum that a magnetizer could radiate to a receptive patient, but also of somnambulists, who according to him had a normal and a 'subliminal personality', which they might activate in a trance. More often than not, a diagnosis was based on intuition rather than knowledge. Van Holthe tot Echten, then, accused physicians of pedantry and laziness: they preferred laughing about something they did not understand to examining it.

Freedom of healing might provide an enormous boost to medical science, Van Holthe tot Echten claimed. In this respect, he pointed to the *Dutch Journal of Medicine* article written by Van Leersum, in which he – as a proponent of medical monopoly – acknowledged that official medicine had borrowed much from popular medicine, such as digitalis, strophantin, cinchona and coca. He therefore expressed the hope that physicians would be prepared to examine everything and to retain the good, even when that involved a healing method borrowed from non-physicians. Van Holthe tot Echten emphasized that he did not look down on medical science and that he did not take pleasure in a fight with physicians. He merely pleaded for the introduction of freedom of healing as a justified principle. He felt that it was warranted to demand that the state be impartial.

It became increasingly clear that the dispute would not be settled, as the arguments were derived from two very different worlds: the legal domain and the medical domain. This becomes evident, for example, in the fervent articles contributed to the issue by the gynaecologist Jan Frederik Selhorst.[29] He described Van Holthe tot Echten as a 'fanatic spiritist' and a 'priest in the temple of darkness and mystery', who should be put under psychiatric observation for the 'glaring nonsense' he talked. Selhorst felt that the debate on the medical monopoly illustrated how scientific expertise was smothered by juridical sophistry.[30] Basically, Selhorst argued that there was a legal monopoly in Dutch society. The favourable reception of the petition, he wrote, could be explained by the fact that government and parliament consisted of laypersons rather than experts. And the same was true of the Central Health Council which mainly consisted of 'office workers' rather than practising physicians. Paradoxically, legal experts were able to exert influence in areas of which they had not the slightest knowledge. While medical science depended on laboratories and hospitals for its development, legal experts – 'who had never held a test tube' – decided on the organization of that science. The downfall of the nation could only be countered by ending the legal monopoly and replacing lawyers by experts from the fields involved. Referring to the upcoming general elections, Selhorst ended his diatribe as follows:

> 'There is a great deal rotten in the State of the Netherlands.' Let it be ended by universal suffrage and if it fails to do so, let a Napoleon *redivivus* come along. *Aux grands maux, les grands remèdes!*[31]

In other words, Selhorst was hoping that the electorate would choose the side of academic medicine. Should that not happen, a dictator was called for to set things right.

It is striking to see that Van Holthe tot Echten was counting on democratic forces as well. At a time when regular medicine only seemed to have an eye for the material and the quantifiable in nature, he made a plea for healing systems based on immaterial phenomena such as magnetic fluid. Observing that most physicians ignored similar phenomena – despite their benefits for the sick – he concluded with the following appeal:

> Let the freedom of Dutch citizens be restored – also their freedom to choose their own way of healing. If the State is willing to regulate this issue, let this regulation be such that knowledge is not seen as the equivalent of healing power and vice versa.[32]

As a lawyer he advocated individual freedom of choice, as a human being he believed in magnetism and reincarnation. In other words, his reasons for co-authoring the petition were not only legally motivated but also of a very personal nature.[33] Because the petition touched on the boundaries of law and medicine it was impossible to settle the dispute using arguments derived from either one of these disciplines. In the debate on freedom of healing the protagonists could only fall back on general cultural notions of body and mind and health and illness. It was precisely the very general dimension of the issue that constituted the petition's broad appeal. That is why 7,700 individuals felt the need to support it by signing and why there was such extensive coverage in the general press.[34]

Modernity and its Discontents

The 'petition movement' found major support among members of the intellectual and political elites in the Netherlands. The physician Pinkhof observed that 'even one of the wisest politicians of our country' had been misled, probably referring to MP De Savornin Lohman.[35] He must also have been irritated by MP Fridolin Knobel, who during one of the first parliamentary debates on the petition had noted that 'we know from experience that there are forces that physicians are unwilling to consider or automatically dismiss as not belonging to their domain'.[36]

It may be somewhat surprising that the protests against the medical monopoly came from society's upper echelons. After all, in the same period there was also a general optimism and belief in progress, to which Dutch natural science had contributed. In a short time span, many new research laboratories were set up and the number of research professors greatly multiplied. By 1913, as many as four Dutch scientists had won the Nobel Prize. Scientists informed each other of their latest results in scholarly societies and at conferences, while they sought to win public support for their cause by writing popular articles and giving lectures across the country. There was, in short, great enthusiasm for natural science in general and medicine in particular. This explains why some have referred to this period as 'the second golden age' of Dutch science.[37]

Why, then, the attack on the medical monopoly? Some physicians argued that the attack reflected resentment among a few. Pinkhof, for one, referred to 'the aversion and hostile approach of the red-black reactionaries in the area of medicine'.[38] Others held the opinion that the movement aimed its arrows at science as such. They identified 'a general dissatisfaction, which is searching for new ways and is perhaps all too eager to believe what is least proven'.[39] Behind the strictly legal reasoning of the petition of the three H's, physicians believed, lurked the wish to pave the way for specific kinds of healers. *Vox medicorum* speculated that this might apply to 'the more mystically based counsel provided by somnambulists, practitioners of spiritualism, Christian Science, theosophists and others'. A few years later Pinkhof noted: 'There is a large group of people today who consult quacks *as a matter of principle*'.[40]

All evidence, however, suggests this type of speculation was misguided: the petition movement was no medical counter-movement, nor did it intend to be one. It seems to have been part of a larger, yet quite amorphous, cultural reorientation. Although the content of the petition specifically reflected a critique of medicine, it was targeted neither at the discipline as such nor at its practitioners. Instead, it was aimed at a particular general attitude, at an overall mentality that merely engaged with the material while disregarding the immaterial, the spiritual, the intuitive and the mystical.[41] This anti-materialist orientation, it should be added, was not limited to laypersons, for academically trained thinkers also supported or joined alternative experiments. These included the physicians Frederik van Eeden and Jacobus van Rees and the mathematician L. E. J. Brouwer. In addition, lesser known physicians gave their support to homeopathy or vegetarianism, fought vivisection, advocated hypnosis as a method of treatment or believed in the miraculous cures at Lourdes.[42] Other physicians displayed an interest in the phenomenon of (auto)suggestion and experimented with hypnosis. Moreover, medical subdisciplines such as psychiatry and neurology began to take shape while psychology was on the rise. The era has been characterized as having a 'zeitgeist that emphasized a sensory and mental awakening'.[43] Most contemporaries, then, were worried not so much about science as such as about its one-sided orientation.

According to Van Leersum, the petition movement was driven by a mixture of blind faith and superstition, ignorance and pedantry, quackery and dissatisfaction.[44] This last qualification deserves closer attention. Undoubtedly there was a certain resentment towards the medical profession, which was seen to be claiming a great deal yet hardly realizing its claims – at least regarding its therapeutic efforts. The dissatisfaction, though, was much more deep-seated and had a different character than was suggested by Van Leersum: it was prompted by anxiety about modern culture, which was increasingly determined by science and technology. Consequently, the need for a reconsideration of all sorts of social and general cultural issues was felt more broadly. The discussions took place in various forms and contexts, such as in several series of pamphlets. One of them was entitled 'Pro and Con on Issues of General Significance' (*Pro en contra betreffende vraagstukken van algemeen belang*); another, 'Vital Questions' (*Levensvragen*), aimed at 'all who are interested in the spiritual struggles of our time', as its subtitle put it. These series of pamphlets suggest the themes that were important to the general public and many of them were controversial. A random selection: spelling simplification, free marriage, the right to strike, women's suffrage and capital punishment, but also naturopathy, animal magnetism, spiritualism, Christian Science, religion and science, hypnotism in medicine, vegetarianism, homeopathy, cures at Lourdes, theosophy, freemasonry and vivisection. Clearly, the Dutch population was exploring epistemological alternatives, looking for new footings in a rapidly changing society.[45]

These series of pamphlets and their various concerns also throw light on the ambitions and frustrations of the petition movement. For some critics of modern society, such as K. H. Beijlevelt, editor of *Friend of Nature. Monthly for the Prevention and Treatment of Disease* (*Natuurvriend. Maandblad ter voorkoming en bestrijding van ziekten*), modern science represented everything they abhorred: rationality, reductionism and alienation.[46] They considered the mere existence of physicians as a sign of alienation: human beings were no longer able to 'know' their own bodies and had to trust the judgement of persons who did not have the power (anymore) to understand life in all its organic unity. Instead, life was deprived of its magic and analysed apart from its natural coherence. Beijlevelt stressed that naturopathy comprised a whole philosophy that was inextricably bound up with a natural diet and a natural way of living. He presented the proponents of this way of living as idealists who pursued 'social reform, in both a material and spiritual sense'. They viewed it as their task to live according to the laws of nature. Each individual's own rational powers pointed the way to such knowledge, but it was at least as much a matter of instinct, which many had lost in modern times. In order to become aware (again) of that latent knowledge, one needed to turn inwards, towards the self. Every human was considered capable of this, because body and mind are 'intimately united'. Those living according to the good laws of nature, then, are bearers of real civilization; those who manage to live in harmony with the self and their social and natural environment will stay healthy.

Other spokespersons involved in this 'cultural reorientation' included people like Felix Ortt, Hendrik Nicolaas de Frémery, J. S. Göbel and Marie Hartman. In countless pamphlets and brochures they tried to interest their contemporaries in vegetarianism, spiritualism, anti-vivisectionism, Buddhism, international disarmament, Christian-anarchism or homeopathy. They hoped that their readers would begin to realize that science and materialism increasingly alienated people from their true selves. The prolific anti-materialist writer Felix Ortt viewed scientific knowledge as subordinate to moral feeling, the latter reflecting the purest form of knowing.[47] Precisely in the domain of morality, however, formal expertise did not exist because morality was 'a matter of feeling rather than reason'. Ortt claimed that there were good reasons to take the arguments of laypersons even more seriously than those of experts, since the former had no stake in a particular field. He underlined his own eclecticism by appealing to Buddha, Saint Francis of Assisi and Jesus to stand by him in his moral doubt. Magnetism was advocated by Hendrik Nicolaas de Frémery, editor of *Future Life* (*Het toekomstig leven*), the journal that in 1914 had published the response of Van Holthe tot Echten to the special issue of the *Dutch Journal of Medicine*.[48] Magnetism assumed the existence of a power that could not be established by objective science, but that could be known through its effects. Each human being was believed to have this power, which by means of specific manipulations could be transferred from one organism to another. Only those who possessed a surplus of vital power could become magnetizers. This quality, then, was an inborn gift that could not be acquired through study.[49] The same was true, according to Göbel, for spiritualism: here too susceptibility and innate talent played a decisive role. Only those who had 'a certain aptitude' could mediate between the world in which we live and 'the "invisible" world'.[50] Such an aptitude was important because spiritualist séances had demonstrated that there was no clear dividing line between the material and the immaterial, that the cosmos was not empty and that life was not just material but eternal and animated. All of this was discounted by regular science. Although science may have produced major insights, it did so at too high a price: the complete disregard of the higher life of the soul. This is why, Göbel argued, there was an imbalance 'between the hunger for spiritual nurturing and that which our era has to offer to people'.[51] In this respect, Marie Hartman occupied the most extreme position.[52] Christian Science held that the so-called outside world was an illusion, a product of our misguided insight. This implied that evil in the world (including sin and illness) was not real, but only consisted of a 'wrong, limited, material *awareness* of the spiritual universe and spiritual man'. Hartman felt that renouncing the belief in sin, illness, death and matter (including the carnal body) was an absolute precondition for 'a process of awakening to people's real, spiritual being in the image of God, Who is Spirit'.[53]

All these various alternative ideologies were not medical counter-movements as such. Rather, they were tied to spiritual or philosophical movements advocating social reform and a new spirituality, comparable to the German *Lebensreform* movement.[54] In so doing, their spokesmen used a language that was peppered with binary oppositions. Purity, naturalness, inborn talent, feeling, spirit and holism were contrasted, respectively, to defilement, science, learned skill, mind, matter and reductionism. The issues of coercion and alienation, which the state and science supposedly forced upon modern individuals, were regularly addressed.[55] Yet the petition movement cannot simply be characterized as antiscientific. On the contrary: its representatives frequently supported the call to look beyond the material and directly visible with notions and analogies derived from the modern natural sciences. Thus magnetic fluid was compared to electrons, ions, atoms and N-rays, which were equally invisible yet assumed to be real.[56]

The critique of science mainly pertained to its one-sided orientation. If scientists were to give up their materialism, they would create a basis for finding natural explanations for what initially seemed irrational or absurd. In this context it becomes understandable that an academically trained lawyer such as Van Holthe tot Echten stood up for the natural talents of the free healer. He contrasted those with the (supposed) book learning of the physician-monopolist that – though valuable – was anything but perfect. The petition movement, it seems, was primarily motivated by epistemological doubt. The attraction of the various alternative ideologies lay precisely in the combination of modern scientific insight and the prospect of a 'return' to a higher, better spiritual life.

These wider implications of the petition were not lost on the Central Health Council. In its advice to Minister Cort van der Linden, it indicated that the subject matter was 'highly complex' and that the Health Council thus considered itself authorized to judge only to a limited degree.[57] It was up to politicians to weigh the many contradictory feelings, considerations and arguments involved – a difficult task indeed, if only because it also implied rethinking the role of the state.[58]

The Political Handling of the Petition

The petition had an important political dimension in that it raised the issue of the relationship between state and society. At stake were the questions raised in the introduction to this volume. They include questions such as whether the state is allowed to interfere with the private lives of its citizens. If so, to what extent (and how) is it responsible for their health and medical treatment? Can health be considered as a civil right and if so, what does that mean? The right to remain free from state intervention or the right to collective arrangements in the field of health care? And how should the responsibilities of state, civil society, the medical profession and individual citizens be delineated?

So how did the petition and its particular proposals influence the political decision process? When preparing the petition, the three Hs decided to use the former liberal Minister Van Houten as main author and figurehead. This was a sensible decision for several reasons. The three were all too familiar with Dutch political mores and it was rather the rule than the exception that members of parliament merely took note of a petition after which they moved on to the order of the day.[59] By capitalizing on Van Houten's stature, the authors tried to ensure that the petition would be treated seriously. In this, they succeeded. No one could defend the petition's political dimension with more authority and persuasion than Van Houten.[60] Although as a down-to-earth rationalist he never engaged in the humanitarian-idealist experiments of his time, he was very committed to the 'liberty' and the 'natural rights' of the patient. In one of his *Letters on Politics* (*Staatkundige brieven*), a series of essays containing his thoughts on Dutch politics, he accounts for the presentation of the petition as follows: 'For as long as the medical legislation has been in force, I have been irritated about the threat of punishment and prosecution against legally unqualified practitioners of healing because it involves a violation of freedom on insufficient grounds.'[61]

He viewed Thorbecke's legislation as *a faux pas*, and an 'unauthorized interference by state authority'. He felt that punishing unqualified healers was indefensible because patients took the initiative in consulting them. Moreover, Van Houten – who had great confidence in science – saw the physicians' passionate response to the petition as a sign of insecurity concerning their own therapeutic powers. This is why he considered a treatment monopoly to be unfair. In the effort to reform Thorbecke 's medical laws, Van Houten – with his independent judgement and solid authority – was precisely the type who was needed to hold his own against the social-liberal Cort van der Linden.

Cort van der Linden's ideas on the renewal of liberalism had been shaped in the 1880s.[62] In his *Direction and Policy of the Liberal Party* (*Richting en beleid der liberale partij*, 1886), he had distanced himself from the classic-liberal tenet of the state's non-interference. Earlier, liberals had assumed that social stability and prosperity would be served by a minimum of external coercion. The individual was expected to pursue self-interest in a rational manner, which would lead to predictable behaviour and therefore to social stability. Having a sense of duty and responsibility was seen as an intrinsic human characteristic; it would prevent liberties from leading to chaos or repression. Cort van der Linden felt that this logic was no longer tenable at the end of the nineteenth century, with its industrialization and large-scale pauperization. This new situation had proven that a sense of duty in the interest of the community had to be exacted. After Cort became a member of government, he practised what he had advocated as a professor of law. As a Minister of Justice in the liberal reform cabinet, with Pierson (1897–1901) he was co-responsible for child welfare legislation and for drafting the Industrial Injuries Law. He also co-signed the Housing Law. The non-interference principle of the liberal 'night-watchman state' transformed gradually – and after 1901 at a faster pace – into a politics of state intervention in society.

Although Van Houten and Cort van der Linden espoused two different visions of liberalism and the role of the state, they were much closer to each other regarding the issue of freedom of healing than might have been expected. Cort van der Linden took a nuanced stance and there are even indications that he agreed with some of the petition's recommendations. Specifically, he made a careful distinction between medical science and medical practice. Already during the first debate in Parliament on the petition in 1914, he articulated his trust in medicine as a science. He valued the critical powers of distinction of science. He had a dislike of fantasy and 'female' capriciousness, which he deemed a danger for social virtue and solidity. According to him, giving free reign to fantasies and passions would have a destabilizing effect on society.[63]

Yet, Cort acknowledged the existence of a reality beyond science: actual medical practice was fickle, a 'dark, infinite space'. It was there, outside the reach of materialist science, that one had to look for the forces that the petition movement thought were there. Therefore, when in 1917 the medical State Committee was set up for the study of the value of unorthodox ways of healing, Cort suggested to its chair that alternative healers be appointed to the committee as well. Presumably, Cort did so on the assumption that much of use could be found in that 'dark space' and that only alternative healers would have the intuition to find it. Pekelharing, however, did not follow up this advice because he felt it to be 'ineffective'.[64] Although the three Hs probably anticipated a titanic struggle between Van Houten and Cort van der Linden, a liberalization of the laws of 1865 seems to have been within reach.

However, things worked out differently. Much time had passed already since the presentation of the petition in 1913.[65] When both reports were finished, it was too late: in the elections of 3 July 1918 – the first after the introduction of universal suffrage – the liberals suffered a very considerable defeat. The number of their seats in Parliament dropped from forty to fifteen. A new confessional cabinet, led by the Catholic Charles Ruys de Beerenbrouck, came into office on 9 September.[66] The new cabinet faced many pressing issues. For one thing, the economy had to be jumpstarted in the wake of the war and social and educational legislation had to be formulated. In the cabinet's first months, moreover, much attention had to be devoted to other issues such as the German emperor's decision to reside in the Netherlands, demobilization and the revolutionary effort of the social-democrat Pieter Jelles Troelstra. Given all this commotion, it is possible that there simply was no time for more debate on liberalizing the medical laws.

It is more likely, however, that the new cabinet felt no need to spend much time on it. Especially in the area of social and medical legislation and state intervention the Ruys de Beerenbrouck cabinet was very ambitious.[67] While Cort van der Linden may have been willing to debate liberalization of the 1865 medical laws with his liberal colleagues, his confessional successors no longer felt such a need, which meant that legislation simply remained in place. Silently, the issue disappeared from the political agenda.

Given all the rhetorical fervour of the preceding five years, this may be called an anticlimax. It becomes understandable, however, when we realize that science and the state were increasingly in need of each other during the first decades of the twentieth century. In a rapidly modernizing world witnessing the rise of civic participation, there was a great need for professionals – physicians among them – to shape society. Faced with the rise and expansion of democratic citizenship, the state could no longer afford to stand by and stick to *laissez-faire* policies. It was realized that the state was expected to intervene. However, it could not do so alone. Scientific experts were needed to shape the public domain in a way that was acceptable to the majority of the electorate. Against this background, there was no time for subtle distinctions between collective and individual medicine, between medical science and medical practice, or between theory and therapy. Because physicians were instrumental in creating new collective arrangements, it was felt that the laws of 1865 remained the best way to frame the Dutch health care system.

4 AMBIVALENCES OF LIBERAL HEALTH POLICY: *LEBENSREFORM* AND SELF-HELP MEDICINE IN BELGIUM, 1890–1914

Evert Peeters and Kaat Wils

The suggestion that public health policies in liberal-democratic Europe have never been a consensual affair is not new. Although such policies implied ever increasing levels of government intervention from the late nineteenth century until the 1980s, the limits of this intervention remained a matter of political and social controversy throughout the twentieth century. At the same time, discourses of public health implied varying ranges of individual responsibility. These discourses were conceptually intertwined with top-down policies, but did not exclude the flourishing of liberal cultures of (medical) self-help. Diverging conceptions of the state and the individual revolved around different conceptions of society – the so-called 'social organism'. Since the individual body's condition, it was believed, ultimately affected the man-made *body politic*, health care became a matter of political *and* personal regulation, informed by philosophies of interventionist utilitarianism and *laissez-faire* alike.[1] In this chapter, the conceptual instability of liberal-democratic health policies will be studied in its early stages, through the example of health reform in *fin-de-siècle* Belgium.

Because Belgium was arguably the most liberal country in nineteenth-century continental Europe, the ambivalences of liberalism became particularly obvious. The guiding principle behind the Belgian constitutional system was the wish to guarantee 'liberty in everything and for all' (*Liberté en tout et pour tous*), which implied a deep-seated suspicion of a coercive state. On this assumption, the only function of the Belgian state was to guarantee the liberties of Belgian citizens. However, the way in which this freedom was defined and organized became the object of a fierce 'culture war' during the second half of the nineteenth century between Catholics and anti-clericals, the latter gathering politically around the banner of liberalism.[2] Whereas the Catholics defended first and foremost the freedom of the traditional Catholic religion of the Belgian population, political liberals promoted the ideal of the free and enlightened individual, who would be the bearer of progress for the nation – even for mankind. Ironically enough, the liberals resorted to the state as the main safeguard of this ideal, which they saw as threatened by clerical attacks. The same state which they suspected of being potentially repressive or coercive had to become the main vehicle of progress and rationality. For this reason, they became the main advocates of compulsory state education, whereas in the economic field their axiomatic belief in 'the liberty of enterprise and labour' turned out to be very persistent. It was precisely on this point that a schism between the 'doctrinaire' and the 'progressive' liberals occurred by the end of the nineteenth century.[3]

If the liberal solutions for education and labour respectively were relatively clear-cut (though opposed), the liberal position in the field of health policy was riddled with ambivalence. As a result, health care became an object of party political dispute only at a relatively late stage. The debate never gained the intensity of the fight over education, nor was it characterized by such a clear-cut divide between Catholics and anticlericals. More than anywhere else, the liberal tenets of individual freedom and progress seemed to be at odds in the field of health care. Should the human body be considered as the most individual of things and therefore something on which everyone could decide autonomously? This position could only be held by those who optimistically believed that the ever more educated citizen would automatically choose the most scientific solutions. In reality, however, scientific medicine (whose capacity to provide effective cures was after all still very limited) did not spontaneously gain a monopoly. Traditional religious beliefs and healing practices remained popular. In order to fight the dominant impact of religion and make the progress of scientific medicine and hygiene widely available, the liberal elites tended to favour some form of state intervention, even though their awareness of this issue developed much later than in the field of education. The degree of state intervention they envisaged could vary from the legal protection of the medical profession to large-scale 'hygienist' programmes. Such programmes involved para-medical matters of 'hygiene' in the first place, such as housing policy, working conditions and alcohol legislation, but also measures such as the building of urban (non-denominational) dispensaries and clinics. Even though Catholic medical doctors sided on many issues with their more vocal liberal colleagues in favour of state regulation, medical hygienism became to a large extent bound up with liberalism and, towards the end of the century, with socialism.

The ambivalences of medical liberalism materialized not only in the 'positive' rhetoric and practice of slowly expanding state intervention. As the medical profession became the object of ever more stringent regulation, medical practice increasingly defined itself through negative demarcation from its 'others'. The emergence of so-called alternative cultures of health from the 1890s onwards, we will argue, was partly a reaction against this tightening-up of medical liberalism. Some reformers turned to the alternative orthodoxy of homeopathy, while others advocated allegedly ancient folk medicine. In this chapter, we will focus upon the Belgian practitioners of classical hydrotherapy and so-called natural healing – an offspring of the natural healing methods (*Naturheilkunde*) practised by medical laymen (*Laienheilkunde*) in Germany.[4]

Despite their public image as 'alternative' and their political and legal exclusion from the medical market, late nineteenth-century alternative cultures of health can be understood as indictors of a tension within the medical mainstream.[5] Their emphasis on individual liberty in medical matters, we will argue, sheds light on the paradox of medical liberalism. They questioned the belief in a medical freedom enjoyed by free citizens that was nonetheless to be protected by a slowly expanding interventionist state.

Medicine and the Liberal State

Throughout the nineteenth century, the liberal Belgian state remained remarkably absent from the domain of medicine. Health care and the regulation of the practice of medicine lay mainly with the local authorities. The national government at first limited its function to the supervision of local policies, the issuing of regulations in situations of crisis such as epidemics, the creation of advisory and decentralized regulatory boards, and the subsidizing of private organizations in the field of public health policy. Competences with regard to health policy were divided between several ministries – Internal Affairs, Justice and War, among others – and priority was given to none of them. An independent Ministry of Public Health was established as late as 1936. Unlike its neighbouring countries, Belgium never adopted a public health act.[6]

With regard to the regulation of the practice of medicine, the Belgian State took over the legal framework which had been set up in 1818 under Dutch rule. Since then, any healer who had not studied medicine at university had been excluded from the practice of medicine. In 1853, a so-called 'interpretative' law (*loi interprétative*) made the activities of non-academic healers illegal, even if they had never (falsely) claimed the possession of a medical degree. The system was similar to the French and diverged from the more liberal regulations in Britain and Germany. The unification of the profession would soon be fostered by a reorganization of the medical university curriculum, which from 1849 on delivered one single medical degree of 'doctor in medicine, surgery and obstetrics'. In the course of the nineteenth century, physicians would increasingly fight against governmental regulation and strive for a system of self-regulation instead. This would finally result in the establishment of a disciplinary professional society, the Order of Physicians, in 1938.[7]

In the field of public health policy also, the Belgian Ministry of Internal Affairs slowly expanded its prerogatives in public health from the 1840s onwards, and started to create other advisory and coordinating boards in the field, a process which further intensified in the 1880s. In 1841, the Royal Academy of Medicine was founded. Throughout the nineteenth century, it effectively advised national government on such issues as prostitution, syphilis, alcoholism and women's and children's labour (even though implementation of the suggested policies was scanty).[8] As a result of the large-scale cholera epidemic in 1848–9, a second advisory board – the Council on Public Hygiene, Conseil Supérieur d'Hygiène Publique – was founded in 1849. After 1870, the government expanded the council's competences, enabling it, for instance, to prepare the first legislation on children's and women's labour. With the creation in 1884 of a government Central Service of Health and Public Hygiene, mandated to regulate, among other things, food and drugs safety, the rudimentary foundations of a Belgian health organization were established.[9]

The members of the above-mentioned committees belonged to a social or intellectual elite of physicians. Mostly wealthy by birth, these hygienists were less dependent on fees than the majority of their colleagues and could invest time in research and membership of scientific associations and advisory boards. Most of them were also active in local scientific medical associations, which had existed since the 1830s or 1840s in larger cities such as Ghent, Bruges, Antwerp, Brussels, Liège and Charleroi. In these societies, interest in questions of public hygiene was strong. Research based on social statistics and, from the late 1860s, experimental physiological research was discussed and stimulated through competitions. An inchoate belief in the possibility of turning medicine into a socially relevant science was fostered by the use which local authorities made of the societies' expertise in times of epidemics. In 1876, a national Royal Society for Public Medicine was founded. This association would soon develop into Belgium's main 'laboratory' of medical statistics, focused on the search for physical and social determinants of illness and mortality.[10]

During the same period, a process of 'politicization' of the field of hygienism seems to have taken place. The first generation of medical statisticians had consisted of socially-minded physicians who were not prominently involved in the ongoing culture war between Catholics and anticlericals. There are indications that the introduction of experimental physiological research, and later bacteriology, into the field of public medicine was paralleled by a growing anticlerical, liberal identification with this project and, subsequently, by a positioning of hygienist physicians on the progressive side of the divide within the liberal political movement. This shift reflected a more general cultural shift towards the natural sciences and their methods. From the late 1860s onwards, natural science became an identifying element in the world view and self-representation of socialists and radical liberal free-thinkers. Science was not only presented as religion's antithesis, but also as the only legitimate basis of knowledge and meaning and as a key to a more human future. During the 1860s, medical materialism was quite popular among politically radical medical students at Brussels University. In the following decades, the field of physiology in particular functioned as the breeding-ground of a culture of scientism in which the topos of an opposition between science and religion was enthusiastically transposed into the topos of a struggle between scientific medicine and religion.[11]

In a city such as Antwerp, where liberals were mostly in power during the last decades of the nineteenth century, a comprehensive hygienist policy was implemented in public schools and elsewhere and quite explicitly identified as a liberal, anticlerical enterprise from which Catholic physicians were to be barred.[12] Of course this type of configuration cannot directly be transposed to the national level. Still, it is clear that on a national level hygienism had become part of the political discourse of progressive liberals and socialists as well. Some of the hygienists were actually elected to Parliament, where they sat with the left-wing members and advocated a social interventionist policy.[13] This policy, they argued, should focus on the improvement of the living conditions of the urban working classes, but would also enhance the well-being of society as a whole. Politicians and physicians had to become doctors of society by preventing disease and cutting away social cancers. The success of hygienism could be read from the large-scale initiatives which were taken in the early twentieth century within both the socialist and the Catholic conglomerate of social organizations (the so-called 'pillars') to set up preventive as well as curative medical services for their members.

Because of the public visibility and cultural success of hygienism, it is tempting to assume that hygienists somehow represented the medical profession and its social aspirations as a whole. In reality, hygienists constituted only a small social and intellectual elite which was often viewed with suspicion by the large group of rank and file doctors. The gap between the urban medical elite and a growing group of doctors working in rural areas or in small towns was enormous. The nineteenth century was characterized by growing numbers in the regular medical market, with a competitive system of unfixed tariffs linked to the patients' income and a flourishing supply of alternative healers. In order to enhance their private income, to set up disciplinary procedures and to overcome internal divisions, physicians had been organizing themselves into local professional associations since the 1830s. In 1863, a national umbrella association was founded. Even at this point, however, professional medical associations did not display the interests of an established profession but rather the struggle of a profession that sought to emancipate itself from the threat of poverty. They cultivated an ambiguous attitude towards the national government, expecting the authorities to punish illegal competitors, but feared in a typically liberal fashion that too much political interference would damage their professional independence.[14]

Even though the social and intellectual outlook and ambitions of hygienists and general practitioners were quite divergent, they did share a concern to consolidate the identity of the medical profession by distinguishing it from its 'others'. In their diatribes against priests and homeopaths, in particular, the arguments of different types of physicians sounded remarkably consistent.[15] In the struggle of professional medical associations against illegal competitors, there seems to have been a certain reality behind the topos of the priestly quack. In rural areas local priests often functioned as healers. More often than not, there was a fine line between fulfilling the pastoral duty of caring for the poor and the sick and acting as a medical healer. Some of them published medical manuals for the poor, with titles such as *Manual of the Sick or Recovery Without a Doctor*. Such manuals constituted a mix of biblical fragments, prescriptions for bodily rituals and natural healing methods. If we are allowed to believe their critics, some priests also organized forms of medical practice in their church sacristy. The authorities hardly responded to these practices. Acquittal from prosecution was often justified on grounds of the urgency of the situation or the non-commercial nature of the actions. A law promulgated in 1853 even declared that there was no legal difference between commercial and charitable motives where illegal medical practice was concerned. Still, even if the clerics gained no profit from their medical interventions, they necessarily deprived physicians of 'their' revenues.[16]

This juridical logic became deeply intertwined with a struggle for therapeutic 'orthodoxy'. The utilitarian project of public health equally encouraged the demarcation of established physicians as supreme guards of sanitary ideas against the spread of 'heterodox' practices and recipes within their own ranks. The development of Belgian homeopathy, for example, testifies to this logic of exclusion. Towards the end of the century, homeopaths were often characterized as the archetypical 'quacks'. Not surprisingly, this condemnation was linked to the active involvement of Catholic priests within the homeopathic movement. As homeopathy was often considered suitable for self-treatment, it easily found its way into pastoral medical lay practice.[17] Priests, nuns, monks and beguines were among the clientele of Belgian homeopaths.[18] As a heterodox medical practice, homeopathy had been introduced to Belgium in the late 1820s with its heyday in the 1870s. The possibilities of its development had been barred, however, by a condemnation by the Royal Academy of Medicine in 1850. This condemnation resulted de facto in the exclusion of homeopaths from the Academy and subsequently from medical boards and committees at the provincial and local level. As the Academy played an important role in the initiatives taken by the national government in the field of public health care, the dividing line between homeopathy and orthodox medicine was established. Homeopaths advocated the establishment of a chair of homeopathic medicine at the public universities of Ghent and Liège and the incorporation of homeopathic medicines in the official Belgian pharmacopoeia, but it was in vain.[19]

The exclusion of untrained priests and heterodox homeopaths helped to construct a professional opposition between (utilitarian) hygienic theorists and physicians on the one hand and 'irregular' competitors on the other. From the beginning, however, this contrast was blurred. Although the 'victims' of medical exclusion resisted the sanitarians' defence of professional interests, their plea for a *laissez-faire* approach was not completely incompatible with regular physicians' preference for professional self-regulation. More importantly, irregular competitors expressed sanitarian concerns about the health of society as a whole. Some homeopathic societies seem to have played a role very similar to that of regular hygienist societies. In the 1890s, for instance, the main Flemish homeopathic society issued a petition to Parliament aimed at prohibiting the use of lead pipes for beer production, in order to prevent lead poisoning. Although there was an ongoing concern about the dissemination of homeopathic knowledge among the masses, homeopaths did succeed in attracting a socially diversified clientele.[20] Efforts made by the advocates of homeopathy at the end of the century to establish public dispensaries for the poor bear witness to this same engagement. On both sides of the homeopathic/allopathic divide, so it seems, concerns over hygiene for society and professional interests became intertwined.

During the nineteenth century, medical practitioners conceived their specific role in society through the double prism of professional ('corporatist') interests on the one hand and governmental health policy on the other. Within their vision of governmental health policy, broader issues of citizenship were also construed. From a hygienist perspective, citizens should not only be able to benefit from collective measures with regard to public health, they should equally be educated in matters of hygiene so as to act responsibly in their own daily lives.

Questioning the Boundaries of the Medical Profession

Towards the end of the century, social and cultural debates around the building of a professional medical identity intensified. The emergence of a broad array of alternative health cultures both challenged and radicalized crucial elements of medical liberalism. People who adopted ideals of German naturopathy very often made a similar 'sanitarian' or hygienic diagnosis of society, as an organism on the verge of degeneration. They did not, however, necessarily believe in the need for state-supported collective action. The cures which *Lebensreform* therapists proposed were neither collective nor disciplinary in nature. Contrary to the proposals of liberal physicians and hygienists, *Lebensreform* therapists advocated a strictly individual reform of lifestyle which the modern citizen had to perform on his own initiative without being forced to do so. The sanitarian ideology of the *Lebensreform* movement produced specific cultures of self-help. This radical conception of individual freedom and responsibility was equally apparent in the alternative 'professional' identity naturopaths upheld. They advocated the free practice of medicine for every individual, trained as well as untrained. They defied all restrictive legislation and criticized the corporatist positions of regular physicians, which they depicted as promoting an egotistical medical 'caste'. Whereas 'orthodox' physicians, so it seemed, mostly defended a liberal vision of society, naturopaths clung to somewhat libertarian beliefs. They heavily criticized professional monopoly and expanding state intervention, both of which had been viewed by hygienists as ultimate safeguards of medical freedom. Since many of the natural healers were either priests or declared themselves to be acting out of their religious convictions as Catholics, this more radical medical liberty was often defended with no less liberal arguments concerning the freedom of religion. In naturopathic discourse, the struggle for complete medical freedom was readily compared to the freedom of religious worship. The latter concept was a watchword that had dominated the culture wars between liberal and Catholic political elites for decades.

In Belgium, naturopathy emerged in the 1890s, mainly inspired by German examples. Naturopathic therapy was centred around the recipes of classical hydrotherapy. This healing system had been reinvented in the German states during the eighteenth century and survived as a heterodox healing method in the medical market of the nineteenth century, which was growing more and more competitive. The fame of mid-nineteenth century healers such as the Austrian Vincent Priessnitz and the Swiss Arnold Rikli helped to turn hydropathy into a European medical peculiarity. From the 1840s onwards, German hydropathy migrated to the British Isles and from the *fin de siècle*, it also gained support in France, the Netherlands and Belgium, mostly through the influence of the Bavarian priest and healer Sebastian Kneipp. In Belgium, a prototypical role was played by the natural healer Frans Jozef van den Broeck. Both his social background and his mode of thought are typical of the general profile of the participants of the Belgian naturopathy movement. Like many of his colleagues in naturopathy, Van den Broeck did not originate from the wealthy urban bourgeoisie, but from a small village in the countryside east of Antwerp, representing the Catholic and provincial petty bourgeoisie. He had worked as a school teacher before entering a career in health reform. By contrasting the modesty of his ancestry with the wealth of some urban physicians, Van den Broeck managed to present himself as a 'man of the people'. In reality, however, his background was fairly typical of many established physicians in the countryside. These rank and file doctors were struggling for their market share in traditional rural areas and inevitably became the bitterest of rivals to quack competitors like Van den Broeck himself.[21]

Like most of his colleagues in naturopathy, Van den Broeck entered the medical market without having obtained a medical degree. Rather, he had studied the works of German hydropaths. In the early 1890s, he had travelled several times to the Bavarian village of Wörishofen, the home base of Father Kneipp. Van den

Broeck had not only undergone Kneipp's treatments, as had many others, but this self-made naturopath had also attended Kneipp's exclusive teaching sessions for a select group of European trainees. Back home, Van den Broeck's practice attracted many hundreds of sick and curious people. It became a point of reference for the handful of naturopaths in Belgium who, like Van den Broeck, hoped to emulate Kneipp's commercial and therapeutic successes. Most of them were active in the Belgian countryside and in provincial towns like Bruges, Hasselt and Namur, although the city of Brussels also welcomed its first hydropathical sanatorium in the 1890s.

After the First World War, Van den Broeck's student Aloïs van Son further developed and institutionalized his medical practice in Antwerp as a 'Hygienic Institute Van den Broeck' with its own monthly journal. Both natural healers were prolific authors of (mainly Dutch-language) leaflets and treatises in which natural therapy was defended and given a theoretical grounding. The practice and ideas of Van den Broeck and his students can be considered prototypical of natural medicine in Belgium.[22] The Belgian naturopathic community remained very small; the clientele of the Belgium-based naturopaths was not big enough to reshape or threaten the general medical market in a significant way. Although figures for the naturopaths' market share are lacking, the fact that only Van den Broeck's sanatorium survived for several decades indicates the fragility of the hydropathical landscape.

How did this alternative culture of health care relate to the emerging discourse of medical liberalism and the physicians' monopoly of medical practice that was contained within it? This naturopathic community tried to define a position that was a clear alternative to orthodox medicine, without being openly antagonistic.[23] Again, the story of Van den Broeck himself is most revealing. In the course of the 1890s, Van den Broeck was prosecuted three times for the illegal practice of medicine. It should be noted that these prosecutions were rather exceptional. When Pol van Waver, a Flemish school teacher and prolific publicist for complete freedom, wrote a leaflet in defence of Van den Broeck in 1899, he could only recount a handful of 'unjust' prosecutions from the 1850s onwards.[24] Van den Broeck acted provocatively at the time of his trial and the judge seemed keen to make an example of a very visible exponent of an illegal practice that was often difficult to discern and therefore to punish. Van den Broeck, for his part, easily turned his lawsuits into a means of propaganda and had little trouble in presenting himself as a 'people's healer' and a rebel against professional physicians. He developed his line of defence in a leaflet addressed to the Belgian Parliament. In it, the naturopath clearly hinted at the ambiguities of medical liberalism in Belgium and even Belgian liberalism as a whole. The priest-like healer who claimed, like Kneipp, to serve Mother Nature and God alike, invoked the constitutional liberties as they were understood by most Catholics in matters of religion and education. The state regulation and intervention that were understood by liberal hygienists as a bulwark against the non-enlightened and non-scientific convictions of the Church were regarded by Catholic naturopaths as a contradiction in terms. Health, like religion, Van den Broeck believed, was a private affair in which no government should ever intrude.[25]

In his leaflet, Van den Broeck explicitly compared his healing practice with a religious service. Healing the sick, he wrote, was an imperative duty to God. This liberty not only applied to non-trained healers, but also to patients. Just as the law should respect the right of citizens to perform 'good and useful acts', he argued, sick people could not be forced by law to be poisoned by medication.[26] In contrast to the medically schooled homeopaths who strove for recognition within officially established medicine, natural healers, who in many cases did not have a formal medical education, did not aspire to official recognition. Instead, they harshly criticized the vast difference between legislation that safeguarded individual liberty of physicians and state regulation, even outlaw status, of all other healers. Although the small number of lawsuits against illegal healers revealed the moderation of Belgian judges, naturopaths could easily refer to the more liberal legislation in Germany and Britain. Unlike the German and British legislators, Van den Broeck and his followers argued, the Belgian legislators had favoured physicians too much. In naturopathic discourse, orthodox physicians were depicted as a homogeneous entity of profiteers who exerted control over the politicians. It became clear that, in so far as the naturopaths' therapeutic identity was dependent on their relationship with the Belgian medical profession, it was based on an oppositional identification. In the publications of natural healers, orthodox practitioners were time and again depicted as a 'caste' of profiteers for whom material profit prevailed over the well-being of their patients. The fight of professional medical associations against cooperative health services, where physicians earned much less than in independent practice, was criticized repeatedly as a mean corporatist defence of material self-interest. On the other hand, they claimed that natural healers had never been driven by material motives. Criticism of the materialist mentality of officially recognized medicine allowed natural healers also to distance themselves from the label of charlatanism. Commercial advertisements for medicines constituted in their eyes the worst form of quackery. As notorious adversaries of medication, they could claim to be uncontaminated by charlatanism and yet distance themselves even further from the medical profession – the biggest sector of 'charlatanism' in the naturopaths' eyes.[27]

From the naturopaths' perspective, medical liberalism as understood by physicians and liberal politicians did not include real medical liberty. In fact, professional associations of physicians stood for a very different kind of liberty. For these organizations, medical freedom consisted in the physicians' freedom to regulate the profession among themselves, with no other state intrusion than the protection of the professional monopoly of orthodox practitioners. The discursive foundation of this professional ideology was the so-called 'liberal medicine' (*médecine libérale*). For these physicians (and their associations), medical freedom could be summed up as the patients' unlimited freedom to choose the regular physician of their preference, the protection of medical confidentiality between physician and patient and the physicians' monopoly over medical practice. The concept of liberal medicine was thus defined by the medical profession as a 'liberal profession' which was to be regulated internally and whose monopoly was to be safeguarded by the state. This ideology paved the way for the absolute physician hegemony over the medical market that became thoroughly established in the decades after the Second World War.

Whereas orthodox physicians asked for state protection against illegal competitors, they also wanted to be left alone with their patients. Disciplinary matters, they said, needed to be arranged amongst colleagues, without the interference of others. Naturopaths, on the other hand, called on the authorities to withdraw from *all* interference in medical practice. They demanded medical freedom for everybody, including untrained healers. The publicist Van Waver passionately defended the individual's freedom to practise medicine even without professional training. He argued that 'science does produce physicians, but these physicians are not necessarily *healers*'. In a provocative manner, Van Waver told his readers that 'medicine needs to serve the people, instead of the people serving medicine'. He urged physicians to renounce their 'privileges'. Van Waver believed that the practice of medicine required a specific talent rather than theoretical study. 'Like poets, healers are not made but born', he wrote. 'Instinct and intuition' were more valuable in a physician than the teachings of the 'faculty'. Van Waver concluded that all too often, medicine was dispensed by individuals 'without any mission or abilities'.[28] The Brussels physician Léopold Dejace, spokesman of the physicians' umbrella organization Fédération Médicale Belge, did not agree. He protested against this questioning of 'the medical monopoly of trained physicians'. Complete medical freedom, Dejace argued, would result in 'anarchy'. If citizens were to experience this anarchy, he wrote, they would understand that the public interest was threatened not by 'a privileged caste' but by 'a hungry horde of charlatans'.[29]

Can the dispute between established physicians on the one hand and the small movement of naturopaths on the other be summed up as a battle between medical liberalism and 'anarchism', as Dejace suggested? It should be noted that the diatribes against 'privileged' official medicine did not hinder naturopaths from recruiting established physicians to their cause. Following Kneipp, who in 1893 had founded the Internationale Verein Kneippscher Ärtze, Belgian naturopaths tried to convince trained physicians to join their ranks. In these attempts to gain respectability, the radical principles of medical liberty were not always consistently upheld. Towards the end of his life, Kneipp himself increasingly stressed the importance of university medical training, in order to weed out the army of self-made men that had spread across Western Europe from the havens of Wörishofen. To the amazement of many hydropaths, Kneipp declared in 1897, during a meeting behind closed doors reported on by the Belgian Auguste Ruyssen, that from now on his method 'could only be practised by qualified doctors'.[30] Ruyssen, who had been one of the first physicians to join the hydropathical movement, confirmed the new marching orders enthusiastically in the Belgian *Kneipp Journal*. The assembled Kneipp doctors, Ruyssen wrote, had henceforth decided to take action against 'the widespread misconception that the Kneipp method could be practised without any thorough prior knowledge of medicine'.

In a similar vein, Belgian naturopaths hoped to include their therapy within a common discourse of scientific respectability, rather than simply to reject the claims of scientific medicine. Van Son's reflections on the ongoing discussions within the medical profession on the desirability of a disciplinary professional society, the Order of Physicians, were significant in this respect. In the 1930s, the Order was the final result of the physicians' striving for the internal regulation of their profession. Van Son was an absolute opponent of the establishment of such a board, which he considered would confirm and reinforce the tyranny which was already dominant within medical circles:

> Their science is *the* science and whoever diverges from it, be it a homeopath, a psychoanalyst, a natural healer or someone else, he may have made the greatest discovery of the century, a discovery which the official school doesn't even dare to dream about – he is a scientific heretic and as soon as the Order of Physicians succeeds in laying its hands on him, they will get him, for sure![31]

Using similar arguments, Van Son not only put natural healing on the same level as homeopathy and psychoanalysis, but also legitimized its claims to scientific status. The official medical profession's concept of science was one of 'erring fathers' opposed to a more progressive form of science, he argued. Although the naturopaths did not waste energy in a vain crusade for the legal recognition of their profession, they remained hopeful that, one day, regular medicine would be forced to recognize the truth and effectiveness of natural therapies. As regular medical doctors – given the 'tyranny' of the professional organizations – did not dare to show interest in natural therapy, natural healers hoped to influence these physicians through their patients, who, they knew, shopped around on the medical market. 'To spread hygienic insights among doctors', Van Son taught in the journal of his institute, 'is the most difficult aspect of our job'.[32]

This radical conception of medical liberty as defended by most naturopaths was modified by their attempts to win over trained physicians and to raise their own respectability. As a result, the naturopaths' alleged 'anarchist' position with regard to the medical monopoly was much closer to the nineteenth-century

Catholic conception of civil liberties in Belgium than to anarchist revolutionary philosophy. Belgian naturopaths not only explicitly referred to freedom of religion in order to legitimize the individual's freedom to adhere to his healing method of choice. The equation of the sphere of medicine with the sphere of religion also implicitly reflected their pastoral conception of the relationship between healers and patients. Van Son himself remembered with regret the distance he had experienced from the trained physicians at his bedside when he was a little boy. He contrasted these memories with the hearty conversations about life, sickness and cures he had had with Van den Broeck as an adult. During these conversations, Van Son remembered many years later, he had learnt to become independent of professional physicians *and* medical outsiders alike.

In a way, this level of patient participation seemed to contradict the modernization of the patient–physician relationship that is said to characterize the second half of the nineteenth century. The professionalization of medicine implied a more distanced and rational relationship between doctor and patient and hence a reduction of the patient's self-determination. Authors such as the British medical sociologist Nicholas Jewson have maintained that a more participatory role for the patient had been typical of an older patient-centred medical culture. This is also what naturopaths claimed. This did not mean, however, that such a pastoral relationship was free of authoritarian traits. The intimacy between healers and patients equally implied a kind of regulation of patients' behaviour. This regulation was not necessarily more lax than that of most contemporary physicians. Here, the detached authority of the professional physician was replaced by the involvement of the priest-like natural healer. In this relationship, the pastor's understanding of Nature's law was not only regarded as admirable, but even as indispensable if the patient wanted to overcome unnatural life.

For naturopaths, the process of healing was equated to a process of conversion. Healers and patients, the suggestion ran, went through this experience together. The vitality of the body in which natural therapists believed was often equated with a mysterious force, with life itself, with a 'universal energy' or with the 'powers of Nature'. In the Catholic discourse of natural therapy, this vocabulary of natural religion was easily merged with references to God, who had created natural harmony, who had stated the equally 'natural' Ten Commandments and who punished severely but fairly all those who sinned with alcohol, tobacco or meat consumption. The pain of healing was a penance, the journey from sickness to health itself a pilgrimage. The patient who read Kneipp's books and followed his advice by going barefoot in his bedroom, plunging his feet in water and letting them dry naturally not only hoped to re-establish the natural harmony within his or her body. They also reconciled themself with the Creator of all things.

The Civic Values of Naturopathy

It has often been argued that hydropathy and natural healing, in so far as they represented specific elements of a broader movement for *Lebensreform*, propagated a flight from modern society. The Dutch historian Jan Romein described these health reformers as sentimentalists, who took refuge from the social upheavals of modernity in the seclusion of individual reform.[33] This contribution, however, seeks to lay bare the political implications of such alternative cultures of health. Their pleas for radical medical liberty, we argue, pushed the paradoxes of medical liberalism to their limits. Whereas these pleas very often remained implicit in the daily routine of the cabinets of natural healers and in their propagandistic writing, they occasionally took a sharper form. In public performances such as Van den Broeck's defence in court, the civic-mindedness of *Lebensreform* became more obvious. From time to time, ambitions to establish a different kind of health policy were explicitly expressed during public campaigns. The most important example of this was the crusade by Belgian hydropaths against compulsory vaccination during the interwar years. In this campaign, civic liberties were not the sole issue. Paradoxically, naturopaths also developed their particular visions about the health of the social organism. Thus it seems they were not always opposed to the hygienists' ambitions to cure society as a whole.

As in all their public stands, natural healers' scepticism towards vaccination was primarily grounded in 'natural' principles. In their view, vaccination, like medication in general, was to be regarded as poisoning the body rather than protecting it. On this issue, natural healers could bolster their position by linking up to a century-long tradition of resistance to smallpox vaccination. In Belgium, this resistance had been particularly strong among the peasantry, but had found occasional support from medical doctors. Bills by medically trained politicians in favour of compulsory vaccination were, until 1946, never accepted by the Belgian Parliament.[34] Although both respectable hygienists and rank and file physicians promoted vaccination intensively among their patients, neither group promoted coercive legislation. The absence of a law which prescribed vaccination was of course applauded by natural healers like Van Son. He nevertheless cautioned against the pressure exerted by most physicians and pointed out to his readers that they had a legal right not to be vaccinated.[35] Again, the naturopathic emphasis on the patient's right to choose and to refuse vaccination contrasted with the mainstream understanding of medical freedom as a patient's freedom to choose among established regular physicians. Instead, the campaign against vaccination hinted once again at complete medical freedom.[36]

Many naturopaths went further. Since they believed that it was not the intrusion of bacteria that made people sick, but rather their own lack of natural resistance, a multi-faceted approach to bacterial diseases emerged within which all kinds of circumstantial factors gained importance. Unsurprisingly, everyday living conditions were among these factors, but naturopaths did not explicitly devise an interventionist social policy in order to address them. When they stressed the impact of the susceptibility of an individual to infections, they not only hinted at the individual's bodily condition, but also referred to the physical environment which possibly caused the imbalance of the body. Hence a statement like '*la question du terrain prime la question du graine*' (the question of the soil prevails over the question of the seed) sought to undermine the cultural status of scientific bacteriology, but also expressed natural healers' belief in the need to transform the dirty, suffocating, artificial and 'anti-biological' city into a salubrious space.[37]

Within a classical hygienist or sanitarian philosophy, this environmental approach had been important too. The whole point of the hygienists' call for collective – public or private – action was to clean up disease-promoting conditions in order to give individuals a proper chance to take care of their own health. However, as early as the 1850s, Belgian hygienists had realized that public health policy could not be effective unless individuals also observed hygienic rules. It would never be possible to eradicate diseases such as tuberculosis or cholera as long as people lacked such habits as washing frequently with soap, using handkerchiefs and eating healthy food. People needed to be convinced of the importance of personal hygiene for the prevention of disease and early death. 'The great struggle against epidemics and all avoidable diseases can be effective only to the extent that the laws of hygiene (cleanliness, moderation, fresh air, sensible diet, hygienic housing etc.) are applied seriously. In addition to general measures, there has to be intellectual, rational and determined individual action, based on both scientific and practical instructions, a Belgian doctor argued in 1850.[38] Hygienists' attention to the impact of individual behaviour only increased after the emergence of bacteriology in the 1880s. The habit of spitting on the ground by tubercular patients, for instance, was now perceived as dangerous. It should, they argued, be replaced by the use of a spittoon.[39]

Natural healers probably agreed to a certain extent with these hygienist programmes, but they chose a different target for their propaganda efforts. Rather than writing for their colleagues about the massive and anonymous group of 'the working class', as hygienists did, they addressed their readers almost personally. Although they shared with hygienists a concern for moderation in human behaviour, their purpose was not to introduce bourgeois ethics to the working classes, but to encourage every individual reader or patient to undergo the bodily experiences they believed to be healing. It was less a question of familiarizing a social group with an ethical code of regularity and self-discipline than of presenting the inner impulses of the soul as the instruments of individual bodily change and personal transformation. In this sense alone can *Lebensreform*'s cultural criticism be seen as a social criticism of modern mass society. Naturopaths, moreover, promoted a very specific type of cultural criticism. It was not the product of systematically developed ideas, but rather the articulation of a physical practice of self-purification. This individualist focus once again reflected the religious background of most naturopaths. As a social group, these petty bourgeois Catholics were foreign to the metropolitan and liberal environment to which most hygienists belonged. Whereas the liberal physicians had advocated moderately interventionist state politics, Catholic naturopaths were sceptical about and sometimes downright hostile towards, government intervention in matters of public health. Practices of conversion and physical reform fitted better with the Christian notions of healing and grace, even though these physical exercises sometimes conflicted with traditional prudery.

With the help of this individualist propaganda and physical exercise, naturopaths seemed to dissociate the logic of self-help from the interventionist programme of hygienism within which the notion of self-help had first originated. The diverging answers offered by naturopaths and *Lebensreform* supporters became most obvious in the very areas that had been crucial for hygienist thinking too. Alcohol was one such area. Vegetarians and natural healers who believed in the necessity of a sober, alcohol-free diet perceived alcoholism quite logically as a huge social problem. Some natural therapists therefore welcomed the temperance associations, their practice of abstinence and their objective of banning alcohol as far as possible from society.[40] They probably applauded the hygienist thinking behind the Belgian law of 1919 prohibiting the sale of distilled drinks in bars and they may even have welcomed the much stricter law that had been promulgated at the beginning of the war. At the same time, however, they stressed the ultimate ineffectiveness of such legal measures, which merely addressed one aspect of a much more complex problem. As long as people consumed meat, for instance, they would inevitably keep longing for alcohol and thus go on producing and consuming it. No external force could replace the work of inner conviction. As soon as someone had decided to take the road of nature, he would not be interested in alcohol any more. Laws were therefore not needed.[41] Nor did it make sense to call bar keepers, as hygienists liked to do, parasites of the social body who undermined the prosperity of the nation.[42]

Natural healers nevertheless did subscribe to hygienists' general diagnosis of modern industrial society as fundamentally sick. To different degrees, both groups were sceptical about urban modernity's capacity to heal itself. More than anywhere else, they believed, disease was located in the city – a conviction for which they found support in their own medical theories. The propositions they put forward in this respect had little in common with the technical language of a classic sanitarian discourse. Naturopaths preferred to hint at a general blueprint for the ideal city of the future, characterized by spacious parks, public hydrotherapeutic installations and fruit trees lining the streets. People should, however, not wait until utopia had become reality. Once again, the main challenge was at the individual level. Clear corporeal prescriptions could be internalized into a way of life: sleeping with an open window, regularly performing breathing exercises, walking. 'Things would go much better in the world if people walked more', the *Kneipp-Journal* stated in 1901.[43] The apparent optimism concerning such recipes could not conceal a fundamental unease about the city. This unease would occasionally give rise to more systematic reflections on the organization of society. According to some, for instance, the spread of a vegetarian diet would lead to a revival of agriculture and so avert the pernicious tendency of rural exodus.[44] Others, however, were tempted by more direct solutions. They tried to build utopian enclaves in the country, in the form of self-sufficient, vegetarian, nature-minded colonies. In the countryside around Brussels and Antwerp, small groups of individuals hoped to prove that the personal fight against meat consumption and the rejection of all kinds of egotism would also bring a better world within sight. Here, the social engineering of hygienist interventionist policy was replaced by a communitarian utopia. Although the two visions referred to very different sorts of 'political' practice, they ultimately appeared as alternative expressions of the same ambition. The emergence of alternative cultures of health did not simply embody an opposition to medical liberalism and hygienism: it also exposed the ambivalences that were contained within them.

PART II: SOCIAL CITIZENSHIP: HEALTH IN THE WELFARE STATE

From the 1840s onwards, many physicians called for social and political reform. As the detrimental effects of industrialization and urbanization became clear, public health schemes were proposed all over Europe, especially after the revolution of 1848. Their implementation was not, however, without problems and contradictions. The reluctance of liberals who refused to abandon the principle of *laissez-faire* was one such problem, but so was ambivalence among physicians. While the physicians as professionals welcomed some degree of protection by the state, they feared subordination to it. Most of all, the implementation of public health policies was hesitant because it proved difficult to reconcile the ideal of freedom with that of equality. Classical 'rights of' (property, free speech) were to be extended with 'rights to' (labour, income, health care), which implied an entitlement. The basic question was always how to organize distributive justice in a way that was acceptable to all members of society. Liberalism had always held that assistance to the sick and the poor should only be a moral obligation for the donor rather than an entitlement of the recipient. Over the course of the nineteenth century, however, governments came to realize that public assistance had become a social necessity to counter epidemics, crime and even revolution. Part II of this volume – roughly covering the period from the mid-nineteenth to the late-twentieth century – is devoted to social citizenship. The period witnessed a transformation from private philanthropy to the intervention state. The 'social' emerged as a domain for professional and state intervention in the lives of needy citizens. The new model of citizenship gradually replaced incidental charity with structural social rights. And even though this was put in place in an attempt to pacify society, it never went uncontested.

In his iconic report on a typhus epidemic in 1848, Rudolf Virchow argued that epidemics were caused by social conditions – like ignorance and poverty – rather than by medical factors. Epidemic disease could only be prevented through education and social reform, which implied an active state. Larry Frohman offers an overview of German responses to the challenges of industrial society, ranging from the medical reformers of the 1850s through the sanitary movement (1860s and 1870s) and the rise of bacteriology (1880s and 1890s) to the early twentieth-century social hygiene movement that was to become an important pillar of the Weimar welfare system. Frohman shows how the right to health became a central element in a broader progressive notion of social citizenship in Germany at the turn of the twentieth century. Countering the standard account of public health in Germany from the Empire to the Third Reich in terms of growing medical control and the rise of racial eugenics, he explores the implications of social citizenship in the field of medical care for its ostensible beneficiaries. For a long time, the social dimensions of morbidity had been marginalized or even ignored. Sickness was believed to be either the result of individual moral failings or to be caused by a bacterium. When around 1900 the bacteriological paradigm entered into a crisis, a new discourse on social rights developed. It led to a new social contract, intended to create a strong nation that could survive in an increasingly competitive world. Frohman argues that the development of social hygiene – and of a broader social perspective on poverty and disease – pointed the way beyond liberal sanitary reform and provided the theoretical foundation for a new positive conception of public responsibility for individual health. At the same time, the development of social hygiene programmes was largely the product of voluntary action at the local level, often in collaboration with local government. Frohman uses the tuberculosis centres and infant welfare centres that developed in the early twentieth century as case studies to throw light on the articulation of this new conception of social citizenship. Neither could have taken off so easily had it not been for the broad support of local voluntary organizations and municipal government. According to Frohman, the success of the social hygiene programmes designed to combat infant mortality in altering the hygienic comportment of the working classes depended as much, if not more, on gaining the informed collaboration of working-class women as it did on disciplining them. He therefore concludes that it is more appropriate to define medicalization during the Weimar Republic as a collective learning process than as a process of social disciplining.

Rosemary Elliot explores the ways in which smoking was incorporated into discourses of health and citizenship in Britain and Germany during both world wars. War represents the apogee of citizenship, she claims. During wartime, citizens are expected to put their individual interests aside in the name of the common good: war therefore makes a good case to study citizenship. There was a marked difference between these two countries in the understanding of smoking and its risks, and during the wars these contrasting attitudes intensified. In Britain, tobacco was seen as essential to keep up morale among the troops. Citizens were urged to save tobacco for 'our lads at the front'. Abstaining from smoking and sending cigarettes to the front was considered to be a patriotic act. In Germany, on the other hand, patriotism was associated with the avoidance of smoking – by both citizens and soldiers – in the interest of racial hygiene and national fitness. In the German context, tobacco was believed to cause hereditary degeneration. It was even argued that Jews had taught the Germans to smoke in order to make money and destroy the nation at the same time. Thus, while in Britain cigarette smoking was linked to soldierly masculinity and creating a positive mood, the German state adopted restrictive policies on smoking in the interests of public health, especially during the Nazi era. Still, Elliot's chapter also contains a warning not to confuse the rhetoric of the state with daily realities. The German tobacco industry succeeded in securing its position by deftly – and successfully – arguing that closing down tobacco companies would not only harm the treasury due to the loss of tobacco taxes, but benefit British and Soviet economies as well. Finally, Elliot asks how these differences can be understood within the context of the current international rhetorical 'war on tobacco'. The transformation of medical and social opinion on smoking has taken place within a relatively short space of time. Nowadays tobacco use is seen to threaten individual health as well as the health of non-smokers and to turn responsible, autonomous citizens into dependent addicts, while treating smoking-related disease increasingly tends to be considered as a misuse of scarce health resources, undermining the financial basis of the welfare state. Smoking raises interesting questions about the relationship between citizenship and lifestyle; the individual and the state, and the role of medical knowledge in assessments of personal and institutional risk.

Whereas previous chapters have focused on somatic medicine – either at the collective or at the individual level – Harry Oosterhuis sheds light on the way psychiatry and mental health care moulded civic ideals in the Netherlands during the twentieth century. While a process of political and social democratization unfolded, the social order was successively disturbed and disrupted by the emancipation of workers, women and religious groups; by two world wars, economic crisis, secularization, the 1960s protest movement and by social fragmentation due to the crisis of the welfare state and the rise of neoliberalism. From the early twentieth century on, in psychiatry as well as in the broader field of mental hygiene and mental health care, psychological definitions of citizenship were advanced in response to the insecurities and concerns provoked by the ongoing extension of political participation among the Dutch people. Social and moral problems were framed as public mental health issues. Expressing their views about the position of individuals in modern society and their possibilities for self-development, psychiatrists, psycho-hygienists and other mental health workers connected mental health to ideals of liberal-democratic and – later on – social citizenship. Thus, they were clearly involved in the modern project of promoting not only virtuous, productive, responsible and adaptive citizens, but also autonomous, self-conscious, assertive and emancipated individuals as members of a democratic society. Oosterhuis maps the development of mental hygiene and mental health care in the Netherlands from the late nineteenth century to the present in order to explore its link to socio-political modernization in general and the changing meanings of citizenship and civic virtue in particular. Over the course of the twentieth century, external pressure by the state to effect democratic stability was no longer called for. Instead, the psychologization of citizenship implied that people should participate in society in a self-conscious and self-controlled way. In the process, citizenship in the Netherlands took on a broad meaning, not just in terms of political rights and duties, but also in the context of material, social, psychological and moral conditions that individuals should meet in order to be able to act according to those rights and duties in a responsible way. Notions such as fairness, social justice, social responsibility, tolerance, emancipation and personal development became elements of the definition of good citizenship.

The revolution of 1848 revitalized the ideals of the French Revolution, reminding Europeans of the fact that the promise of democratic rights and liberties and social justice had not yet yielded much tangible result. The poverty and epidemics caused by the ongoing process of industrialization and urbanization created a sense of urgency that would ultimately transform citizenship. For a long time, state intervention had been directed to the poor only. After the Second World War, with the rise of the welfare state, the population as a whole became the target of its increasing interference.

5 THE RIGHT TO HEALTH AND SOCIAL CITIZENSHIP IN GERMANY, 1848–1918

Larry Frohman

Health is both a positive end in itself and the foundation of the entire spectrum of other goods that flow from the ability of healthy individuals to engage in productive labour. And in nineteenth-century Germany the debate over the right to health was part of a much broader debate – one that was simultaneously medical and political – over the causes of ill-health, especially the relation between poverty, work, sickness and personal morality. From the 1848 revolution to the end of the Empire, the vigour with which a right to health was defended was directly related to the extent to which sickness was regarded as a specifically *social* problem. In the following pages I would like to use the intertwined histories of social medicine and the right to health to make two sets of arguments: one concerning the methodological problems involved in thinking about the relationship between medicine and politics; the other concerning the actual interplay of medicine and politics in the shaping of the German state from 1848 to the founding of the Weimar Republic.[1]

The main point argued here is that, although medical sciences may have evolved according to their respective disciplinary logics, public attitudes towards these sciences and the willingness to translate medical knowledge into public health policy did not depend only – and perhaps not even primarily – on the assumed scientific validity of such knowledge. Public health policies also depended on the extent to which the epidemiological and hygienic practices prescribed by these sciences were believed to be compatible with prevailing ideas concerning both individual responsibility for sickness and the role of the community in assisting the sick and needy, as well as the ability to find ways of providing these services in ways that would uphold rather than undermine the responsibility of the recipient. In the first part of this chapter, I will argue that the various schools of public health that dominated public thinking on the topic between the 1848 revolution and the turn of the century were able to maintain their dominant position because their understanding of the causes of both individual sickness and epidemic disease operated according to the same moral logic and political rationality as the broader habitus of the liberal middle classes. On the one hand, they framed their arguments in such a way as to make sickness and poverty appear as the result of diverse moral failings on the part of the afflicted individual and consequently regarded deterrence as the best means of promoting personal responsibility and individual health. On the other hand, they abstracted the individual from his social and material life-worlds and conceptualized sickness in such a narrowly medical or natural scientific manner that this deviation from the normal state of health could not be used as the basis on which to make rights claims with regard to the larger community. However, although bacteriology had come to dominate both medical theory and public health practice in the 1880s and 1890s, around the turn of the century a growing awareness of the explanatory limits of the bacteriological paradigm gave rise to a renewed emphasis upon the social and environmental causes of disease. In the second section of the chapter I will argue that the breakthrough of the new discipline of social hygiene in the years leading up to the First World War went hand in hand with the emergence of a new Progressive conception of social citizenship, which regarded public intervention to ameliorate the differential, socially-determined impact of disease upon the labouring classes not as a threat to individual responsibility and initiative, but as the precondition for their realization. It will be argued that it was this medico-political synthesis that ultimately provided the theoretical underpinning for the rapidly expanding network of preventive social hygiene programmes that became one of the pillars of the Weimar welfare system.

The question, however, is whether the preventive social welfare programmes that evolved to give substance to the social right to health enhanced the personal well-being of the target populations or simply opened the door to the more intensive surveillance and control of these persons. In the final section, I will argue – with reference to programmes to combat tuberculosis and infant mortality – that these programmes did, in fact, enhance the health and well-being of the intended beneficiaries and that, although German physicians and social reformers may have harboured dreams of a far-reaching transformation of the hygienic comportment of the working classes, the success of the preventive project depended as much, if not more, on gaining the informed collaboration of working-class women as it did on disciplining them.

For two decades now, the standard account of public health in Germany from the Empire through the Third Reich has been Paul Weindling's significant 1989 study.[2] In this work, Weindling argued that the history of health, medicine and welfare in Germany should be viewed in terms of the rise of a form of state-sponsored eugenic medicine, which progressively subordinated the rights of the individual to those of the *Volk* and the race. The narrative that follows, which draws on my own work on the German welfare system, differs in important respects from that of Weindling.[3] Here I would like to suggest that his account of the rise of illiberal, eugenic state medicine captures only one aspect of a much more complicated story. The Wilhelmine years saw the development of a dense network of preventive social welfare programmes, which aimed to give substance to the new Progressive social contract by ensuring that the labouring classes – and especially their children – developed into the industrious work-ers, patriotic citizens, brave soldiers or caring parents upon whom the strength of the nation and its position in a competitive global system were believed to depend. These programmes received their theoretical legitimation from social hygiene, rather than eugenics or racial hygiene. They were primarily the product of voluntary initiative by the diverse reform groups active at the local level. And the benefits that they provided were real and cannot be reduced to a form of manipulative social imperialism. While the roots of Weimar and Nazi eugenics can be traced back to the Empire, this was not the only game in town. Nor was it the most important one before the end of the 1920s, when the Great Depression and the Nazi seizure of power altered the political rationality of public health in a way that enabled eugenics to supplant social hygiene as the medico-political foundation of the German state.

Public Health, Citizenship and the State in Germany, 1848–1900

Although Germany had a long tradition of absolutist medical police, the starting point for German thinking on public health, the rights of the citizen and the role of the state in the new bourgeois society taking shape across mid-century were the ideas of the left liberal or radical democratic 'medical reformers' Rudolf Vir-chow (1821–1902), Salomon Neumann (1819–1908) and Rudolf Leubuscher (1822–61), who all believed that a right to health had to be a central element of a democratic polity.

In Britain, Edwin Chadwick's (1800–90) sanitary project was founded on the belief that disease was not caused in any direct sense by destitution or overwork, and the exclusion – under the auspices of a miasmatic understand-ing of contagion and sickness – of these factors from the domain of medical knowledge and public intervention made it possible to regard the question of public health as one of human waste and foul odours, whose systematic flush-ing from the urban environment could eliminate disease without weakening the principles of individual self-reliance.[4] In contrast to the liberal-utilitarian British sanitarians, the German medical reformers (so named for the journal *Medicinsche Reform* published by Virchow and Leubuscher during the 1848/9 revolution) placed the nexus of poverty, work and health at the centre of their thinking on the social question. As Neumann explained on the eve of the 1848 revolution, 'it is and will remain uncontestable that poverty, need and misery, though not identical with death, sickness and debility, are nevertheless the inex-haustible springs from which they flow along with their inevitable bedfellows prejudice, the absence of culture and stupidity'. Since health was the foundation for work, property and all of the higher pursuits of civilized man, Neumann maintained that the state, whose *raison d'être* was to promote the development of the natural capacities of its citizens, had to take a direct interest in the health of its individual citizens.[5]

Virchow argued in a similar vein that the government had 'the obligation to guarantee to the working man not merely his subsistence but also the opportunity of creating his livelihood by his own efforts. A reasonable political constitution must establish the unquestionable right of the individual to a healthy life'.[6] Both he and Neumann viewed medicine as an essentially social science dedicated to disentangling the complex connections between sickness and social conditions, and his prescription for improving the health of the labouring classes pivoted more on political and social reform than on specific medical measures. For exam-ple, in his *Report on the Typhus Epidemic in Upper Silesia* (1848), Virchow argued that both the endemic nature of typhus in the region and its epidemic spread were attributable to the cultural and material impoverishment of the population. The cure, he insisted, was to be found in democracy, education and the material and social progress that would follow once individuals were freed from the state of ignorance and dependence in which they had been held.

This focus on the social etiology of disease did not disappear entirely after 1848. For example, in 1859 Friedrich Oesterlen (1812–77), the author of the first German handbook on hygiene, wrote that

> if, for example, people only eat insufficient quantities of poor food, if you put them in narrow, filthy rooms and apartments without light and air or close to overflowing drainage ditches, graves, privies and the like, if you ensure that they are exhausted by excessive labor, if you burden them with cares, hardship and misery of all kinds, then there will soon be a surfeit of disease-causing agents that can be set off by any spark.[7]

However, the political reaction of the 1850s did make it more difficult to draw from this theoretical account of the origins of sickness the same conclusions regarding the rights of the individual and the role of the state as the medical reformers had done a mere decade earlier.

One of the other leading theorists of public health in the post-revolutionary era was Lorenz von Stein (1815–90). Stein's theory of public administration was inspired by Hegel's conception of the state and its bureaucracy, and his theory of public health grew out of his broader social philosophy. Stein's rationale in making individual health into a matter of public concern was twofold. On the one hand, he argued that the failure to protect the unpropertied against this tangible form of social inequality threatened again to set in motion the dialectic of socio-political revolution that had been the driving force in European politics since the French Revolution. On the other hand, Stein's arguments also reflected a historical awareness of how the increasing density of urban life had established new forms of interdependence among the urban population. Public concern for the health of the individual, Stein wrote, begins at the point

> where the actions of one individual impair, destroy or perhaps even enhance those external conditions on which the health of another person depends. The health and sickness of the individual is thus removed from its previous individual sphere ... and, in addition to that which the individual does or neglects to do in order to maintain his own health, the life of the community thus becomes the condition for the sickness and health of all its individual members.[8]

While individuals should be held responsible for their own health as far as possible, the 'absolute value' of individual health, Stein argued, could not be held hostage to the possession of the property necessary to secure this value on a strictly private basis. The community had, therefore, to recognize its obligation to 'render the protection of life and health independent of the lack of property'.[9] However, despite his agreement with the medical reformers that social inequalities were revealing formal citizenship rights to be a hollow promise, Stein's conservative Hegelianism led him to see the solution not in a revolutionary assertion of citizenship rights, but in paternalistic social reform designed to demonstrate the commitment of the monarch and his officials to stand above and mediate between the essentially conflicting interests of civil society.

In the decades after 1848, the belief in the integral connection between health, poverty and citizenship that had informed the work of the medical reformers was substantially attenuated by the two schools that dominated thinking on the question in the second half of the century: sanitary reform and bacteriology. Although sanitary reform and bacteriology were quite different programmes, what they had in common was that they both framed the question of disease in such a way that it denied those individuals who were unable to live in accordance with the prevailing norms of individual hygiene any firm basis on which they could demand communal action to restore or maintain their health and well-being.

Public health (*öffentliche Gesundheitspflege*) emerged in the 1860s and 1870s as a coherent domain of scientific knowledge and social action. The central figure in this movement was the Bavarian chemist Max von Pettenkofer (1818–1901), who in 1865 was appointed to the first professorship of hygiene in the Germanies. Pettenkofer had first made his reputation in the 1850s with a study of cholera, which he then expanded into a general theory of epidemic disease and its prevention. Pettenkofer's epidemiology represented a variant of the localistic, anti-contagionist school, which attributed disease to infectious miasmas generated by filth and dirt. Where Pettenkofer went beyond prevailing beliefs was in identifying a causal mechanism: the fermentation or decay of human excrement and other biological matter caused by changes in the water level of the soil in which these wastes were deposited.

Pettenkofer's work provided what was widely recognized at the time as a compelling scientific justification for the broad set of public policies that marched together under the flag of sanitary reform. Since disease was caused by miasmas produced by the chemical interaction of waste and water, the mission of sanitary reform was to cleanse the city of organic waste, drain away the stagnant water in which this material could fester and improve ventilation to prevent the dangerous accumulation of infected air. These efforts to compensate for the rapidly increasing density of urban life gave rise to a lengthy catalogue of measures that defined the scope of sanitary reform and urban planning for the remainder of the century: first, the construction of water filtration plants, sewer systems, streets and surface drainage systems to supply the city with an adequate amount of clean drinking water and flush away accumulated human, animal and industrial waste, and, secondly, the regulation of housing, land use, food quality, working conditions, slaughterhouses and markets.[10]

Like Stein, the sanitarians also focused on the growing interdependence of rich and poor within an increasingly insalubrious urban space, and they were willing to invest massively in urban infrastructure between the 1860s and the First World War.[11] In his influential account of the welfare state, Abram de Swaan has examined this sense of interdependence by viewing it as the expression of a modern social consciousness that embodies the form of reflexive solidarity appropriate to that dual process of collectivization and individual self-disciplining described by Norbert Elias.[12] But the problem with de Swaan's account is that it leaves out both political context and the diverse discourses – cultural, religious, economic, medical – that determined how the individuals engaged in the social reform field understood and then sought to respond to these interdependencies. The policies of the sanitarians cannot be said to have substantially expanded the social rights of the poor, at least in the short run. Nevertheless, their solution to the contemporary urban problem enjoyed broad public support because their diagnoses of the causes of sickness and the remedies they proposed were consistent with the common sense of the middle classes and the National Liberal politicians who dominated political life in most of the nation's cities. Although the benefits of clean water and sewage systems were theoretically available to all, the sanitarians regarded the decision to take advantage of this infrastructure as a matter of individual insight and will, and, consequently, they continued to regard popular enlightenment as the most appropriate means for elevating the hygienic culture of the labouring classes. However, such an approach glossed over the ways in which real social inequalities limited the social capacity of the poor to change their way of life – and it did so in a quintessentially liberal manner that made sickness appear to be the result of individual moral failings that would be rewarded by public health programmes designed directly to assist these persons. It is no accident that, in the English context, Chadwick had been the intellectual architect of both the deterrent poor laws and sanitary reform.

This moralization of sickness and the corresponding blindness to the impact of social inequalities on individual health was reinforced by the growing prestige of both the natural sciences and the professionals who practised them. The middle decades of the nineteenth century saw great advances in chemistry and biology, and the public health movement increasingly came to define hygiene as applied physiology, that is, as the investigation of the metabolic interaction between the human body and its natural environment.[13] In this way, hygiene was transformed into an experimental science focused on such issues as respiration and the ventilation techniques and requirements needed to prevent the vitiation of air, the role of clothing and shelter in regulating the heat exchange between the body and the environment, the amount and kinds of foods required to meet the basic nutritional needs of the body, and the decomposition of the human body and its excreta. Productivity (*Leistungsfähigkeit*) became the measure of individual health, and, as Carl Reclam (1821–87) wrote in 1869, the task of hygiene was to quantify the 'natural physiological needs' that had to be met if the body were to function at its optimal level.[14] However, this reduction of health to abstract labour power tended to transform workers into the passive objects of biopolitical management via the state and the market. Moreover, the laboratory isolation of the individual from the world within which he lived and laboured served to bar inquiry into the causes of unequal or insufficient access to these physiological minima and hopelessly blurred the questions of how demands for more adequate resources might be legitimated and to whom claims for redress might be directed.

Both the social dimensions of morbidity and mortality and any rights claims that might derive therefrom were marginalized even further by the rise of bacteriology, which focused on the pathogenic microorganisms discovered by Louis Pasteur (1822–95), Robert Koch (1843–1910) and their students.[15] The bacteriological paradigm that triumphed during the 1880s and 1890s maintained that infection invariably followed from the invasion of the human host by these parasites and that the only truly effective way to combat contagious disease was to destroy the sources of infection and thereby break the chain of transmission. Humans figured in bacteriological thinking primarily as walking petri dishes and as the 'carriers' of disease, while the commitment to a deterministic specific etiology led bacteriologists to deny that the poverty and filth that had loomed so large in the imagination of both the medical and sanitary reformers could play any autonomous role. As Koch wrote in 1888, epidemics are never caused

> solely by dirt and garbage, by the effluvia of people living on top of one another, by hunger, poverty and deprivation, not at all by the collective factors that are generally lumped together under the expression 'social misery', nor by climatic factors, but rather only by the spread of the specific disease-causing germs whose multiplication and propagation can certainly be enabled by these factors.[16]

Social Hygiene and the Progressive Social Contract

Although it would continue to dominate state-level public health policy until after 1918, by the turn of the century the bacteriological paradigm had entered into a crisis from which it would only emerge in a substantially altered form. While the failure of Koch's tuberculin therapy and the inability to develop an effective vaccination against tuberculosis may have tarnished his public image, the discovery of both healthy carriers and the environmental omnipresence of tuberculosis germs, together with the statistical documentation of the disproportionate incidence of epidemic contagious disease among the labouring classes, struck at the explanatory heart of the bacteriological paradigm by loosening the postulated connection – logical, inevitable, direct – between invasion of the body by a pathogenic microorganism and the subsequent development of a specific disease. However, the resulting explanatory gap in the bacteriological paradigm was soon filled by the idea that the differential impact of specific pathogens on different persons could be accounted for by their individual 'constitutions', which could explain the relative success or failure of such persons in resisting the invasion and multiplication of disease-causing germs. The problem was that the character of individual constitution could be explained in both hereditarian and social terms, and at the turn of the century both the social hygienic and eugenic traditions forked off from this common constitutionalist response to the limitations of bacteriology.[17] The issue was further complicated by the fact that the recognition of how social factors could limit the scope of a narrowly bacteriological explanation of disease did not necessarily imply a commitment to any particular political position. Ferdinand Hueppe (1852–1938) is a case in point. Although Hueppe was a military doctor who had studied with Koch, his criticisms of the bacteriological paradigm ultimately led him to claim that 'hygiene is as a social art called forth by social distress and it must and will, therefore, always be social hygiene if it is to exist at all', though this insight did not lead him to abandon his conservative nationalist politics.[18]

How, then, did social hygiene come to provide the theoretical foundation for a social right to health?[19] As a form of medical knowledge, social hygiene stood and fell on its ability to disentangle the individual threads that made up the complex skein of social causality at work behind the widely-noted statistical correlations between 'sickness and social conditions', to use the title of the summa of the pre-war social hygiene movement.[20] But the success of the new discipline was due not only to its theoretical claims, but also to the fact that the preventive and curative measures it prescribed could be seen as giving substance to the new conception of social citizenship that was being articulated during these years. While deterrent poor relief and public health had regarded the poor as a burden on and potential danger to society, the period from the 1890s through the First

World War saw the birth of a new discourse on welfare and social rights that increasingly regarded the labouring classes as a precious national resource, while dependence, sickness, delinquency and criminality were seen to entail costs to the entire nation that could no longer be tolerated in the age of intensified national rivalries. Building on these new attitudes towards the labouring poor, Progressive social reformers began to articulate a new social understanding of need, which provided the socio- and medico-scientific rationale for the inversion of the political rationality of deterrence in the name of a new social contract in which the needy would enjoy more expansive social rights to those preventive and curative social programmes that would put them in a position where they would be able to fulfil the more extensive social duties expected of them. In this way the political rationality of Progressivism flowed together seamlessly with the social hygienic account of the relation between sickness and social conditions to form a new medico-political synthesis, which began to take shape in the pre-war years, which expanded exponentially during the war, and which was finally institutionalized during the Weimar Republic.

The most important theorist of social hygiene in the years leading up to the First World War was the former student of Gustav Schmoller (and later Social Democrat) Alfred Grotjahn (1869–1931). Although Grotjahn's work exemplifies in many ways the overlap of the social and hereditarian dimensions of constitutional hygiene, here I would like to focus on the social strand of his work. In his 1912 *Social Pathology*, Grotjahn argued that, in order to understand the connections between sickness and social conditions, social hygiene had to focus on how these conditions increased the predisposition towards disease among certain groups of individuals, how they immediately caused sickness, how they spread disease, and how they influenced the course and outcome of a disease. Grotjahn's point here was that sickness and poverty were attributable primarily to social forces rooted in the structure of industrial society, rather than individual fault or failing, as liberals had long insisted. His account of the diverse ways in which individual health was influenced and constrained by social forces beyond individuals' control represented a systematic response to both the bacteriological neglect of the social world and the operative assumption underlying Pettenkofer's vision of public health: that society was composed of discrete individuals whose 'normal' physiological qualities and natural needs were identical and thus capable of being studied in abstraction from the real social conditions under which they lived. Lastly, Grotjahn considered social hygiene to be both a descriptive and a normative discipline because the mere knowledge of the differential impact of social conditions on the health of the different social classes contained within itself a self-evident imperative to provide those preventive social welfare services that would elevate the 'hygienic culture' of those groups who suffered disproportionately from the existing organization of society and thus enable them to enjoy more fully those advances in medicine, hygiene, nutrition and domestic culture heretofore reserved for the middle and upper classes.[21]

It was, however, Adolf Gottstein (1857–1941) who in the pre-war years most clearly teased out the ways in which social hygiene supported the right to health. In a 1908 essay Gottstein, whose criticisms of the bacteriological establishment had blocked his career path and forced him to earn a living first as a private practitioner and then as municipal physician and municipal councillor in the Berlin district of Charlottenburg, argued that the new political importance of personal health was transforming the nature of medical assistance for the poor from an act of charity to an act of social policy undertaken by the state in order to reduce the costs of sickness and other social problems that could no longer be tolerated:

> Even care for the sick is no longer provided simply out of sympathy with their misfortune, as was once the case. Rather, we take into account the material harm to the community caused by the presence of a large number of sick persons, whose debility and inability to work can be expressed numerically in terms of the economic burden on society that they represent. In the same way, the protection of the healthy from the threat of disease is now based on social policy considerations. In view of the steady decrease in the birth rate in German cities and the transition from an agrarian to an industrial society, the value to the community of each productive individual in the economic and political struggle with other nations increases to such an extent that the common interest obligates us to take steps to ensure that our young generation is as large, healthy and productive as possible.[22]

The question, though, is whether such policies were intended to benefit the nation or enhance the rights of its individual citizens? For Gottstein, the answer was both – if only because the cultivation of healthy, strong and productive workers and soldiers for the nation could not be separated from the tangible improvements in the health, nutrition, longevity and overall well-being of the concrete individuals who made up the community. As Gottstein explained, the task of social hygiene was not simply to determine the obligations that the individual had to assume in the name of the public good, but also 'to secure and, to the extent possible, increase, the rights of the individual, who, as a member of the community, is in danger of being oppressed by it'.[23] In this way, Gottstein and the social hygiene movement more generally, circled back to the arguments on behalf of a social right to health that had first been advanced by the medical reformers of 1848, but with the difference that advances in applied physiology and bacteriology now provided both a better scientific account of the connections between sickness and the social conditions of poverty and a firmer foundation for preventive action to combat sickness and the poverty with which it was often linked. Nothing symbolized the recognition of this new relationship between health and (social) democracy better than the 1919 appointment of Gottstein as Ministerial Director in the Prussian Medical Administration, replacing Martin Kirchner (1854–1925), who had played a pivotal role in the institutionalization of bacteriology since the turn of the century.

When seen from this perspective, then, the history of public health in Germany culminates not in Nazism, but rather in the democratic welfare state that was constructed between the turn of the century and the Great Depression as social reformers struggled to find the best means of providing those preventive social welfare services that were necessary to give substance to the social rights upon which the Progressive social contract depended. It was only the political calamity of 1933 that gave retrospective plausibility to the foregrounding of eugenic medicine and its anti-democratic proclivities as the dominant feature of the medical history of the previous decades.

Social Hygiene, Citizenship and the Question of Social Discipline

The two most important preventive social hygiene programmes in early twentieth-century Germany were those created to combat tuberculosis and infant mortality. Tuberculosis and the respiratory illnesses and gastrointestinal infections grouped under the rubric of infant mortality were far and away the largest killers in Imperial Germany, and their decline accounted for the greatest part of the dramatic drop in the national mortality rate from the 1880s through the interwar years. This decline was attributable both to improvements in medicine and nutrition and to the development of new forms of social intervention, which brought knowledge of medical advances into the homes of the labouring classes and taught them to use this knowledge to take advantage of the opportunities of a healthier life made possible by the preceding decades of sanitary reform.[24]

The most important innovations in this domain were the tuberculosis welfare and infant welfare centres (*Tuberkulose-* and *Säuglingsfürsorgestellen*) and the outreach and educational programmes they sponsored. Beginning around the turn of the century, these centres evolved rapidly as the practical embodiment of the logic of prevention, and by 1920 or so it was possible to speak of something approaching a seamless network of such centres covering the urban areas of the country. The history of these programmes mirrors the complex relations between state and society – at both the national and local levels – during the Wilhelmine years. Tuberculosis and infant welfare programmes were, as Weindling and others have argued, one of the preferred domains of social intervention by conservative notables, who hoped that such initiatives would help stabilize an Empire whose national political structures were growing increasingly sclerotic. For example, the Empress Auguste Victoria Hospital, which was the organizational centre of the official infant protection movement, was established in 1905–9 by a group of highly placed conservative notables at the urging of the empress herself. Similar initiatives led to the formation of state-level associations for infant protection in Prussia, Hesse, Hamburg and other states, and in 1909 these notable associations came together to found the German Association for Infant Protection. The German Central Committee for the Prevention of Tuberculosis was similarly dominated by members of the conservative medical establishment.[25]

However, the reach of these organizations only extended so far and neither the tuberculosis nor the infant welfare centres would have spread so quickly if they had not enjoyed broad support at the local level from both the voluntary sector and municipal government – groups whose ideas coincided only to a small degree with those of these conservatives. Until the First World War, the principled refusal of the national state to assume direct responsibility for the provision of social assistance meant that the cities remained both the primary site for social politics and the primary providers of health care and other social services for the substantial portion of the population who were not covered by social insurance. This had two important implications. First, although the German poor laws obligated the cities to provide only the barest existence minimum and to do so only under the most stringent, socially stigmatizing conditions, this focus on deterrence was complemented by a universal belief in the value of personal social engagement for building bonds across classes and assisting those deserving poor whose legitimate needs could never be met by a rigorous system of deterrent relief. Such social engagement on behalf of philanthropic and charitable goals was regarded as just as integral a part of the liberal conception of citizenship as the act of voting itself, and, as a result, the philanthropic landscape of Wilhelmine Germany was characterized by the proliferation in every city and town of voluntary associations, which represented the entire spectrum of religious and political beliefs and which competed with one another to combating the many facets of the social question – and to do so in ways that corresponded to their respective understandings of the nature of need.

Secondly, the limited role of the central government also meant that the parameters of social policy were determined primarily by the balance of power at the local level, by the freedom of voluntary associations to act even in the absence of majority support for any given programme and by the expectation that public support – either in the form of municipal subsidies or the engagement of interested notables – could ultimately be expected for successful voluntary programmes.[26] Throughout the Empire, local government was dominated by the National Liberals and municipal health and welfare administrations were often led by socially-engaged liberal city councillors, who had first-hand knowledge of the socio-economic causes of poverty and disease. After the lifting of the ban on the Social Democratic Party in 1890, liberal sensitivities to such problems were heightened by the growing political voice of the urban working classes.[27] Moreover, in many of the nation's largest cities, as well as in the smaller cities in the south-western part of the country, greater electoral support for the left liberal parties directly translated into even more progressive municipal policies. However, in other areas the dominance of conservative industrialists gave municipal social policies – as well as the maternal counselling, infant welfare and tuberculosis programmes sponsored by these employers – an entirely different cast.[28] In short, although the early initiatives of conservative notables may have stimulated action at the local level, local reformers did not simply implement in an unthinking, automatic manner commands that came down from above. Rather, local associations and authorities enjoyed a great deal of autonomy in the domain of social policy, and the programmes that they adopted to combat tuberculosis and infant mortality always reflected the priorities of local decision-makers and their understanding of the social problem.

Philanthropic associations had long provided an outlet for the energies of middle-class women, and the tuberculosis and infant welfare centres developed within a dense web of local associational life. In many instances these centres evolved out of existing associations, and the professionalization of what was coming to be known as 'social' work played a pivotal role in reorienting the work of these women from traditional charity towards preventive social welfare. Moreover, these associations were often supported by local government in ways that complicated the public–private distinction almost beyond all recognition. What happened in many cases was that local government ultimately chose to provide financial assistance to social programs that had been established by voluntary associations, but that did not have adequate financial resources to meet the demand for their services.[29] In some instances, local government would simply provide annual subsidies to these associations. In others, local government simply took over programmes that had been set up by voluntary associations, and funded them out of discretionary funds allocated outside the poor relief budget, though the cities often continued to depend on voluntary associations to meet the diverse ancillary needs of the people who visited the centres. In still other cases, local authorities might agree to provide the office space for the welfare centre and/or pay the salaries of the physicians who worked there, with the social workers who were responsible for visiting the needy in their homes remaining in the pay of voluntary associations. Since the danger of coercion and stigmatization was always much closer to the surface in the work of the tuberculosis centres than in that of the infant welfare centres, this latter arrangement was regarded as particularly beneficial because social workers in the employ of voluntary associations were more likely to be able to gain the trust of afflicted individuals visitors dispatched by the local health office.[30] Such decisions were facilitated by the fact that the local officials who made such decisions were themselves often either members of these associations, married to the women who ran them or closely connected to these women through local social networks. In this way they mediated between the public and the private/voluntary dimensions of social engagement.

As I have argued elsewhere, the years between the turn of the century and the First World War witnessed the broad acceptance within the social reform community of a new understanding of the social question that located the causes

of poverty, sickness, delinquency and unemployment more in the social structures industrial civilization – and the ways in which they shaped the life-world
and everyday experience of the underprivileged – than in failings of individual
character or morality, and it was this social perspective on poverty, rather than
eugenic concerns, that provided the theoretical bases for the work of the tuberculosis and infant welfare centres. The goal of the welfare centres was to oversee
and assist the entire needy population, not to provide differential treatment to
different sections of the population based on their perceived racial value; their
preventive labours would have been incomprehensible, if not counterproduc-
tive, from a eugenic perspective. While the war led the national state to expand
financial support substantially for these programmes, the centres themselves
remained in the hands of local government and local associations, and neither
these wartime subsidies nor post-war developments led to any fundamental
change in their approach to combating tuberculosis and infant mortality.

Although the shift from deterrence to prevention provided a positive
rationale for public intervention that appeared to outweigh the dangers long
associated with pauperism, the realization of this preventive project required
greater latitude for intervening in the private sphere than could be sanctioned
by classical liberalism. Perhaps the most important question is how did these
preventive social hygiene programmes affect the freedom and welfare of their
ostensible beneficiaries? Taking tuberculosis as an example, if infectious expec-
torations were the means by which this *Volkskrankheit* perpetuated itself, then
the logical first step in breaking its grip was to survey the general population,
seek out the quite literally hundreds of thousands of sources of contagion and
destroy them by treating each case in the appropriate manner. This was the mission of the welfare centres, whose guiding principle was

> to track down and attack (*Erfassen*) [the sources and victims of infection]. Before
> anything is done, all cases under consideration must be surveyed and classified
> according to the nature of the proposed measures, which extend from the simplest
> enlightenment all the way to sanatorium treatment ... It is only through the centers
> that the war on tuberculosis is approached from the epidemiological perspective of
> combating epidemic disease rather than that of curative treatment or the restoration
> of the labor power. Consequently, observation and diagnosis are not restricted to
> curative measures for the afflicted individual, but also embrace his entire surround-
> ing environment. [The centers] weave a net in conjunction with all the other offices
> charged with hygienic observation of the population and their primary goal is the
> systematic and timely discovery of all sources of contagion and their neutralization.[31]

Since the prevention of both tuberculosis and infant mortality depended on
the early identification of needy and endangered populations, their education
and timely medical treatment, the outreach strategies developed by the centres,
which focused on seeking out those they wished to target, encouraging them to

visit the centres, and monitoring their conditions in a continuous, systematic manner, represented an important extension of the administrative capacity of the early social state. The immediate goal of both the tuberculosis and infant welfare centres was to persuade their respective target populations to visit the centres so that potential medical problems could be caught early and treated while the prognosis was still good. Once there, physicians and social workers would have – at least temporarily – a captive audience. However, a one-off visit would only have minimal impact on the health of the endangered individual and that of the nation, and the rationalization of preventive care depended on finding a way to maintain regular contact between the welfare centres and their target populations. To achieve this goal, the centres relied, on the one hand, on house visits by social workers – on the basis of information gleaned from a variety of sources – to working-class women, who were almost always the first point of contact. On the other hand, the centres also relied on a wide variety of incentives to encourage regular visits and thus facilitate more continuous surveillance of the population. In addition to helping needy families secure financial assistance and providing such things as spittoons, disinfectant and baby formula, the most important incentives offered by the centres were free medical examinations, recommendations for sanatorium treatment (for those who met the criteria), and the various premium programmes that were adopted in many cities to encourage mothers to nurse their infants.

The social concerns of the welfare centres and their roots in the social hygiene tradition helped define their goals and distinguish their work from that of hospitals, clinics and sanatoria. They were quite explicit that their primary aim was to protect the healthy, not to cure the sick or help the poor, and they were concerned with the latter only insofar as their sickness was a source of danger to others. The social problems of tuberculosis and infant mortality were constructed primarily via the representation of working-class women as ignorant of the basic principles of modern hygiene and infant care and therefore as negligent with regard to their maternal duties. 'The enemies', wrote Arthur Schlossmann, the founder of the influential Association for Infant Welfare in Düsseldorf and one of the leading figures in the infant protection movement, are 'ignorance and indifference'.[32] However, this was not a congenital indifference that forever marked them off as an irredeemably different racial other, but rather one bred of the lack of education and understanding of how – thanks to the advance of medicine and hygiene – things might be done differently, and why. From such a perspective, the obvious solution was to educate working-class women in the latest scientific advances in infant hygiene, nutrition and care and then to ensure that they drew the proper conclusions from this education. Within this pedagogical discourse, the counterpart of such rhetoric of disempowerment was (at least potentially) a rhetoric of entitlement in the form of a social right to health and to the advice and assistance that would put these women – once they had been awakened to a new hygienic consciousness – in a position to care for their children in accordance with the principles of modern hygiene; only then could they be held to the higher standards of civic responsibility that were the counterpart to these expanded social rights.

In a very similar way, the war on tuberculosis also depended on enlightenment, the informed collaboration of the needy and endangered, and the development of a solidaristic consciousness that all persons are individually and collectively responsible for the well-being of the community. Since sanatoria were not an effective means of combating epidemic disease and since compulsory institutionalization was not a viable political option, isolating the sick to break the cycle of contagion and infection meant less their physical removal from the family than what might be called outdoor isolation or the 'sanitization of the tubercular family in its own home'. This involved educating both the sick and the healthy on the nature of infection and the basic rules of hygiene required to protect themselves and others from the disease so that the sick would no longer pose a danger to the population within which they lived. The family was the alpha and omega of prevention because tuberculosis was most often spread by living or working together for a sustained period of time in an enclosed space with someone who already had the disease, and it was thus within the physical and social space of the family that the sick had to be isolated. The contagious nature of the disease meant that where there was one person with advanced tuberculosis, other family members were often affected as well, and the logic of prevention dictated that they, too, be made the object of preventive surveillance, solicitude and enlightenment.

The question, though, is how to conceptualize these efforts to alter the behaviour of the poor. The relationship between physicians and social workers, on the one hand, and the populations they targeted, on the other, have often been described in terms of social disciplining or medicalization. Such processes refer to both the discursive construction of need and the idea that welfare programmes based on this knowledge had to be intrusive, coercive and repressive because this was the only way to bridge the gap between the middle and the working classes and thereby impose upon the latter the rational lifestyle and cultural values of the former – buttressed as they were by the elitist authority of sciences. However, it is not clear how accurately the strong version of the social discipline paradigm described what was actually happening in the tuberculosis and infant welfare centres, whether these administrative knowledges were directly and logically translated into disciplinary control over working-class families, whether social reformers aspired to such control, or whether they in fact needed to rely on coercion and discipline to achieve their preventive goals.

I would argue that hygienic enlightenment was the key to the success of these preventive social hygiene programmes, not only because suasion was the only way to ensure that the needy and endangered internalized these new ideas and put them into practice in their everyday lives, but also because the welfare centres had little capacity to coerce people into acting in accordance with their wishes or to discipline them for failing to do so. The real issue is not so much whether the physicians and social workers who worked in the tuberculosis and infant welfare centres tried to get something out these people, but rather the terms of exchange between the two. The basic purpose of these programmes was to encourage needy women to behave in certain ways, and it would have been self-defeating for these programmes to have made their terms of eligibility so harsh as to discourage people from taking advantage of the assistance they offered. As with infant welfare, anti-tuberculosis programmes succeeded to the extent that the working classes perceived them as offering something that they valued on terms with which they could live: medical treatment (which came at the recommendation of the welfare centres, even though it was not provided by them) and advice on how to keep themselves and others healthy. However, these were things that the working classes had to *learn* to value, and it is perhaps more accurate to speak here of medicalization as a collective learning process than as a process of social disciplining. Thus, unless we are willing to insist that all attempts to influence the behaviour of others are nothing other than surface manifestations of a deeper, cunning logic of social discipline that undermines the rights of individuals in the name of their emancipation, then we need to take seriously the role of hygienic enlightenment and social learning and to approach the history of the welfare state in new ways that are capable of better capturing the expanded social rights that flowed from the combination of enlightenment, conditional incentives and social discipline embodied in these programmes.

6 FROM TOBACCO IN THE WAR TO THE WAR ON TOBACCO: SMOKING IN BRITAIN AND GERMANY FROM *c.* 1900 TO 1945

Rosemary Elliot

By the end of the twentieth century, international epidemiological evidence on smoking and passive smoking and the risks which they posed to the individual and the community respectively were widely accepted. Indeed, tobacco use provided one of the key foundations of the new public health, with expert knowledge, an evidence base, advocacy groups and central government pressure combining with a lifestyle focus on individual behaviour to move anti-smoking campaigns beyond a peripheral concern to centre stage. While the new public health put the onus on the individual to take responsibility for their health status as a mark of citizenship, state and non-government organizations and initiatives seeking to guide people to make the correct choices mushroomed. National education and policy programmes became a matter of international concern, with cross-European initiatives and global developments, such as the World Health Organization's Framework Convention on Tobacco Control.[1] Countries which lagged behind or did not wholly subscribe to the anti-smoking ethos were castigated in the medical and public health press. For example, talking about slow European progress on smoking policy in 2002, the director of English anti-smoking organization Action on Smoking and Health, was quoted as saying, 'Europe is moving at the speed of its slowest ship, Germany, and that ship has got the tobacco industry on the bridge'.[2]

In the narrative which developed in the early 2000s, Britain was seen to be at the forefront of developments in anti-smoking advocacy, while Germany was seen as much more liberal and even blocking legislation. This was explained by historians and public health commentators alike as the legacy of anti-smoking propaganda in the Third Reich, the influx of US Virginian cigarettes through the occupation period and the influence of the tobacco industry in the latter decades of the twentieth century.[3] Thus, engagement with the new public health, an international phenomenon, was shaped at a national level by historical factors. It is on some of these historical factors that this chapter will focus.

The role and prominence of smoking within the new public health is merely one in a series of incarnations of smoking which can be located in changing understandings of health and citizenship. From the gentleman smoker of the nineteenth century who exercised rational control and moderation in his tobacco consumption through to the health conscious non-smoker of the late twentieth century, tobacco use or avoidance has long been connected with ideals of what constitutes a healthy body, with implications for the positioning of that body within the state and society as a whole. There have been multiple understandings of tobacco use, dependent on who was smoking, their gender, class and race and how these were perceived.

Such multiple understandings of smoking have also operated at a national level – the most obvious example being in Britain and Germany during the Second World War, as this essay will show. In Britain, tobacco use was tied to patriotic discourses of citizenship as civilians were urged to send tobacco to troops at the front as a symbol of their commitment to the war effort and related to this, their desire to protect democratic freedoms. In Germany, on the other hand, anti-smoking campaigns were orchestrated at state level and the avoidance of smoking was constructed as a patriotic duty for racial health within the context of the National Socialist dictatorship.

Despite the widespread association of the Nazis with anti-smoking propaganda by the end of the twentieth century, in large part a result of the successful work of Robert Proctor and others, anti-smoking policy in Germany was not the creation of the National Socialist regime. Proctor refers to early anti-smoking movements within Germany and the concomitant rise of medical research on smoking, but gives less attention to the relationship between the two trends by the early 1930s, when the Nazis assumed power.[4] As this chapter will show, the existing early twentieth-century German anti-smoking movement saw the Nazi takeover of power as an opportunity to further the anti-smoking cause. This contrasted to the situation in Britain where people sought to distance themselves from punitive anti-smoking measures, seeing them as part and parcel of an extremist racial ideology which had taken hold within a dictatorship. Nonetheless, these divergent paths developed from a similar history: eugenic anti-smoking discourse was evident in both Britain and Germany in the earlier twentieth century. Here it will be argued that the different paths taken by Britain and Germany in the 1930s and 1940s can be explained both by the political make-up of the respective states and the position of smoking within them. A key factor was the relative strength of the anti-smoking movement in the interwar period: in Britain, it had all but vanished, whereas in Germany, it was gathering momentum.

These differences became marked by the outbreak of the Second World War, as noted above. In Britain tobacco use was tied to patriotic discourses of citizenship as civilians were urged to send tobacco to troops at the front as a symbol of their commitment to the war effort and related to this, their desire to protect democracy. In this context, a rebuttal of anti-smoking measures demonstrated British smokers' position within a democratic liberal state. In Germany, on the other hand, *not* smoking was constructed as a patriotic duty. However, anti-smoking discourse was not the only tenet of tobacco policy in the Third Reich. The provision of tobacco for the troops was as important in Germany as it was in Britain. This suggests a need to disassociate the rhetoric around smoking from the economic, political and social realities.

In the immediate post-war period, anti-smoking groups in West Germany continued to operate as NGOs, pushing health in relation to tobacco policy onto the agenda at a federal level, in a way that was absent in Britain at that time. The need for revenue from tobacco taxation, the desire to rebuild and protect the domestic tobacco industry and the role of tobacco in international trade all meant that health concerns were outweighed by economic and political concerns in post-war West Germany. Thus, as I have argued elsewhere, debates around smoking and health need to take into account economic concerns and the role of the tobacco industry in promoting these arguments in the immediate post-war years.[5]

Smoking and Liberal Citizenship

There is ample literature on the positioning of smoking within bourgeois liberal culture in the Victorian period. The act of, and language around, smoking reflected the tenets of liberal citizenship. Both Matthew Hilton and Jarrett Rudy have convincingly shown the ways in which tobacco use was cultivated as the outward symbol of rational thought and individual autonomy in Britain and Canada, respectively.[6] Gentleman smokers exercised choice in the blends of tobacco they consumed, they educated themselves about tobaccos and smoking products through a range of literature and they were part of a wider culture which saw tobacco use as conducive to intellectual and creative pursuits. In Britain, moderation was seen as key: an 1856 article in the *Lancet* described moderation as no more than one or two pipes a day and no smoking before breakfast.[7]

Crucially, this rational consumption of tobacco was demarcated along class and gender lines, reflecting the extent to which political rights and civic participation were still exclusive to wealthy men. In English-language literature, working-class and poorer smokers were criticized for squandering scarce resources on tobacco, for idleness when smoking and for polluting the atmosphere with tobacco smoke.[8] Here, smoking was seen to work against self-improvement and responsible citizenship. Youth smokers, that is, those who had not yet gained maturity, were portrayed as too immature, physically and mentally, to cope with nicotine. For women, smoking was taboo: a lengthy editorial, also in the *Lancet*, which referred to 'the man who smokes', was not just linguistic convention, but reflected the prevailing social norms.[9] Female smoking was associated with deviance from ideal feminine norms and criticized on medical and biological grounds, as well as moral ones.[10] Like young people, women were thought unable to exercise the level of rational thought and responsibility to moderate their tobacco intake. Tobacco use was seen to have a negative impact on reproduction and birth and on breastfeeding.[11] Indeed, women were urged to exercise their superior moral virtue in persuading husbands, sons and other male relatives not to smoke.[12]

Similar discourses can be found in Imperial German literature through the nineteenth century. Smoking belonged among men as befitting their public position in social and political life, but was frowned upon among women. Concerns about smoking and reproduction were also evident.[13] Of course, in both Britain and Germany, it is likely that women smoked behind closed doors and in the literature of the time, there are examples of prominent women who dared to smoke in public.[14] But it was not until the early twentieth century that visual images of female smokers began to appear in advertising in both Britain and Germany and then such images represented a challenge to existing social norms.[15] While anti-smoking literature did feature concerns about smoking among women in Germany, the real focus of anxieties was young people. At its inception in 1910, the German Anti-Tobacco League argued for legislative measures restricting smoking among young people (under 16s) and the sale of tobacco to this group. Parallels can be seen in the Anglo-American context, where campaigners such as Lucy Page Gaston and her brother, Edward Page Gaston, sought to dissuade boys from taking up smoking. Such campaigns were couched in the language of liberal citizenship, as smoking was seen to erode personal autonomy and freedom, condemning its users to a lifetime of nicotine abuse. However, the language of eugenics had already begun to creep in.[16]

Smoking in the First World War

From the early twentieth century onwards in Britain and Germany, tobacco brands were increasingly promoted within discourses of nationalism and, in the British context, Empire.[17] It was not necessary to smoke to be a good citizen, but in nineteenth and early twentieth-century Britain, tobacco played its part in creating the particularly masculine public arena in which citizenship could be demonstrated. It is no accident that, as women increasingly staked a claim to a role in the public sphere and access to full citizenship, the cigarette provided a powerful and contested symbol of those claims.[18]

Against this background, war represented the apogee of citizenship; as civilian men were called on to defend their country and civilian tensions were – on the surface at least – papered over in the quest for national unity in the face of a common enemy.[19] The extent to which fighting for one's country was an autonomous choice was variable in the First World War: in the early months in Britain, many men did join up in a rush of patriotism, but as the war progressed this slowed to a trickle, leading to ever greater social coercion and, ultimately, state coercion in the form of conscription.[20] In the Second World War, conscription was introduced almost immediately and while conscientious objection was always an option, it was one with social consequences.[21] This contrasted with the situation in Germany where conscription had been in place throughout the Imperial period.[22] In Britain, the language of citizenship gained unprecedented currency as a means of encouraging individuals to participate in the war effort, promoting a sense of national unity and identity, dissuading people from non-civic behaviour, such as shirking war duties, and attempting to heighten morale. To a certain extent, being a good citizen was synonymous with patriotism, but with the growing expectation of a post-war welfare state and social entitlements, this patriotism was imbued with a sense of reciprocity.[23]

In Britain in both wars, tobacco smoking was linked with a particular form of soldierly masculinity: demonstrating and creating strength and courage, endurance and male bonding. Indeed, it was the experience of the First World War which arguably cemented the cigarette's popularity among men, establishing the rather more feminine tobacco article as the favourite over the more masculine pipe and cigar.[24] This was the result of both astute marketing by cigarette manufacturers and a grassroots shift in smoking tastes. In practical terms, the cigarette was the most convenient, quickest and effective way of consuming tobacco on the Front line.[25] In letters home, published in the *British American Tobacco Bulletin*, a weekly communiqué for troops at the Front and staff back home produced by the cigarette manufacturer of that name, cigarettes featured centrally in the men's experiences of war. In a letter of May 1915 published in the bulletin, for example, J. W. Spearman explained his high cigarette consumption.

> In the trenches we smoke the whole time, except the few hours we snatch for a snooze and during the time we stand to, just before dusk and dawn. I never relished a smoke so much as when in the trenches; it keeps my mind off the snipers and controls my language when the bullets whizz by.[26]

The ethos through much of the correspondence was one of maintaining composure through whatever hardships might be faced, but cigarettes also provided a chance to escape from hostilities, in one's mind if not in reality.[27] Cigarettes were widely perceived as a democratizing force: officers and privates could and did, share cigarettes, as did members of different battalions.[28] More sensationally, tobacco manufacturer Players received a number of letters from soldiers claiming to owe their lives to the physical presence of cigarettes or tobacco around their body. One soldier, a Mr G. Dowell, wrote in December 1914 enclosing a tin of

Players tobacco. This had, he said, saved his life as it had stopped some shrapnel when it was in the pocket of his serge trench coat.[29] A similar letter in December 1916 from another soldier described how a Players cigarette tin, which he had been using to store his soap, had also stopped a shrapnel bullet.[30] Cigarette packets also came in useful for holding together torn one franc notes and several soldiers wrote to British American Tobacco and Players enclosing examples of these.[31] In these many different ways, cigarettes and tobacco became an integral part of day to day life in the Forces. The trade press described cigarettes as 'chief of all creature comforts [for] our lads in service': the 'our' indicating that, while it was the lads laying down their lives, they belonged to a wider community with a common purpose.[32]

This latter comment indicates a further role of the cigarette in citizenship: collecting and sending cigarettes to 'our' lads in service helping to create the sense of united community. In December 1914, for example, people in Glasgow held a 'Tobacco Day', collecting money to send to the troops. They collected over £1,700 and 'liberal' donations of cigarettes and tobacco. The day was rounded off with a fancy dress procession by torchlight, which suggests that the day also served as a diversion from everyday life.[33] The desire to buy cigarettes for loved ones in the armed forces also brought more women into the traditionally male sphere of the tobacconist's. The transgression that women's entering the tobacconist's represented was justified by the fact that they were doing it for the war effort. A correspondent in the *Tobacco Trade Review* noted that 'the women folks, whatever their personal feelings with regard to tobacco itself, are only too glad to purchase comfort for those who know what relief the weed brings'.[34]

However, while women were incorporated into the lexicon of patriotic citizenship through the purchase of cigarettes, tobacco consumption itself remained highly gendered. Smoking was seen as a necessity of war-time life, but only for those fighting for their country. When conscription was introduced in 1916 as part of Britain's move towards total war, the link between fighting for the nation and citizenship was reinforced. As part of the country's move towards total war, the government also took control of the task of supplying tobacco and cigarettes to the troops, at times importing tobacco at the expense of other goods to protect morale.[35] Civilians, particularly women, were asked to reduce their consumption in order that 'Tommy' (the informal name for a private in the British army) might be adequately supplied. In response, one woman wrote that she would gladly give up her cigarettes for the troops, but asked why exempted men, 'men who were not doing their bit', elderly men and 'in fact all men who were not in hospital or at the Front' were not also being asked to do their share.[36] The answer lay in the fact that smoking was still perceived as a masculine habit and women were deemed to be encroaching on male privilege by smoking. Despite the fact that many women were in the field of military action or performing vital services back home, female smokers were presented in the press in two ways. The first was as society women who smoked in ladies' clubs and hoarded cigarettes to the detriment of the troops, the second was as 'good time girls' who fraternized with the troops and smoked as part of a constellation of behaviours which pushed the boundaries of respectable femininity.[37] Neither construction suggested that women needed or deserved cigarettes in the way men were seen to.

In the British context, manufacturers were thus successful in claiming nationalist rhetoric and associating it with smoking, exploiting the prevailing ethos of patriotic citizenship and the popularity of cigarettes to indirectly dispel any concerns about smoking's negative effects on youth and the future of the race. As a result, concerns and anxieties around youth smoking largely disappeared in the First World War. In Germany, the situation was more complex. Manufacturers sought to create a specific German identity for cigarette brands, which fused heroism and nation in the symbol of the soldier at the front, for example, with names like 'Deutsche Helden' (German Heroes) and 'Reichsadler' (Imperial Eagle). Military and naval imagery was also frequent.[38] This contrasted with the heavy emphasis on oriental names and imagery in the late nineteenth and early twentieth centuries, when manufacturers were keen to position their products as exotic, semi-luxury goods.[39] In the early twentieth century, English and French names had also proliferated, but with the outbreak of the war, these were changed to, or made to sound more, German.[40] Such Germanization of brand names was not confined to cigarettes and illustrates the extent to which the consumption of goods became tied up with national identity as a means of demonstrating patriotism.

In Germany, however, concerns around smoking, particularly its impact on young people, remained. Smoking among young men was seen to have a detrimental impact on their physical readiness for military service and this was confounded by moral concerns about youth culture generally. In 1915, the Reich Interior Minister wrote to the *Länder* about smoking and other worrying behaviours such as young people visiting cinemas, clubs and cafes, reading trash literature and hanging about at night. Such behaviours were seen as a manifestation of a lack of discipline and paternal influence as many fathers and male teachers were fighting in the war. This letter was prompted by a petition from the German Anti-Tobacco League who sought a prohibition of smoking among young people.

Alongside the concerns already listed, the German Anti-Tobacco League was also concerned about the future of the race. Anxieties focused on young men, again showing the parameters of smoking at that time. There were also nationalist concerns, for example, a letter from the Württemberg Minister of the Interior at the end of 1915 referred to the money going overseas when young people smoked tobacco: 'as tobacco for cigarettes comes from abroad, the money [spent on cigarettes] goes there as well' ('*Da der Tabak für die Ciga-*

retten aus dem Ausland stammt, fließt das Geld auch dorthin').[41] The question of a complete ban on smoking among young people was raised in 1915, but a ban for the duration of the war was considered more practical. Nonetheless, concerns about smoking among young people and a general drift into wayward-ness lingered after the end of the First World War. During the early years of the Weimar Republic, concerns were exacerbated by fears about mass culture, particularly given the influence of cinema.[42]

Thus, moral and medical concerns mixed with nationalism in interwar German youth protection discourse. Such concerns were gendered and focused more or less exclusively on young male smokers. Women were urged not to smoke on economic grounds – an understandable emphasis given the turbulence of the Weimar period – but also to use their 'natural' influence in the family to dissuade male relatives from smoking.[43] In much of the writing, the problematic compo-nent of tobacco was seen to be nicotine – this was recognized as addictive and also seen to damage heart function and circulation.[44]

Smoking in the Second World War

By the interwar period in Germany, discourses around smoking, like alcohol con-sumption, were linked to wider concerns about hereditary degeneration, which explains why youth smoking was seen as particularly problematic. Nicotine was understood to have a negative effect on reproduction and future generations. Thus, the Baltic-German physiologist, Gustav von Bunge, cautioned:

> one forgets that the youngest and most sensitive organism is the germ cell [*Keimzelle*] ... Therefore we need to question whether regular smoking among adults also dam-ages the germ cell. Looking at chronic alcoholism would suggest that it [nicotine consumption] does.[45]

Bunge was writing under the auspices of the German Anti-Tobacco League and it is clear that their concerns about degeneration allied with the broader con-cerns of the medical profession about racial hygiene. The League was headed up by Fritz Lickint from 1931 onwards. Lickint was a prominent researcher into the health effects of smoking and one of Germany's leading critics of tobacco use. He substantially reorganized the League's journal and doubled the length of it. It is clear that members of the League saw the Nazi takeover of power in 1933 as an opportunity to further their cause. An editorial in 1933, under a picture of Adolf Hitler, proclaimed:

> The Führer of our new state lives free from tobacco. All opponents of tobacco will realize this with sincere pleasure. It is also the first time that a German Chancellor of the Reich is a non-smoker and can make decisions over the fate of our *Volk* uninflu-enced by nicotine and other social drugs [*Genußgifte*]. With this, we can hope for the

first time, that our voice will be heard in government, after years and decades in which it has been practically impossible to even get a cautionary article into the daily press ...

No wonder we have not yet succeeded in making the population aware of such important requirements as a tobacco-free upbringing and education for children and young people.

Now finally the time has come for us to arrive on the scene! The first step should be a prohibition of smoking among young people.[46]

The focus here was again on smoking among young people, which was justified on the grounds of ensuring they achieved their full potential. An article in the same edition focusing on health education aimed at young people referred also to 'the need to create an undamaged, free, new Germany from the embryo upwards' and also drew on contemporary understandings of hereditary biology, continuing: '[it] must be our aim for the future to reproduce our German Volk not only in the context of a pure race but with reference to the hygiene of the germ cell [*Keimhygiene*]'.[47]

Thus, already in 1933, there was a clear emphasis on hereditary biology and racial hygiene in anti-smoking material which pre-dated the inception of the Reich Agency Against the Dangers of Alcohol and Tobacco (Reichsstelle gegen die Alkohol- und Tabakgefahren) in 1939. Indeed, the Reich Agency had formerly focused on alcohol only, which suggests that tobacco came to the fore as a concern for the National Socialists relatively late on. The impetus for greater concern was arguably the publication of Lickint's extensive volume on smoking and health, *Tabak und Organismus*, in 1939, the same year as Franz Müller published one of the earliest epidemiological studies making the connection between smoking and lung cancer. Subsequently, the field was taken up by scholars at the Scientific Institute for Research on the Dangers of Tobacco (Wissenschaftliches Institut zur Erforschung der Tabakgefahren) in Jena, which was founded in 1941 and funded partially by Hitler.[48] Research carried out there looked at various topics, but the subject of smoking and reproduction carried the most weight in terms of racial hygiene.[49] Lickint argued, for example, that 'the quality of smokers' descendants is as important as the quantity' and quoted another piece of work which suggested that, on account of nicotine poisoning, 'the germ plasm [*Keimplasma*] of the German people would be fundamentally altered, indeed irreversibly, in ten to twelve generations'.[50] Preventing this damage was seen as a patriotic duty. To quote Lickint:

Whoever loves his people and his Fatherland, cannot, in my opinion, pass over the question of smoking. All the foregoing reasons, be they economic, medical, moral or any other, lead in the end to the demand that the fight against all dangers of smoking must be the first patriotic duty![51]

In this argument, abstaining from smoking was constructed as the act of a good citizen, in order to preserve the health of the German people, with health configured at a racial and national level as well as an individual one.

The deployment of anti-smoking discourse within the context of nationalist and racist policies meant that the tobacco industry was constrained in what it was able to do to market the product in Germany. The restrictions on advertising tobacco and tobacco consumption among women, as well as the anti-smoking campaigns which mixed racial hygiene with medical warnings against smoking have been well-documented.[52] The point here is that the industry had its hands tied and could not openly increase its market out of the exigencies of war, in the way that its British counterpart was able to do. Nonetheless, as early as 1939, cigarette manufacturers were lobbying the Nazi Party to protect their position. In a lengthy letter to the Commission for Economic Policy of the National Socialist Party (Kommission für Wirtschaftspolitik der NSDAP), tobacco magnate Phillip Reemstma employed the language of nationalism and collective good to position himself and, more importantly, the product his factories produced, as integral to the survival of the German race. He argued that the key role of tobacco in the economies of the Orient made tobacco consumption a question of '*Ostraumpolitik*' which spoke to the Nazis' expansion plans in Eastern Europe. If Germany stopped buying produce from countries such as Turkey, Greece and Bulgaria, these countries would, according to Reemstma, very quickly turn to Russia, as the only other country who could provide an adequate market for their tobacco. He put this in stark terms: without the possibility of selling tobacco in Germany, Turkey would very quickly become a Russian colony. The effects in Greece and Bulgaria would not be much different. Further, if German manufacturers were to close down, the other main companies supplying German demand would be British American Tobacco and two Greek companies, Richard Greiling and Kyriasi Frères. In other words, Reemstma stated, 'tobacco trade and import policy from the Orient would be decided in London'.[53]

Further, Reemstma suggested that closing cigarette factories would not advance Germany's war effort, saying that cigarette manufacture was less labour intensive than producing other forms of tobacco goods, such as cigars and thus closing cigarette firms would not free up that many workers for the war effort. He also faced arguments about the detrimental effects of nicotine head on by arguing that cigarettes contained the lowest amount of nicotine of all tobacco products. This lengthy letter was just the start of a campaign by cigarette manufacturers against anti-smoking propaganda and restrictions on smoking. Reemstma's arguments neatly tied together discourses of nationalism with Germany's trade and foreign policy in the Second World War. Clearly, smoking policy was not only connected to discourses of health and citizenship, but was a question of economic policy and international trade. Further, as the war progressed and tobacco shortages became more acute, economic concerns arguably determined tobacco policy more than concerns about health.[54]

Economic issues remained important in the post-war period, when German tobacco manufacturers found themselves in competition with the influx of US manufactured Virginia cigarettes. In the debates which surrounded tobacco taxation in the early 1950s, West German manufacturers were keen to promote their product as key to the economic and social rebuilding of the state. The West German government was also keen to maintain revenue from tobacco taxation and to rebuild links with Oriental tobacco growers for trade reasons.[55] Discourses around health did not disappear from the agenda, being taken up by the German Agency against the Dangers of Addiction (*Deutsche Hauptstelle gegen die Suchtgefahren*), a non-government organization made up from the abstinence and anti-smoking agencies who had previously come together in the Reich Agency Against the Dangers of Alcohol and Tobacco, established under the National Socialist regime.[56] However, concerns about health were outweighed by fiscal and economic necessity: smoking was constructed as integral to the recovery of West Germany.

Discourses positing smoking as integral to the success of the country were apparent in Britain throughout the war and replicated the situation in the First World War. By the Second World War, the parameters of citizenship had shifted to incorporate women, providing that they conformed to prevailing ideals of respectability.[57] Unlike in the First World War, the machinery to establish conscription was implemented almost immediately, food rationing was introduced and the entire country was mobilized for total war. Women as well as men were registered for war work and could be legally compelled to participate, extending civic responsibility to both sexes.[58] Opportunities for women to take on men's jobs and roles extended to cigarette smoking: women in the forces and in the NAAFI (Navy, Army and Air Force Institutes) were provided with cigarette supplies in the same way as men, while some munitions factories provided their workers with a ration as an incentive to productivity.[59] Independent financial income meant that women had the financial means to buy cigarettes, continuing a trend apparent in the interwar period, while the presence of American GI's after 1942 meant a plentiful supply of gifts of cigarettes, nylons and lipsticks for their British girlfriends.[60] Tobacco consumption rose among both sexes as female smoking was legitimated, to a certain extent, by the shared experience of war.[61]

The legitimacy of female smoking within extending parameters of citizenship remained limited since provision of tobacco and patterns of consumption were still gendered, albeit less obviously, at government, social and individual levels. There was a discernible hierarchy of perceived need, from military to civilian, men to women. The fact that troops needed cigarettes was seen as axiomatic: male military personnel were given an allowance of fifty duty free cigarettes a week, women being given twenty-five.[62] Cigarette funds were set up almost immediately and endorsed by the Secretary of State for War, Leslie Hore-Belisha.[63] Gift parcels sent by relatives and friends to troops at the Front and to British and Allied POWs were also exempt from duty.[64] It is also worth noting that enemy POWs were given cigarettes in their rations, although at thirty-five cigarettes per week the numbers were less than those given to male British and Allied troops.[65] Nonetheless, both the removal of duty on cigarettes and the provision of cigarette rations to POWs suggest that providing tobacco and facilitating smoking was seen as a necessary expense of war.

Ordinary British civilians, however, found their tobacco supplies much reduced, although the government, in conjunction with manufacturers, instituted a number of schemes to protect the supply and distribution of tobacco. These included pooling schemes, lifting restrictions on the amount of tobacco which could be cleared through Customs and Excise and a system of rationing wholesalers on the basis of past trade.[66] In April 1941, the President of the Board of Trade authorized clearances to be increased by 20 per cent, saying, 'in war conditions smoking must be regarded as an essential rather than a luxury and as important for the maintenance of morale as tea and beer'.[67] But civilian provision was never at the expense of the military: when supplies became particularly tight at the end of 1944, further reductions were made in civilian provision to ensure that ample supplies were available for troops fighting in France.[68] This continued a trend of aiming to cut civilian consumption throughout the war by increasing taxes and making appeals to the public to cut consumption.[69] Such appeals incorporated the central ideal of much war-time commentary, namely self-sacrifice in the interests of the national cause. Recognizing the addictive nature of tobacco and the difficulty of cutting down, London newspaper *The Times* drew on the rhetoric of citizenship and the war effort, drawing a parallel with military endeavour – 'Whichever plan the good citizen adopts (in reducing tobacco consumption), he will have days of hard fighting before him'.[70]

The shortage of the more popular Virginian tobacco was particularly severe for political reasons and Britain was also committed to supporting the neutral countries of Greece and Turkey by importing their tobacco.[71] Turkish cigarettes became the butt of popular humour, while the government tried to persuade women to smoke them by running information campaigns promoting Turkish cigarettes as the glamorous choice.[72] Certainly, handmade Turkish cigarettes had been the choice of the few society ladies who smoked in the late nineteenth century, but these probably bore no relation to the much despised 'Pasha' cigarettes of the Second World War.[73] The feeling that women were smoking what was rightfully men's was never articulated at a government level, but it persisted among some members of the public: in June 1941, the issue was raised at Parliamentary Questions, it being alleged that some tobacconists were refusing to sell women cigarettes, while a similar situation was reported in the Edinburgh newspaper, the *Scotsman*.[74]

Discourses opposing the centrality of tobacco to the military and civilian population in Britain were marginal, but echoed the language of citizenship. Critics of smoking argued that tobacco use affected physical fitness among troops; while others suggested that the use of valuable shipping space to import tobacco was to the detriment of the nutritional needs of the community as a whole.[75] However, such criticisms were countered by the dominant rhetoric of patriotism, emphasizing the primacy of the war effort: it was felt that troops could not be asked not to smoke when they were fighting for their country, ready to sacrifice their lives for the good of the nation. Equally, the enormous revenue generated by smokers was seen as 'a worthy contribution to the national war effort'.[76] Further, in Britain, as in Germany, concerns about taxation in the post-war period affected the extent to which an anti-smoking argument was made. The small National Society of Non-Smokers, which had been founded in 1926 and employed Temperance rhetoric infused with eugenic concerns about the future of the race, concentrated more on campaigning for smoke free public spaces and helping people to quit by the post-war period.

The German anti-smoking campaigns were reported in the British press as part and parcel of the wider drive towards racial hygiene, which had the effect of detracting from any reasonable core to the argument – thus, the *Scotsman* in 1938 reported that Julius Streicher 'Germany's notorious No. 1 jew-baiter ... blamed the Jews for introducing tobacco to Germany'. In a reported speech, Streicher claimed that 'Nicotine is the greatest poison of our nation ... Jews taught the Germans to smoke in order to destroy the German nation and to make money'. Such remarks were so obviously tainted by anti-Semitism that any underlying medical rationale was lost.[77] At the same time, the German anti-smoking drive was seen to crack down on reasonable enjoyment - *Genußmittel* was, for example, translated as 'enjoyment poisons'.[78] The British medical press also reported on German research on smoking and health, but stopped short of offering any judgement or recommendations based on this.[79] The consensus remained among the medical profession that moderate smoking was not harmful and that the smoker, assumed to be male, was well able to make up his own mind how to proceed in the face of medical disquiet.[80] The social imperative to smoke also remained strong: correspondence in the *British Medical Journal* attests to doctors' desire to advise their patients without impinging on their social inclination to smoke.[81] So, while there was an awareness of German anti-smoking campaigns in Britain and some anti-smoking sentiment in Britain itself, the dominant discourse was of acceptance and rationalization of the risks, in a way which echoed classic liberal discourse.

Conclusion

The common thread which runs through discourses about smoking in both countries is the positioning of smoking within the masculine sphere and discourses of rational behaviour and moderation during the nineteenth century. By the early twentieth century, the influence of eugenics had become apparent, re-casting male privilege into racial terms: female and juvenile smoking was portrayed as harmful to the future of the race. In Germany, such discourses fed into and were augmented by the widening acceptance of racial hygiene and increasing trust in scientific and medical expertise which posited the dangers of smoking. The healthy citizen was one who, conscious of his duty to state, nation and race, abstained from smoking. In Britain, in contrast, eugenic discourses did not overtake the prevailing classic liberal doctrine of individual freedom and personal choice in relation to tobacco use, despite some awareness of the health risks of smoking. By the late 1930s, moreover, German anti-smoking campaigns had become discredited because of their association with the more extreme manifestations of racial hygiene. Where anti-smoking sentiment was visible in Britain, it was in the context of smoke free public space – an argument which pitted the rights of the citizen to clean air against the freedom of his fellow citizens to smoke.

Nonetheless, in both countries during the first half of the twentieth century, smoking was also constructed not just as an individual choice, but as an action which fed into prevailing, if opposing, discourses of nationalism and what created a good citizen. The tobacco industry sought to capitalize on nationalistic discourses in both countries, by and large successfully. It was only once such nationalistic discourses were superseded by the international claims and, indeed, pressures of the 'new public health' that domestic economic and political imperatives could be more effectively countered.

7 MENTAL HEALTH AND CIVIC VIRTUE: PSYCHIATRY, SELF-DEVELOPMENT AND CITIZENSHIP IN THE NETHERLANDS, 1870–2005

Harry Oosterhuis

As a product of nineteenth-century bourgeois society, psychiatry developed in a dynamic between social-political integration and exclusion. Into the twentieth century, institutional psychiatry fulfilled two functions: a medical one (care and cure), which gave priority to the interests of patients and a social-political one (segregation), which was geared towards freeing society of the nuisance and danger associated with the insane. Of these two, the most prominent function varied depending on a given country's political constellation. From around 1840 various Western European countries adopted legal regulations for the institutionalization of the insane. Within the margins of the constitutional state, these regulations served to protect citizens against random deprivation of freedom and to allow for effective admission procedures to ensure public order as well as medical treatment for mental patients. The hospitalized insane fell under special jurisdiction and state supervision, which implied a suspension of their civic rights. The liberal contract society assumed autonomous individuals who were capable of serving their own rights and interests while respecting those of others. Liberalism linked citizenship to rationality, autonomy and responsibility, which were precisely the qualities mental patients had to do without. Mental incapacity counted in fact as the opposite of citizenship as it had been articulated on the basis of the ideals of freedom and equality since the American and French Revolutions.

The relationship between institutional psychiatry and liberal-democratic citizenship was 'negative' or 'exclusive' in the sense that hospitalization in an asylum generally required legal certification and therefore the loss of basic civil rights. In the course of the twentieth century, however, a more 'positive' or 'inclusive' connection between psychiatry and citizenship was established in two ways. Firstly, the last three decades of the last century saw a growing recognition of the civil rights of the mentally ill, reflecting a shift from values associated with maintaining law and order to values associated with mental patients' autonomy and consent. Secondly, from the early twentieth century on, in psychiatry as well as in the broader field of mental health care, psychological definitions of citizenship were advanced. Expressing views about the position of individuals in modern society and their possibilities for self-development, psychiatrists and other mental health workers connected mental health to ideals of democratic citizenship. Thus, they were clearly involved in the liberal-democratic project of promoting not only productive, responsible and adaptive citizens, but also autonomous, self-conscious and emancipated individuals.

This chapter focuses on the development of mental health care in the Netherlands from the late nineteenth to the early twenty-first century in order to explore its relation to socio-political modernization in general and changing meanings of citizenship in particular. Citizenship took on a broad meaning, not just in terms of political rights and duties, but also in the context of material, social, psychological and moral conditions that individuals should meet in order to develop themselves and be able to act according to those rights and duties in a responsible way. On the basis of the four different ideals of self-development that I identify, my account is divided into four periods: 1870–1945 (self-development through social adaptation); 1945–65 (guided self-development); 1965–85 (spontaneous self-development); and 1985–2005 (autonomous self-development).[1] In the last section I will elaborate several general characteristics of Dutch mental health care in its socio-political context.

Self-Development through Social Adaptation, 1870–1945

In 1848 the liberal constitutional state was established in the Netherlands. With the granting of fundamental liberty rights all Dutch citizens became equal citizens before the law. Voting rights, however, were limited to the upper classes whose members met the liberal criteria for active citizenship: economic independence, paying taxes on property and education. The masses were excluded from political participation. In the last decades of the nineteenth century, however, the exclusive political citizenship of the liberal bourgeoisie increasingly came under pressure. In part as a consequence of industrialization, growing geographical and social mobility and the emergence of mass politics and a civil society, disadvantaged groups like the working class, women and religious groups that had been excluded, began to make themselves heard. Reform-minded liberals became convinced of the need to integrate these groups into the political nation and to solve the 'social issue' by extending the role of the state in society. If classic liberalism started from the self-reliance and diligence of individuals while seeking to minimize state intervention, social-liberals acknowledged that the individual opportunities for self-development depended not only on talents and will power, but also on changing economic and social circumstances and the general risks of life. Collective social insurance was considered necessary to protect the socially weak from disaster and to create such conditions that those lagging behind might also improve their social position, which in turn would render them eligible for full citizenship.[2] The process of political democratization, which in 1919 led to universal suffrage, was gradual. The striving for emancipation of disadvantaged groups was mainly geared towards social integration on the basis of middle-class values, which now were less tied to social position and took on a more general significance as civic virtues that applied to all members of society. Self-control, a sense of order and duty, social responsibility, a proper balance between individual independence and community spirit, an industrious and productive existence and family values acted as cornerstones of the democratized middle-class ideal of citizenship.[3]

The emergence of mass society caused mounting concerns among the upper and middle classes regarding the dominance of irrational emotions and drives, which would lead to unruliness and social disintegration. Divergent behaviours, ranging from drinking, gambling and other forms of 'low entertainment' to sexual licentiousness, child abandonment and crime, became the target of interference and intervention by both voluntary organizations and the state. The question behind this was whether all individuals had the necessary rational and moral qualities to meet the demands of modern society and to act as responsible citizens. What mattered was not just the resolution of social wrongs and misfortunes like poverty, illness, backwardness and exploitation; it was equally important to achieve a productive and virtuous life for everybody. As society's democratization progressed, it was deemed all the more essential to elevate the lower orders morally and to inculcate in them a civil sense of responsibility and decency. In pleas for a national-level education of the people, 'character formation' was central. Apart from politicians, social reformers and moral entrepreneurs, the proponents of this social-moral activism were found especially among the professional groups that were gaining influence and self-awareness, such as physicians, teachers, youth leaders, social workers and, later, mental health workers.[4]

It was against the backdrop of social-political modernization that from the late nineteenth century asylum-doctors began to break the isolation of their professional domain and seek to expand it. The leading members of the Dutch Society of Psychiatry, founded in 1871, were liberal and positivist-minded physicians who considered science and social conscience as crucial for progress. Despite their focus on scientific medicine, they not only pointed to the biological causes of insanity and nervous disorders. They also blamed the spread of mental disorders on certain harmful behaviours and social-cultural influences, such as pauperism, poor hygiene, immorality, alcoholism, bad upbringing and the hectic pace of urban life. New clinical entities such as neurasthenia, moral insanity and criminal psychopathy and the assumed danger of degeneration provided psychiatrists with arguments to expand their intervention domain from asylums to society at large. They thus aligned themselves with social hygiene, in which the effort to prevent people from falling ill through reform of their living conditions and way of life was centre-stage. To counter the debasing influences of modern society that were considered to undermine people's nerves and mental well-being, psychiatrists pointed to the relevance of self-control, will power and a sense of discipline.[5]

Between the First World War and the early 1940s, the groundwork was laid for the psycho-hygienic movement and a national network of outpatient mental health care provisions, which developed independently of the mental institutions and which were staffed by psychiatrists as well as other physicians, teachers, psychologists, lawyers, social workers and clergymen. The professional domain claimed by these psycho-hygienists was wide: it stretched from family-life, sexuality and education to work and leisure, alcoholism, crime and the social rehabilitation of mentally ill, mentally disabled and psychopathic individuals. The psycho-hygienic ideal materialized in a growing number of counselling centres for alcoholics, pre- and aftercare services for the mentally ill and retarded, child guidance clinics, centres for marriage and family problems and institutes for psychotherapy. In these facilities psycho-hygienists mainly adopted social, moral-didactic, pastoral and psycho-dynamic approaches rather than biomedical or eugenic ones.[6]

The psycho-hygienic movement was rooted in a more broadly shared cultural pessimism about the harmful effects of the rapid changes in society, as well as in the optimistic belief in the potential of scientific expertise to solve those problems. They viewed modernization, marked by fragmentation and disorientation, as the major cause of the increase in mental and nervous problems. A rising number of people would have trouble keeping up with the complexity and fast-paced lifestyle of industrialized and urbanized society. This trend could be contained, psycho-hygienists argued, by taking preventive measures, such as treatment of the early stages of mental and behavioural problems so as to prevent them from becoming worse. Fearing cultural decay and social disintegration, they repeatedly stressed the significance of spiritual values and a sense of community.[7] The psycho-hygienic doctrine basically fitted in with efforts to 'civilize' the people. In the nineteenth century, these activities had been promoted by the liberal bourgeoisie, but from the turn of the century they became entangled with confessional as well as socialist politics aimed at furthering the emancipation and national integration of their constituencies. This effort indeed suggested an optimistic belief in the perfectibility of mankind, even though such vision was frequently couched in a more or less conceited moral-didactic paternalism. With their particular understanding of public mental health, psycho-hygienists closely aligned themselves with the paradigm of an orderly mass society that was based on the unconditional adaptation of the individual to middle-class norms and values. In their view, responsible citizenship required the development of 'character': self-control, will-power, social adaptation and community spirit.[8]

Guided Self-Development, 1945–65

In the 1940s and 1950s, Dutch outpatient mental health care facilities expanded rapidly. Their growth was strongly advanced by worries about social disruption in the wake of the German occupation and liberation by the allied forces. Because the war and Nazism epitomized the cultural pessimism of the psycho-hygienists, in the post-war years their doctrine won more support among politicians and other influential groups. Various forms of misconduct and presumed lack of ethical standards – idleness, juvenile mischief, lack of respect for authority, but also family disruption, growing divorce rates and sexual license – were considered serious threats both to the moral fibre of the nation and public mental health. The leitmotiv of this widespread anxiety was the observation that uncontrollable urges had gained the upper hand. It was widely felt that in order to rebuild the devastated country in unity and to ward off the new threat of communism, the people's moral resilience should be strengthened. Again, the insistence on self-discipline served to underline the importance of responsible citizenship in a democratic mass society as well as in the emerging welfare state.[9] In their striving for a mental recovery of the Dutch people, psycho-hygienists displayed a great sense of mission. Through the use of medical-biological metaphors – society viewed as body, the family as vital organ, the individual as cell, social wrongs as pathologies and problem groups as nuclei – social and moral problems were framed as public mental health issues. The notion of mental health was turned into a comprehensive concept that was tied to the prevention of war and totalitarianism and the realization of a better world.

The development of mental health care was strongly influenced by the specific ways in which the experts in this field interpreted social transformations. When the moral panic about the disruptive effects of the war faded around 1950, they began to focus in particular on the potentially harmful influences of ongoing modernization. The 1950s brought a new and vigorous economic dynamic, based on great confidence in science and technology. Large-scale urbanization, industrialization and infrastructural innovation had far-reaching effects on people's social relationships and everyday life. Spatial and social mobility rose sharply, allowing more individuals to evade the paternalism and social control of small communities, the church and their families. A steadily increasing prosperity provided more material security, and class differences and other hierarchical relationships gradually lost their edge. Increasingly, the new dynamic of everyday life was at odds with the still prevailing bourgeois and Christian norms and values with their clearly defined dos and don'ts.[10]

In the views that psycho-hygienists articulated about these developments, cultural pessimism reverberated. Its essence seemed basically unchanged: the mental and moral development of man was out of step with the ongoing economic and technological progress.[11] Like other intellectuals, they argued that modernization caused society to be dominated by instrumental rationality and materialism, which jeopardized moral and spiritual values. Their critique focused on the so-called mass-man, the embodiment of all evils that accompanied modernity. He was lonely and uprooted, had no fixed norms and values and no longer felt any ties to religion, tradition or community. He let his life be dictated by his unconscious drives and emotions and showed no regard whatsoever for moral authority. His inner emptiness was shown by his flight into material consumption, popular entertainment and sexual gratification. This rudderless man, critics argued, undermined social solidarity and democratic citizenship. They argued in favour of social planning and a normative education of the people, so as to prevent democratic mass society from degenerating into either anarchy or dictatorship. Although rationalization was regarded as one of the main causes of the cultural crisis, at the same time there was great confidence in the possibility of reforming society with the help of the social and human sciences. That is why sociologists as well as psycho-hygienists believed they had a major task to fulfil.[12]

Initially, mental health workers stressed the need for a fixed collective morality and the social adaptation of the individual and they looked for solutions in moral-pedagogical measures.[13] In the 1950s, however, their defensive stance towards modernization made way for a more accommodating approach. More and more they acknowledged that restrictions and coercion only affected the outer behaviour of people while leaving their inner self untouched. What in the late 1940s was still seen as lack of moral strength, in the 1950s was increasingly explained in psychological and relational terms. Personality flaws, developmental disorders and unconscious conflicts, caused by defective education and poorly functioning families, it was now believed, constituted the underlying causes of deprivation and misbehaviour. The older moral-didactic discourse about the need to develop 'character' was beginning to give way to a psychological argument around the development of 'personality'.

The belief that social-economic progress was inevitable, brought about a new perspective on the task of mental health professionals. The results of preventive psychiatric treatment of allied soldiers during the war, the psycho-dynamic model and new (American) psychosocial methods such as social case-work and counselling, raised expectations about the potential of psychiatry and the behavioural sciences to shape people's mental make-up. Inspired by the World Federation of Mental Health, psychiatrists underlined not only that prevention and treatment of mental disorders mattered, but also that it was crucial to improve mental health in general and thus ensure maximal opportunities for all citizens to develop themselves in a wholesome way. Apart from offering support to those who struggled to keep pace with modernization, it was argued that mental health workers should also enhance the mental attitude and abilities individuals needed to function properly in a changing society. Thus the pursuit of a more dynamic and flexible adaptation took the place of frantic attempts at restoring morality and community spirit. It was now believed that new social conditions required a redirection of norms and values and that individuals should be granted more scope for self-development.

Leading psycho-hygienists began to present themselves as guides who prepared people for the dynamism of modern life by spear-heading the effort to change people's mentality. Inspired by phenomenological psychology and personalism, which stressed personality formation, they now identified 'maturity', 'inner freedom' and 'self-responsible self-determination' as basic elements of mental health. Such mental qualities were the opposite of impulsive behaviour; they entailed inner regulation, which would guarantee that people did not need external pressures to lead a responsible life. It became the individual's task to pursue optimal self-development and grow into a 'personality'. The mentally healthy were not those who uncritically subjected themselves to rules, but those who achieved a certain measure of inner autonomy in relation to the outside world and at the same time thoughtfully adapted to social modernization.[14] If individuals were to be able to decide on their own how to shape their lives, scrupulous self-examination was needed to ensure that their intentions were conscientious and based on good grounds. People were assumed to follow their own conviction, but they were also considered to do so in line with social expectations involving a morally responsible mode of life, as articulated by mental health workers and other expert leaders. Individuals could only develop their personality in a meaningful way if they were able to internalize social norms and values in an autonomous self. By fostering constant reflection on individual conduct and motivation, mental health care would reinforce the conditions for civil and political involvement and thus for maintaining and deepening democracy.[15]

The ideal of citizenship promoted in the 1950s and early 1960s can be characterized as 'guided self-development'. It was geared towards social-economic modernization, which required more individuality, flexibility and mobility. Self-identity used to be a product of given and more or less stable social categories, such as class, religion and family background, but it increasingly became a product of personal qualities and preferences. This individualization was understood as an inescapable effect of modernity, but in an effort to avoid social disintegration, psycho-hygienists considered it essential to offer guidance and add normative standards, as a counterbalance to the individual's growing freedom.

Spontaneous Self-Development, 1965–85

Psycho-hygienists believed in controlled modernization and guided self-development under the supervision of a morally inspired and professionally trained elite. Their patronising approach was characteristic of the post-war period of reconstruction, but from the mid-1960s it came under attack. In the ensuing decade the Netherlands changed from a rather conservative and Christian nation into one of the most liberal and permissive countries in the Western world.[16] Secularization as well as growing prosperity and the expanding welfare state caused more and more people to break away from established traditions and hierarchical relationships so as to enhance their independence and individuality. Various protest movements loudly voiced their concern for democratization, liberation and self-determination. The control of emotions and the individual's adaptation to society were no longer considered signs of social responsibility, but as the repression of the authentic self.

The ideal of spontaneous self-realization paved the way for emotional self-expression and assertive individualism, which together with the democratization movement rocked the foundations of Dutch society and its mental health care system as well. If individuals had previously been expected to comply with the social order, now society itself had to change to facilitate optimal self-actualization and fulfilment of democratic citizenship. The 1848 constitution had provided the Dutch people with basic civil rights, the introduction of universal suffrage in 1919 had made them into citizens in the political sense and the post-war welfare state had guaranteed their material security. Now, some psycho-hygienists argued, the time was ripe for taking the next step in this continuing process of emancipation: the settling of immaterial needs in order to advance personal well-being for everybody.[17]

Embracing some of the basic tenets of the protest movements and anti-psychiatry, mental health workers increasingly voiced self-criticism. A growing number of them were trained in the behavioural and social sciences and they demanded attention to the social causes of mental distress. The therapeutic treatment of individuals with the aim of adapting them to society became subject to debate. Instead, people needed to be liberated from the coercive 'social structures' that restricted their spontaneous self-development. Welfare work and political activism seemed more helpful to realize this objective than psychiatry and mental health care. However, whereas institutional and medical psychiatry were forced on to the defensive, in the 1970s the psychosocial and especially psychotherapeutic services increased more than ever in size and prestige. The very dissatisfaction with medical psychiatry prompted new pleas for alternative and better mental health care, like therapeutic communities and more psychosocial outpatient facilities.[18] Their growth was facilitated by the welfare state: more and more collective social funds guaranteed broad access to mental health care. The prevailing trend between 1965 and 1985 was a substantial increase in and scaling-up of services with steadily growing numbers of clients. In the early 1980s, the various outpatient facilities merged into Regional Institutes for Ambulatory Mental Health Care, which were aimed at a broad spectrum of psychosocial problems and psychiatric disorders.

The 1970s were the heyday of psychotherapy, which, psychiatrists apart, was practised increasingly by psychologists and social workers in a growing number of public psychotherapeutic institutes. Although critical mental health care workers blamed social evils for psychological problems, psychotherapy focused on the inner self. A growing number of people began to seek psychotherapeutic help for all sorts of discomforts or personality flaws that bothered them and that previously were not regarded as mental problems. Both therapists and clients strongly believed that psychotherapy would liberate individuals from inhibitions and limitations, advance their 'personal growth' and improve the quality of their lives.[19]

While engaging in heated debates on the political implications of their practice, mental health experts widened their professional domain to include welfare work, a sector that experienced enormous growth in the 1970s. Together with social workers, they undertook the task of encouraging clients to become aware of their true needs and selves. As one psychiatrist explained, personal unhappiness should not be viewed as an individual fate, but as a social evil that could be remedied.[20] As some experts emphasized, countering prejudice and advancing tolerance was part of the broader effort to improve the quality of social relations and to 'democratize happiness'.[21] Some psychiatrists and other psycho-hygienic experts put controversial issues on the social agenda and played a crucial role in public debates. Already in the 1950s and early 1960s, some leading psycho-hygienists contributed significantly to changing the moral climate in the areas of family, marriage and sexuality. In the 1960s and 1970s, psychiatrists also stood up for the recognition of the mental suffering of war victims and other traumatized people, the self-determination of patients and a de-penalization of euthanasia, abortion and drugs.[22] Mental health experts revealed themselves as inspired advocates of personal liberation in many sensitive areas. In this way, they contributed to the implementation of rather liberal practices, certainly from an international perspective. In so doing they drew on the 1960s culture of liberation and democratization, but they also followed in the footsteps of the reform-minded psycho-hygienists from the 1950s. By raising issues that had earlier been largely avoided, they sought to break taboos and put an end to hypocrisy, thus paving the way for more openness, understanding and tolerance. To achieve this, so they explained, a sense of responsibility and deliberation, conscientious positioning, a sincere and open-minded exchange of arguments and a willingness by people to respect each other was required. As psychiatrist R. H. van den Hoofdakker wrote: 'in a world of emancipated and independent human beings' there was only one way to overcome outmoded ideas and habits and that was 'talking, talking, talking'.[23] Rules and laws should not be rigidly applied, but discussed and sensibly interpreted. Emphasizing the 'debatability' of an issue – which in the Netherlands became a major norm serving as the basis for policies of channelled toleration – was essentially the opposite of being noncommittal as well as outright permissive. Making sensitive issues debatable was inextricably bound up with the belief in a fully democratized society. Only self-reflective and socially involved citizens empathized with others, did not shy away from unpleasant truths, regulated their emotions and were capable of making rational considerations and – through negotiation and mutual understanding – arriving at balanced decisions. From a psychological and ethical perspective, this psycho-hygienic ideal of citizenship made great demands on people's competence.

Autonomous Self-Development, 1985–2005

Until the late 1970s, there was great faith in social engineering as a way to change society in directions that would allow individuals to liberate themselves. However, the practice of social planning, which was self-evident during the post-war era of reconstruction as well as in the social-democratic reform policies of the 1970s, conflicted with society's increasing individualization. The socially critical dimension of spontaneous self-development eroded when the pursuit of social reform was increasingly replaced by the values of the 'me-generation', stressing an inner-directed, independent self. At the same time, the welfare state was under attack, mainly because its costs had risen tremendously, but also because critics argued that collective services nullified people's sense of responsibility and self-reliance. Around 1980, welfare work in particular was singled out as a target: rather than enlarging people's self-autonomy, it would make them dependent.[24] The generous public funding of psychotherapy was also criticized: psychotherapists were accused of making good money by serving a privileged clientele, while neglecting psychiatric patients with serious disorders.

As a consequence of neoliberal politics of deregulation and privatization, the emphasis shifted from public welfare to the self-reliance of citizens in the community and in the market. Autonomous self-development of independent individuals on the basis of their talents and efforts, with a minimum of interference from government or welfare agencies, came to be the new standard of good citizenship. However, the crisis of the welfare state, which led to a downsizing of social work, hardly affected mental health care; on the contrary, it saw more expansion in subsequent years, although its focus changed. Further growth of the outpatient sector in particular was stimulated by the effort to develop community care for psychiatric patients, which became a governmental priority. Moreover, efficiency, rationalization, standardization and a partial re-medicalization of psychiatry as well as market incentives and account of costs and benefits took the place of the ideals of the 1960s and 1970s.

The government and some psychiatrists repeatedly argued that the main outpatient facilities, the Regional Institutes for Ambulatory Mental Health Care, were geared one-sidedly to clients with minor psychological afflictions, which would cause a boundless increase in the demand for mental health care. Instead, the treatment and care of acute and chronic psychiatric patients should become a priority, also to keep the number of admissions to mental hospitals as low as possible. Only patients who were unable to get by in society without hurting either others or themselves were considered to be eligible for hospitalization. Others should be cared for in halfway and outpatient facilities so as to allow them to function as much as possible as regular members of society. In the late 1990s, to improve the co-operation between psychiatric hospitals and the out-patient services, the government pressured them to merge in comprehensive mental health facilities that offered intramural as well as extramural care. All of this marked a break with the historical constellation of mental health care, which since the 1930s had been divided between clinical psychiatry for serious mental disorders and a psychosocially oriented outpatient sector for a wide spec-trum of milder problems.

The 'socialization' of mental health care, as this policy was termed, echoed some of the democratic ideals of the 1960s and 1970s, such as the need to coun-ter the isolation of psychiatric patients, improve their self-autonomy and respect their civil rights. The paternalistic for-your-own-good criterion in the Insanity Act of 1884, which until then had justified involuntary institutionalization, was replaced by a new mental health law in 1994. It formulated strict criteria for forced hospitalization against the will of patients, namely when they pose a danger to themselves or to others. This law, which restricted the possibility of certification and loss of civil rights of the mentally ill, as well as some other new laws on patient's rights, sealed the increased recognition of the individual integrity and responsibility of the mentally ill. They regained, so to speak, their status as citizens, an aim that since the 1970s had been championed by the criti-cal patient's movement.

One of the basic motivations for the policy of socialization was that although psychiatric patients were limited in their autonomy and judgement, they should not be excluded in advance from either their rights or their duties as citizens. The measure by which they would be able to realize themselves as more or less inde-pendent citizens, partly relied on a mental health care system that guaranteed the mentally ill were not isolated from the rest of society. In practice, however, the citizenship of psychiatric patients caused problems all the time and was con-tested in the 1990s. Critics pointed out that the emphasis on empowerment entirely ignored what in effect constituted the essence of mental illness: the lim-ited power to self-determination and the loss of the basic and taken-for-granted patterns of social interaction. Fragile psychiatric patients were in need of secu-rity, protection and a simple and quiet life shielded from the dynamic of society. As long as the defining qualities of citizenship were agency and active social par-ticipation (especially by having regular work), the mentally ill and handicapped were at best consigned to the category of marginal citizens.[25]

Also, the positive evaluation of self-determination was questioned because it allowed the mentally ill with serious behavioural problems to refuse psychiatric treatment – even if they were unable to take care of themselves, caused social trouble, or were aggressive. From this perspective socialization soon ran up against its limits. The striving for social integration and employment rehabilitation of psychiatric patients was complicated under increasing pressure on social cohesion in (sub)urban neighbourhoods and the ever greater demands of the labour market in terms of proper training, social skills, performance and flexibility, which many patients were unable to meet. It also became clear that from the late 1980s the tolerance of the Dutch population towards disturbing conduct of mental patients decreased as direct confrontation with them in everyday life increased.[26]

The downside of the policy of socialization was the social isolation of some patients, their abandonment and poverty, and also the nuisance caused, for instance, by the homeless, mentally ill and alcohol or drug addicts.[27] Pleas for more coercion in social-psychiatric care as well as new experiments in outreach care for unwilling and unreachable mental patients, put ideals of emancipation and self-determination into perspective. Basically, these lacked any relevance to those suffering from serious disorders, who were incapable of living on their own, who could not assert their needs and who lacked the capacity of self-reflection as to their abilities and limitations. For these patients, social reintegration was no real option: they were living proof that mental illness and full citizenship were hard to reconcile.

The optimism that since the 1950s had prevailed in the psycho-hygienic outpatient services regarding the possibility of stimulating individuals in terms of their self-development, had in part been facilitated precisely because there was a strong tendency to keep patients with serious psychiatric disorders out of these facilities. Emphasizing their identity in terms of welfare, the psychotherapeutic institutes, centres for family and marriage problems and child guidance clinics, catered to a clientele with a variety of psychosocial and existential problems and focused on the improvement of their social functioning and assertiveness. A socio-psychological perspective and various talking-cures had set the tone in these facilities. Clients were expected to have some capacity for introspection, verbal ability, initiative and willingness to change and this automatically excluded the mentally ill.

However, when in the 1990s, in the Regional Institutes for Ambulatory Mental Health Care, social psychiatry was prioritized and ever more of these services merged with psychiatric hospitals, the emphasis shifted to people with serious and incurable mental disorders and the ideal of personal change and emancipation was replaced by the more modest objective of limiting or alleviating mental suffering and control its symptoms as much as possible. Notwithstanding the increasing use of psycho-pharmaceuticals, various social, psycho- and behavioural therapies remained in use in mental health facilities, but they were less directed at personal growth than at the acquisition of social and practical skills to cope with life, for better or worse.

Yet in another way the 1960s and 1970s ideology of individual liberation and emancipation was called into question. Under the influence of ever-expanding mental health care consumption and of epidemiological research showing a high frequency of psychic disorders among the population, the social dimension of mental disorders again attracted attention in the 1990s.[28] Studies were made of the causes of the assumed rise in the number of mental problems and the measures needed.[29] The message of the subsequent reports and policy recommendations was ambiguous. On the one hand, the experts explained that the rising demand for professional care was partly a result of the widened care supply, greater public familiarity with it, a declining tolerance regarding all sorts of inconvenience in life and an increased trust in the possibility of treating complaints professionally. On the other hand, the tone of these reports betrayed the resurfacing of cultural pessimism. They pointed to an array of social developments likely to trigger psychic problems: the fast pace and intensity of social change; individualization; the pressure of achievement-oriented society; unemployment; the deprivation among ethnic minorities; and the diminishing sense of social security and safety. There was much emphasis in particular on the assumed loss of shared norms and values. One of the reports suggested that precisely in the densely populated and urbanized Netherlands individual freedom and tolerance could not flourish without a high degree of social cohesion. Inasmuch as policy advisors issued proposals for boosting public mental health, they tended to revert to remedies from the past, such as a strengthening of civil society and collective values and norms and more robust government policies that balanced individual freedom with limits and rules.[30] Evidently, in mental health care the optimistic view of society, in which self-responsible citizens tried to solve problems together in mutual interaction, had been replaced by concern about the loss of community spirit and public morality.

The citizenship ideal that had been promoted in mental health care since the 1960s was called into question more broadly. In the 1990s, politicians and intellectuals – not only Christian-democrats and conservative liberals, but also social-democrats – took stock of the legacy of the 1960s and 1970s and concluded that it was largely a negative one. The anti-authoritarian celebration of individual liberation, they argued, had degenerated into egoism, a lack of self-restraint, an erosion of social responsibility and an exaggerated assertiveness that was exclusively based on rights rather than duties. The welfare state had resulted in calculating behaviour and improper use of benefits. These developments had to be countered by a downsizing of social security arrangements, moral regeneration and the restoration and revitalizing of a sense of civic virtue.[31] The taboo on coercion and duties began to recede, for instance regarding efforts aimed at the reactivation of the poorly educated unemployed as well as at the integration of migrants. At the start of the twenty-first century the concern for the weakening of social cohesion and the degradation of the public domain mingled with fear for the loss of national identity through rising ethnic diversity, continuing European integration and globalization.

Discussion: Democratic Citizenship and Psychological Self-Development

The link between the democratization and psychologization of citizenship, illustrated here by following the development of mental health care in the Netherlands, is part of a more general historical process in the Western world. In traditional systems of political domination, which subjected people by coercion and force, whether they accepted it or not, their inner selves were generally irrelevant. The need to shape individuals and make them internalize certain values and behaviour-patterns became greater the more a society was democratized. If in the nineteenth century citizens were largely judged on external factors (such as status, sex, economic independence and tax liability), in the twentieth century, when adult suffrage was established and the welfare state softened the contradiction between formal political rights and social-economic inequality, the formation of a proper mentality gained prominence. Democratic citizenship presupposes a sense of public commitment on the basis of individual autonomy, self-determination and self-direction; citizenship can hardly be reconciled with subordination and dependence. It is in democratic societies, in which the social order is basically founded on the consent of individual citizens rather than external constraint, that the inner motivation of the citizen is considered of crucial importance. A democratic social order can only be maintained if individuals are capable of using their basic liberties in a responsible way. Ironically, the pursuit of individual self-determination goes hand in hand with gentle but persistent pressure on people to open their inner selves for scrutiny by others and to account for their urges and motivations, for example to mental health experts.

Against this backdrop, the Dutch developments are hardly unique. In Britain also, for example, from the 1920s on, mental health provided a paradigm to articulate in psychological terms a secular ideal for self-development as the basis for responsible democratic citizenship. In the United States the mental hygiene movement linked together the ills of modern society and the malaise of individuals, and mental health experts used theories of personality development to show how they could contribute to the formation of robust and self-reliant democratic subjects. In Germany it was especially at the time of the striving for fundamental reforms in psychiatry in the 1960s and 1970s, when the Nazi past was critically used as a spectre, that mental health care acquired a strong political dimension. Against the complicity of psychiatry in the atrocities of the Third Reich, a democratic counter vision of mental health care emerged, based on a conception of citizenship that stressed political awareness, independence of mind and the social rights of the infirm and indigent.[32]

What was often missing in these countries, however, was an extensive network of public outpatient facilities to underpin the rhetoric about mental health and citizenship with concrete care-providing practices. In the Netherlands, models of psychological self-development were not mere abstract theories: in the practice of outpatient mental health care these ideals materialized. From the 1950s on, in various facilities clients were encouraged so be self-reflective about their conduct and motivations, initially in private life, but also with respect to their attitude in the public domain.[33] The psycho-hygienic movement and the outpatient services were more enduring, more broadly distributed and more generously funded in the Netherlands than in Britain, Germany or the United States.

Another striking element of the Dutch outpatient sector was its broad orientation. It not only comprised social psychiatry in the sense of outpatient care for the mentally ill, but already from the 1930s and 1940s on it also included various counselling centres for problem children, marriage and family related issues, psychotherapy and alcohol and drug addiction. This broad orientation is in part accounted for by the fairly early differentiation between institutional psychiatry and the outpatient sector as well as a strong psychosocial (rather than biomedical) focus of the extramural facilities. In other European countries the institutional and public mental health sectors were more exclusively geared towards psychiatric patients, while there was also a closer link with the domain of (poli)clinical psychiatry.[34]

In the twentieth century, the mental hygiene movement and the outpatient sector successfully established themselves in the Netherlands. The notion of mental health, which heaped together a host of problems in and between people, caught on and it linked various social domains and appealed to various groups. The notion of health care evoked associations with medicine and hygiene, while 'mental' – the Dutch *geestelijk* also means 'spiritual' – referred to psychic features as well as religious, moral and cultural values. Thus it was possible to establish an explicit connection with the strong charitable tradition in the Netherlands and the bourgeois civilization offensive, which in the form of a moral-didactic ethos was adopted by both confessionals and socialists. The ideal of mental health tied in with the need to articulate public morals and the belief in the perfectibility of society.

The modernization of Dutch society and the evolving concepts of democratic citizenship provided a socio-political context for the pursuit of mental health, whereby cultural pessimism and an optimistic belief in society's progress balanced each other. In this light, it is possible to identify a turning point in the mid-1950s. In this decade the defensive response to modernization was exchanged for a much more accommodating stance. In reflection on citizenship there was a shift from unconditional adaptation to established values and norms ('character') to individual self-development ('personality'). People's personal experience and their inner motivations came to be centre-stage and therapeutic treatment and social integration were definitively prioritized over coercion and exclusion. In the years between 1950 and 1965, by building on the ideal of guided self-development, mental health care hooked up with social-economic modernization: individuals had to shape their personality, develop their autonomy, be open for renewal and, in a responsible way, achieve self-realization. In the late 1960s and the 1970s, mental health workers embraced spontaneous self-development as a core value, thus legitimizing the need for personal emancipation. Subsequently, in the neoliberal 1980s and 1990s, they viewed their clients as autonomous and self-responsible citizens, whose freedom to make choices as members of a pluralist market society was highlighted. At the close of the twentieth century, however, cultural pessimism recurred with regard to the self-determination and autonomy of some groups, such as the mentally ill.

The national government generally kept a low profile regarding the organization and implementation of mental health care and the articulation of civic virtues. At least until the late 1960s, when it began to play a more active role, the state mainly left these issues to voluntary organizations or local government. Models for self-development and citizenship were hardly imposed from above by the state, but they were developed and enunciated by leading groups in civil society itself. Mental health care played a major part in the articulation of the psychic dimension of personal as well as public life, but the spread of a psychological *habitus* among the Dutch population also took place as an effect of more general social developments. Psychologization, a change of mentality characterized by a combination of growing individualization and internalization, was connected with the democratization of social relationships, changed manners and authority structures, the shift from social coercion to self-control and the increasingly subjective way of fashioning personal identity. People's conduct was increasingly seen as a reflection of personal wishes, motives and feelings.[35] It was more and more common for people to talk about themselves or others in psychological terms and to refer to mood or feeling as a way to legitimate their behaviour.

In the Netherlands, which used to be essentially conservative and Christian, the cultural revolution of the 1960s was more sweeping than in other countries because it coincided with rapid secularization. In few countries was control and coercion from above banned so comprehensively as in the Netherlands.[36] The ensuing moral or spiritual vacuum was partially filled by a psychological ethos; from the 1960s on mental health care, psychotherapy in particular, expanded at an unprecedented rate. The strongly developed democratization of public and everyday life replaced hierarchy and social coercion with individual emancipation and informal manners. To find the proper balance between assertiveness and compliance, people needed self-knowledge, subtle social skills, empathy and an inner, self-directed regulation of emotions and actions. What mattered in a democratized and information-ridden new social dynamic, in which formal rules were replaced by negotiation and self-regulation, was a strongly developed mental resilience and understanding of the drives and motivations of others. Thus, the interactions between people and the ways in which they evaluated each other became determined more and more by psychological insight. Tensions and conflicts between people had concrete ramifications for their inner life, on account of which mental pressures could mount and the chances of their suffering from serious doubts, fears and uncertainties increased.

With their emphasis on self-reflection and raising sensitive issues, mental health experts articulated new values and offered a clear alternative to the outdated morality of dos and don'ts. Talking was their preferred strategy for solving problems, which not only linked them with the Dutch culture of negotiation and consensus, but also with the practice of everyday life of many people. From the 1930s the largest segment of the working population has been active in the services sector. It is a sector in which social interaction and communications have increasingly grown central.[37] In the densely populated and highly urbanized Netherlands, therefore, proper social functioning depended much on personality traits associated with verbal and communicative skills and subtle emotion-regulation. Finally, the strong inclination towards psychologization is also tied to the specific ways in which, in the Dutch culture of consensus, social and ethical issues are addressed by experts. Their expertise is frequently called upon because their supposedly objective professional stance neutralizes social conflicts concerning sensitive issues. In the articulation of policies on euthanasia, sexuality, birth-control, abortion and drugs, for example, experts such as physicians, psychiatrists, psychologists and social workers had a large say. They generally contributed to formulating practical solutions that are both pragmatic and well-considered and that focus on individual conditions and motivations.

In the last two decades, however, confidence in the possibility of motivating individuals through considerate, 'soft' psychosocial support towards self-guidance and socializing them in such way that as full citizens they automatically integrate in an egalitarian and democratic society, has subsided. As a result of the emphasis on the market and growing rationalization and commercialization, individualization has become increasingly characterized as competition and the need to perform, rather than as liberation and immaterial well-being. The neo-liberal ideal of citizenship elevated (economic) autonomy to the highest good. Those lagging behind, many of whom depended on the shrinking welfare state and/or belonged to ethnic minorities, were seen as problem cases and increasingly treated by coercion so as to activate them towards social participation and self-reliance. For these groups, the emphasis shifted from rights to duties. Dependence on the welfare state and a lack of social integration – on account of unemployment, educational disadvantages, insufficient language skills or certain religious (as in, Islamic) values – came to be more or less at odds with full citizenship. The view that citizenship was not a given entitlement, but had to be earned once again began to make headway, but in this construction more was expected from education, employment, entrepreneurship, didactic instruction and a hardening of criminal law than from the psychological subtleties of mental health care.

PART III: NEO-REPUBLICAN CITIZENSHIP: HEALTH IN THE RISK SOCIETY

The late twentieth century witnessed a revolution that affected the Western welfare state at its core. After a century of growing state intervention, it was increasingly felt that the state had become almost omnipresent, taking care of citizens from cradle to grave. Particularly after the Second World War, state intervention increased due to aging populations, the rise of chronic disease and improved technological possibilities. This led to spiralling costs, but also – critics argued – to dependent and calculating citizens as well. Therefore, the situation triggered two kinds of response: one economic, one moral. First, it was felt that the welfare system was no longer affordable in a competitive global economy. The neo-liberal revolution of the 1980s, initiated by British Prime Minister Margaret Thatcher and American President Ronald Reagan, and later copied by other Western European states, advocated that the state withdraw from the social domain. Collective arrangements were being reconsidered, reformed, abolished or 'left to the market'. The second, moral response to the crisis of the welfare state felt that civic responsibility – necessary to sustain the welfare state – was crumbling; therefore, citizenship needed to be redefined. It was argued that the emphasis should shift from collective solidarity (organized by the state) to individual responsibility (embodied by citizens), and from passive entitlement to active participation. Neo-republican citizenship entailed major shifts in the health care system. By reframing disease as a risk that could (and should) be managed by adopting a healthy lifestyle, the 'new public health' addressed citizens as autonomous, reflexive and competent persons, responsible for the destinies of their own lives. In some ways, this was the reversal of a process that had started in the nineteenth century. For that reason, the new public health is not without its critics.

In his contribution to this collection, Martin Powell tests the thesis of a shift from social liberal to neo-republican citizenship outlined in the general introduction to this volume. The transformation of the British National Health Service (NHS), initiated in 1979 by the Thatcher Conservative government, might be seen as symbolic of this shift. Therefore, it seems a perfect case study to test the thesis. Powell argues that although there have been changes in the NHS after 1979, there were important continuities as well. State-owned and tax-funded, the NHS is generally considered the centrepiece of the British welfare state. The rhetoric of the NHS promised access to health care as a more or less unqualified right of British citizens. However, even the 'classic' NHS (1948–79) was never fully compatible with the Marshallian ideal of social citizenship. It did not, for example, treat all medical claims; patients were clients rather than citizens, and rights were determined by professional opinion. The system combined formal generosity with tight control over the consumption of services. After 1979, the 'new' NHS patient never developed into a full neo-republican citizen. Neo-republican citizenship is a mix of neo-liberal and communitarian values that shift the balance from rights and entitlements to responsibilities and obligations. During the 'new' NHS period (1979 onwards), some of these elements – such as rational and autonomous consumer choice in a transparent market – can be found. However, none of them were fully developed. For example, there has been no wholesale privatization of the NHS, and for most of the period it was health authority managers rather than patients making the choices. Moreover, while post-1979 governments were keen on creating greater civic participation, health boards tended to be composed of professionals with business skills rather than of engaged and responsible citizens. Both Conservative and New Labour governments favoured greater conditionality: rights should be earned, while the emphasis on lifestyle led to victim blaming. Finally, policy statements such as *The Health of the Nation* and *Our Healthier Nation* have been published, and strategies such as healthy living campaigns and smoking bans put in place, but their importance and consistency have varied. Powell concludes that, in the British case, the thesis outlined in the introduction is partial and limited: the modern NHS patient is not a full neo-republican citizen.

Klasien Horstman takes position vis-à-vis the introduction as well. She addresses a problem that many contemporary Western societies are facing due to the shift in morbidity patterns from infectious to chronic diseases, which took place over the course of the twentieth century. While social citizenship and state intervention were relevant in an era in which contagious diseases were the biggest killers, they do not seem effective in a time when 'lifestyle diseases' constitute the dominant threat. At first sight, countering the risks of smoking cigarettes, drinking alcohol or eating too much fat seems to be a matter of individual choice. However, since lung cancer, cardiovascular disease and obesity constitute a financial burden on society, governments tend to point to the risks of an unhealthy lifestyle, urging citizens to take responsibility for their lives. In the 'new public health', the emphasis has shifted from changing the environment towards changing people's lifestyles. In the twenty-first century, leading a healthy life has become a matter of risk management in an uncertain world. The dangers of modern life are everywhere. The new public health sciences framed a 'healthy lifestyle' in such a way that responsible citizenship implies complying with the advice of public health experts. Horstman argues that their rationalistic style has led to 'expertocracy' and to paternalism in disguise – in short: to *quasi* neo-republican citizenship. While epidemiological and technocratic knowledge abounds, the voice of citizens is not heard. At the same time, by elaborating three case studies (public youth care, health promotion at work and vaccination programmes), Horstman shows that citizens are not easily disciplined into 'proper' health behaviour. As it turns out, citizens do not easily identify with the ideals of public health experts; nor do they comply with their blueprints. Citizens tend to ignore the advice of public health experts. Horstman concludes by arguing that too much is expected from scientific expertise. Instead, public trust may be regained by replacing the language of technocratic steering and control by a language of interactive learning, thus allowing for pluralism and diversity.

This raises the issue of whether citizens have the democratic right to lead unhealthy lives, the question being whether they are still entitled to the benefits of collective health insurance when they do. Ine Van Hoyweghen argues that predictive medicine covers new ground in the old debates about individual responsibility and accountability for health. Modern probabilistic epidemiology has contributed to a situation in which problems of health and disease have become problems of health risks, shifting the focus from symptoms and treatment of disease to pre-symptomatic diagnosis and preventive management of potential risk. Thus, new definitions of health and disease lead to new conceptualizations of citizenship and to a redistribution of responsibilities between citizens, health care institutions and the state. This goes to the heart of the basis for good citizenship and how this articulates with membership of – or exclusion from – the insurance pool. Private health insurance may be qualified as a normative technology. In producing risk categories, insurance companies regulate behaviour by excluding some and mandating the conditions of inclusion for others. When life insurance companies were set up at the end of the nineteenth century, the issue of medical selection was often the subject of public debate. Since then, medical underwriting has generally been accepted as a regular procedure in insurance, while medicine's gatekeeper role in insurance has rarely been questioned. The rise of predictive medicine and technologies like genetic testing has, however, prompted new debates on risk selection in insurance. In an attempt to open up these debates, Van Hoyweghen analyses the ways in which insurers are using predictive medicine for risk assessment. Having undertaken ethnographic fieldwork in the underwriting departments of Belgian insurance companies, she demonstrates how insurers highlight predictive lifestyle health information in underwriting and how individual responsibility for health risks has become the gold standard for assessing eligibility for membership of the insurance pool. In doing so, she is pointing to a potential danger of preventive medicine: by broadening its scope to the *prognosis* of illness in the future, it may contribute to increasing exclusion from insurance, undoing the democratization process in insurance which has been linked to ideals of social citizenship, while putting increasing numbers of people in danger of being ranked as second-class citizens.

The neo-liberal revolution and the shift towards neo-republican citizenship that we are witnessing today not only have social and economic dimensions, but political and moral ones as well. As developments unfold, there have been gains and losses. While it may be considered beneficial that people are challenged to think afresh about their role as citizens with an awareness of their rights and duties, the decline of the welfare state has resulted in a crisis of citizen confidence in democracy and the state.

8 NEO-REPUBLICAN CITIZENSHIP AND THE BRITISH NATIONAL HEALTH SERVICE SINCE 1979

Martin Powell

The British National Health Service (NHS) was created by the Labour government under the Minister of Health, Aneurin Bevan in 1948.[1] It is generally classified as a 'Beveridge' as opposed to a 'Bismarck' health care system: state-owned and tax-funded, rather than insurance based, offering health care free at the point of use to all. Unlike some of the Nordic and Southern European state systems, it is based on central rather than local government and local administrative bodies tend to be appointed rather than elected, with the centre having top–down authority over local bodies.[2] At first sight the principles of the NHS – comprehensive, universal and free care that is provided equally to all[3] – appears to fit well with citizenship. Many arguments link social democratic or Marshallian citizenship to the welfare state. For example, according to Gosta Esping-Andersen, 'Few can disagree with T. H. Marshall's proposition that social citizenship constitutes the core idea of a welfare state' and 'the outstanding criterion of social rights must be the degree to which they permit people to make their living standards independently of pure market forces'.[4] As the NHS is often seen as the centre-piece of the welfare state, it has been claimed that it represents social-democratic citizenship.[5] There are many linkages of citizenship to health care and to the NHS.[6] Thus Ian Greener draws on Marshall in his account of 'citizenship at the creation of the NHS',[7] and Brian Salter discusses Marshall, noting that 'within welfare state citizenship, health care rights play a central role'.[8] David Marquand points out that the right to medical care sprang from citizenship pure and simple, all being eligible and the costs paid for from general taxation.[9]

Michael Moran argues that rights to social citizenship have two distinguishing features: they are 'universal' entitlements, claimable under impersonal eligibility rules by all people called citizens; and the quality of entitlements bears no relation to individual income or wealth. 'Health care citizenship' might thus be summarily defined as the right to health care for all citizens free at the point of treatment.[10] Moran writes that the rhetoric of the NHS promised access to health care as a more-or-less unqualified right of citizenship. De-commodification occurs where access is entirely a right of citizenship independent of market location or contribution history, with Britain as an example of de-commodified entitlement. The language of citizenship is nowhere mentioned in the establishing legislation, but when Marshall gave his famous lecture on citizenship one year after the foundation of the service, he plainly was thinking of the NHS when characterizing social citizenship as a set of equal entitlements for all citizens to a 'guaranteed minimum' of service.[11]

As explained in the introduction to this volume, there are different types of citizenship and citizenship is often qualified.[12] Moreover, the users of health services have been conceptualized in a variety of ways beyond citizenship.[13] Many accounts see the user as a client in the context of professionalism. Talcott Parsons's 'sick role' sums up the relationship between professional and client: the professional has expert knowledge and the passive client should be compliant. Clients are often portrayed as 'pawns' – as relatively passive figures in thrall to a professional expertise.[14] The term 'health care consumer' is contested,[15] since consumers are generally seen as having choice.[16] However, Charlotte Williamson argues that to see health consumerism as purely a commercial phenomenon is a narrow and limiting perspective. In other words, rather than being polar opposites, the line between 'citizen', 'consumer' and 'client' is blurred; users may best be regarded as hybrids having elements of each term.[17]

A major thesis outlined in the introduction to this volume is that there have been moves in health care from the social-liberal and social-democratic citizenship of the late nineteenth to mid-to-late twentieth century towards neo-republic citizenship, which is a mix of neo-liberal and communitarian values that shift the balance from rights and entitlements to responsibilities and obligations. Similarly, Stephen Harrison and Ruth McDonald claim that until about 1980 Marshallian citizenship, with a stress on rights, was dominant in the NHS, but that there has been a more recent shift to 'active communitarian citizenship', a complex mix of communitarianism, republicanism, community development and consumerism.[18] This chapter examines this thesis for the British NHS in the period since 1979. It is claimed that while it has some validity, it is subject to major caveats. This is because social-liberal citizenship did not fully characterize the 'classic' NHS before 1979 and that neo-republican citizenship does not fully characterize the NHS after then. The chapter examines citizenship in the 'classic' NHS (1948–79) as the analytical template of social-democratic citizenship before exploring the neo-republican citizenship thesis for the period since 1979 under the Conservative (1979–97) and New Labour (1997–2010) governments.[19]

Citizenship in the Classic NHS

It can be argued that citizenship in the classic NHS was passive in two senses. First, citizens were largely passive right-bearers rather than active citizens.[20] NHS patients had 'rights' but few responsibilities. Moreover, 'rights' were qualified in a number of ways. Marshall claims that benefits in the form of a service have the characteristic that the rights of the citizen cannot be precisely defined. The qualitative element is too great. A modicum of legally enforceable rights may be granted, but what matters to the citizen is the superstructure of legitimate expectations. For example, it may be possible for every citizen who wishes it to be registered with a doctor, but it is much harder to ensure that his ailments will be properly cared for.[21] Marshall claims that equality of persons is compatible with inequality of incomes provided the inequality is not too great. He insists that doctors should regard all their patients and school teachers all their pupils, as deserving to be treated with the same care: 'And that is as near as I can get to a demonstration of what I mean when I speak of a qualitative equality of welfare that can co-exist with a quantitative inequality of income'.[22]

Moran points out that Marshall's phrase of the 'guaranteed minimum' exactly catches the double edge of the entitlements offered by the NHS: the 'guarantee' catches the historic generosity of Bevan's reforms; 'minimum' catches what is less often declared – that the guarantees were tightly circumscribed and that the NHS combined formal generosity with tight control over the actual consumption of services. A uniquely generous philosophy went with parsimonious practice. The tension between formal generosity and the reality of tight control lies at the heart of the politics of consumption in the United Kingdom.[23] Indeed, as Moran stresses, 'pure' citizenship services are rare and no Western country offers the right of health care citizenship.[24]

Moreover, Marshall is also clear that individual rights must be subordinated to national plans, with expectations representing details in a design for community living rather than individual claims that must be met in each case when presented. He later considered that almost any benefit or service that is really designed to satisfy a particular individual need must include an element of discretion. For example, in health care, a patient may sue a doctor for gross negligence, but not simply for refusing to prescribe the treatment asked for.[25] Discretion exercised in this way, however, does not make a right inferior in quality to other rights.[26] The NHS tends to be in line with Marshall's argument that individual 'rights' are not enforceable. While citizens are entitled to be registered with a GP, it is the professional rather than the patient who decides on treatment. While citizens are entitled to visit the GP, they leave their rights at the surgery door, with the professional or 'street level bureaucrat' deciding on treatment on the basis of clinical judgement. The NHS was born in an era when doctors' authority and expertise was revered and their decisions were rarely challenged. There was no need to seek patients' views because doctors knew what was best.[27] The Secretary of State remains responsible for providing or promoting a 'comprehensive' health service and the courts have largely decided against individual and enforceable rights to treatment even for life-saving drugs.[28] Brazier notes that although patients enjoy a cluster of legally enforceable rights, they tend to be collective rather than individual and it is extremely dubious whether there is in the United Kingdom any legally enforceable right to health care on demand. The courts will intervene to protect the individual interest in the collective right only in the most exceptional and restricted circumstances. Again and again the English courts have in effect declared that 'doctor knows best'. The courts take refuge in professional opinion, in effect leaving doctors holding the baby (although some recent decisions have supported patients).[29]

Secondly, the classic mechanism of liberal and social-democratic citizenship is the (collective) 'voice'. Greener links citizenship with voice and participation, but records that at the creation of the NHS, there were few mechanisms by which user voices could be involved in policymaking or implementation.[30] According to Marquand, citizen control through voice remained weak. The social citizenship state did not feel like a citizenship state at all. The British were not and never had been, citizens of a state with the rights and duties that go with citizenship; they were subjects of a monarch, with a subject culture that had little or no place for active and participatory citizenship.[31] As the Labour politician Richard Crossman put it in 1952, there had been no effort to encourage participation in the welfare state.[32] Citizens had little voice in the NHS beyond electing national Parliaments every five years. Local health organizations were appointed by the Minister of Health rather than elected, with Aneurin Bevan arguing for Parliamentary accountability in the NHS.[33] In both senses of the term, then, health care users in the classic NHS appeared more like passive clients than active citizens.[34]

Neo-Republican Citizenship in the NHS?

As highlighted elsewhere, neo-republican citizenship is a mix of neo-liberal and communitarian values that shift the balance from rights and entitlements to responsibilities and obligations. This section gives a brief and partial sketch of policy relevant to citizenship since 1979.[35]

The Thatcher Conservative Government of 1979 attempted to make the NHS more 'business-like' in a number of ways such as subjecting ancillary services to compulsory competitive tendering (CCT), commodification of the optical market and introducing general management and performance indicators.[36] CCT involved putting the 'in-house hotel' services such as catering, cleaning and laundry out to tender, where private companies would compete with the existing 'in-house' suppliers to win the contract. People on low incomes requiring spectacles would no longer receive 'NHS frames' (a basic, standard style) but would receive vouchers with which they could 'shop around' with different providers, who would compete for their business. A single 'general manager' (on the chief executive officer model of the private sector) replaced the 'consensus management' of making decisions by committee. As standard private sector measures of performance, such as profit and share value, were not applicable to the NHS, general managers required performance indicators such as length of stay in hospitals as a (crude) measure of efficiency. The 1989 White Paper *Working for Patients* broadly continued these broad themes of markets and consumer choice. One of its objectives was 'to give patients ... greater choice of services'.[37] It introduced a 'purchaser/provider split' where health authorities and General Practitioner Fund Holders (GPFH) would 'shop around' to purchase treatments from providers (such as NHS hospital trusts). The rhetoric was that in this 'internal market' the money would follow the patient. In addition to greater choice within the NHS, it was intended to make it easier for people to get treatment in the private rather than the state sector. Tax relief on private medical insurance for certain groups reduced the cost of private treatment, allowing more people the choice of 'going private'. With John Major replacing Margaret Thatcher as prime minister, the Conservatives introduced the Citizens' Charter initiative. The Patient's Charter aimed to specify standards of service for 'the rights and standards' patients could expect to receive.[38] Finally, the Health of the Nation strategy focused on preventive strategies to achieve health gain, including setting national targets.[39]

Within a few months of its landslide election victory of 1997, New Labour introduced the 'third way' to the NHS with a system based on neither the old centralized command and control systems of the 1970s nor the divisive internal market system of the 1990s but based on partnership and driven by performance.[40] New Labour claimed to have abolished the 'internal market' with collaboration replacing competition, but rather recast it onto a longer-term basis with the purchaser–provider split still very much in place. It introduced institutions such as the National Institute of Clinical Excellence (NICE) and the Commission for Health Improvement (CHI) at the national level. NICE was a body that examined the cost-effectiveness of treatments and aimed to abolish the 'post-code lottery' (local inequalities) from the NHS.[41] CHI was in all but name an inspectorate. At the local level, Primary Care Groups and Trusts (PCG/T) replaced GPFH and health authorities as the commissioning or purchasing bodies. On the provider side, NHS Trusts were set up. However, some commentators argue that central performance management increased the 'command and control' that the third way was meant to abolish.

The replacement of Frank Dobson with Alan Milburn as Secretary of State in 1999, seems to mark a change of direction, with the NHS Plan and related subsequent documents returning to the more consumerist approach of the Conservatives, which New Labour claimed to have abolished only a few years earlier. 'Investment and reform' stressed that the NHS would benefit from large injections of resources but would in return need to 'modernize'.[42] Specific initiatives included NHS Foundation Trusts, Independent Surgical Treatment Centres (ISTC), a concordat that allowed NHS patients to be treated in private hospitals, a range of alternative ways to contact the NHS such as NHS Direct and NHS Walk-in centres.[43] New hospitals were built under the Private Finance Initiative (PFI) scheme.[44] Choices to book hospital appointments were rolled out in stages under the 'Choose and Book' scheme, with 'free choice' (of all hospitals, including private hospitals) fully introduced from April 2008 for all patients who require an elective referral. Individual budgets (IB) were introduced in social care.[45] These allowed individual citizens to take control of their care by using state finance to purchase packages of care. A different strand of policy focused on public health, setting a range of targets including reducing health inequalities and later stressing individual rather than government responsibility for health.[46] The Darzi reports of 2007 and 2008 set out a range of initiatives to ensure that 'quality' was at the heart of the NHS, including stressing choice, 'personalized care', 'polyclinics' and pilots of personalized budgets.[47]

This brief policy chronology has shown many changes over a short period of time, with variations both between and within governments. However, there are also key continuities. Ironically, the Conservatives talked up an individual 'retail' market, but largely failed to deliver one, while New Labour initially promised to abolish the internal market, but then delivered a 'retail' and 'external' market.[48] There appear to be few signs of the collaboration and partnership central to New Labour's 'third way' but broadly a movement from an initial 'command and control' system towards a 'divisive' market, more radical than the one criticized by Labour in the 1990s. The next sections examine the dimensions of neo-republican citizenship.

The Market and the State

The first dimension concerns the state and the market. Neo-republican citizenship would move the boundary towards the market and privatize risk. Privatization takes many complex forms. While there have been many moves towards the market such as increasing charges for patients ('commodification') and encouraging private medicine, there has been no wholesale privatization of the NHS, despite many commentators 'crying wolf' since 1979. The major concerns are that Foundation Trusts may be the thin wedge of the privatization door and that the NHS leases rather than owns new hospitals built under PFI from private companies that have brokered expensive, long term and poor deals for the NHS.[49]

There has been limited privatization of risk for the majority of the most expensive parts of the NHS such as hospital in-patient treatment. However, there has been some privatization in risk in some areas. The most severe short-term effects felt by citizens are in the field of continuing care where many people feel angry and powerless that they have to pay for 'social' care that they considered was part of the 'cradle to grave' social rights paid for by their taxes. Despite Tony Blair's claim in opposition that he did not want his child to grow up in a country where old people were forced to sell their houses to pay for their care and the setting up of a Royal Commission to examine the issue, New Labour ignored its majority report on the grounds of affordability. The Majority Report was largely introduced to provide free personal care in Scotland, but some reports regard the Scottish system as unaffordable.[50] New Labour revisited this issue in 2009 and pledged to set up a 'National Care Service'. The Green Paper 'Shaping the Future of Care Together' remarkably failed to contain a reference to the 1999 Royal Commission, with the Commission seemingly erased from history as if it had never happened. The document set out a vision underpinned by national rights and entitlements. However, unlike the NHS, the NCS was not to be tax-funded. This option was ruled out (in bold letters) because it placed a heavy burden on people of working age. It is just as well that Bevan did not take this view for the NHS in 1945.[51] The Personal Care at Home Bill was introduced in Parliament in November 2009 as the first step towards setting up a new National Care Service. It was claimed that this first step, which would cost £670 million, would help around 400,000 people with the highest care needs and guarantee free personal care for 280,000.[52]

Another issue has been NHS dentistry. In some parts of the country it is difficult to find an NHS dentist, with a survey by the consumer magazine *Which?* finding that three million people had been unable to see a NHS dentist, while a further 4.5 million had abandoned even trying. This has resulted in some people being forced to go private, become a 'dental tourist' overseas or resort to 'DIY' (Do It Yourself) dentistry, sometimes from the household tool-kit. The NHS has a target to ensure that all patients are able to see an NHS dentist if they wish by 2011 and ministers will consult on whether access should be made a legal right, but critics dismiss these plans as not worth the paper they are written on.[53] Another area of concern has been the availability of new and expensive drug treatments. Here there has been a debate on 'co-payments' since there have been cases of clinicians advising some expensive (mainly anti-cancer) drugs that have not been approved by NICE. Patients have bought these drugs themselves but this resulted in them being de facto excluded from the NHS and having to finance *all* their care. The 'cancer Czar' Mike Richards was asked to write a review, which resulted in these patients being accepted within the NHS.[54]

New Labour wished to see a more plural system, with more care provided by private and third sector providers, bound together by more state regulation.[55] The main debate was whether or not it matters where care takes place. Commentators such as Julian Le Grand argue that patients do not care whether treatment takes place in public or private hospitals so long as it is free at the point of use, timely and of high quality. While there has been a shift in the balance of state and private provision, there has been less of a shift in terms of state finance in that the state will pay for care in facilities of private and third sector providers. This is related to the debate on regulation in the mixed economy of health care. It has been argued that if standards are clearly monitored by regulators, then the location of care (public or private) is of no great significance.[56] In contrast defenders of the 'traditional' NHS stress the importance of the 'public sector ethos' of state care.[57] However, recent media exposures of private care homes and excess deaths in Stafford hospital suggest that the Healthcare Commission (now Care Quality Commission) will find it difficult to ensure high quality care for all through regulation.[58]

Regulated Consumerism

The Conservative governments of the 1980s wished to encourage people to 'shop around' for GPs and to choose private care. However, although there was a large increase in the discourse of consumerism and choice, this does not necessarily mean that users had more consumer mechanisms. Harrison and McDonald note that the NHS quasi-market, though accompanied by a good deal of rhetoric about choice and closeness to patients, provided few mechanisms to procure this. Perri 6 states that there is very limited direct consumer choice in the NHS.[59] The 1990 reforms appear not to have greatly increased choice as the market was largely a 'mimic market' where patients followed the money rather than money following the patients. In other words, health authority managers made choices on behalf of patients by making contracts with providers on grounds of cost-effectiveness. The inconsistencies in the 1990s Conservative approach to the consumer and continued resistance to strands of consumerism, suggests that the citizenship regime promoted by the Conservatives was not fully consumerized and so more neo-liberal in words than in deeds.[60]

Indeed, it is possible to argue – at least in principle – that the Conservative internal market reforms saw a *reduction* in choice for most people in that they lost their theoretical right to be referred anywhere, instead being referred to where the health authority managers had placed their contracts. Alain Enthoven, sometimes credited or blamed for the internal market, considered that on the scale from Soviet planning (0) to the textbook free market (10), the 'internal market' was about a '2'.[61] In some ways, then, despite the rhetoric, the period saw an increase in power to managers, where the logic of bureaucracy trumped the logic of either markets or professional paternalism.

John Major's Patient's Charter saw some 'soft' consumerism such as moves towards individual hospital appointment times and some limited guarantees on waiting time at hospitals and for those whose treatment was cancelled. However, Margaret Brazier notes that the right to health care on the basis on clinical need in the 'Patient's Charter' is 'pure rhetoric'.[62] Critics argue that the apostrophe is important: it was a Patient's (individual) rather than a Patients' (collective) Charter, or a Consumer's rather than a Citizen's Charter. However, it was not a strong consumer mechanism. Despite the language of rights and their careful differentiation from those elements patients could 'expect' only, charter rights were not legally enforceable.[63] Salter claims that the Conservative government favoured the concept of consumerism rather than citizenship, with policies increasing rather than reducing rights, but for consumers rather than citizens.[64]

New Labour introduced choice in a number of dimensions in the NHS. Its prime concern was waiting times and the reduction of waiting lists culminating in the eighteen-week waiting target. However, it also delivered choices about professional and access channel (NHS Direct; NHS Walk-In Centres). Recent policy tended to favour choice mechanisms over those of trust, voice and command.[65] In other words, it was assumed that individual patients were best placed to drive performance improvements rather than trusting the professionals, listening to collective voices, or forcing top–down performance management by bureaucrats. Commentators have pointed to a 'return to the market', although – as we have seen – New Labour's market is stronger than that of the Conservatives.[66] New Labour claimed that patients wanted consumer choice but this has been disputed.[67] However, it should also be noted that there have been strict limits on some choices such as that to choose single rather than multiple vaccine, as for example of measles vaccine as opposed to the measles, mumps and rubella (MMR) vaccine. Some choices, such as referral to complementary medicine, appear to have declined under New Labour.[68] It was only towards the end of New Labour's term in office that the most radical forms of (consumer as chooser) consumerism of individual choice and individual budgets were introduced. However, many people did not wish to choose; the take up of choice was fairly limited, with many people 'choosing' the local hospital or relying on their GP to 'choose' on their behalf. Few researched the available information on alternative providers in order to be active choosers. A study reported that about half of the patients recalled being offered a choice of hospital or treatment centre, with only 4 per cent using the NHS Choices website.[69] Moreover, 'choice' might conflict with the government's 'evidence-based policy' agenda. It has been argued that including homeopathy as an option in the Personal Budget scheme was 'ill conceived' if it meant that consumers could spend state money on 'ineffective' treatments. This meant that in terms of 'opportunity cost', the effectiveness of state finance was reduced as money was spent on ineffective rather than effective therapies.[70]

Trust in professionals was questioned after the scandal at the Bristol Royal Infirmary, where a high level of deaths in operations on young children was allowed to continue for a long period. This suggested that the professionals could no longer be allowed to regulate themselves and since then the regulation of the medical profession has become increasingly important. Angela Coulter argues that the Kennedy Report on events at the Bristol Royal Infirmary, 'After Bristol', was a 'defining moment in the history of the NHS' as its previously secretive, professional, inward-facing culture was seen to be unsuitable for a modern service.[71]

Citizenship and (In)equality

The language of 'rights' continues to be important under both Conservative and New Labour governments. However, 'rights' in both New Labour's NHS Constitution and the Conservative's Citizen's Charter include a mix of existing entitlements (such as the 'right' to sue a provider for negligence) and vague non-enforceable aspirations (such as the 'right' to be treated with respect).[72] Under proposals that some commentators saw as 'future-proofing' the NHS against a Conservative government in 2010, Labour offered a new 'legal right' to go to another public or private provider if the NHS failed to provide their routine treatment within eighteen weeks or an initial specialist cancer consultation within two weeks. However, these rights could be regarded as 'less robust' than had been suggested after it emerged that PCTs would only have to take 'reasonable steps' to find alternative providers.[73]

The Conservatives did not place a high priority on reducing health inequalities or 'health variations' as they were termed. Health inequalities did not feature in the 'Health of the Nation' (1992).[74] New Labour initially set aggregate health gain targets but rejected health inequalities targets in 'Our Healthier Nation', which were introduced in the 'NHS Plan'.[75] However, despite a range of initiatives, health inequalities in terms of social class appear to have increased since the targets were set.[76]

Turning to health care, New Labour introduced *National* Service Frameworks (NSFs) and the *National* Institute for Clinical Excellence (NICE) in order to increase the 'national-ness' of the service and reduce the 'postcode lottery'.[77] However, here too, progress in reducing geographical inequalities was problematic and there are continuing post-code lotteries in a number of services.[78] For example, despite the 'national cancer strategy', survival rates a year after diagnosis continue to show a 'post-code lottery' with lung cancer patients in Herefordshire more than three times as likely to die within a year of diagnosis compared to lung cancer patients in Kensington and Chelsea.[79] Moreover, it is difficult to discuss 'national' aspects of service provision as most writers argue that political devolution to Northern Ireland, Scotland and Wales has resulted in greater differentiation between the nations.[80] There was a further debate around how an increase of individual choice would impact on inequality. Le Grand argued that increasing choice might reduce inequalities, while other commentators claimed the opposite, but there is little solid empirical evidence on this issue.[81] As Rudolf Klein concludes, 'more than 40 years after its birth, the NHS had yet to offer everyone with the same level of service'.[82] It remains clear that the NHS – perhaps the most 'national' of all services in the United Kingdom – fails to deliver services on the basis of 'need not geography'. The NHS has never been, and could never be, a *perfectly* equitable service.[83] More thought is needed on which variations are unacceptable and how much variation should be tolerated.[84] Given that perfectly uniform services are not possible, how much difference can exist before citizenship is undermined?

Citizenship: Participative and Conditional

Both Conservative and New Labour governments have favoured greater 'participation', although the term lacks a clear definition. However, while public and patient involvement (PPI) policy has seen many twists and turns of policy, the degree of participation among citizens is far from clear. The Community Health Councils (CHCs) were set up in 1974 to 'represent' the community with citizens appointed to reflect local interests. They have seen mixed results, with most commentators claiming that these community 'watchdogs' lacked teeth and were largely muzzled.[85] The Conservatives broadly replaced representative accountability with managerial accountability, arguing that appointed health boards should not be 'representative' of the community, but instead be composed of individuals with business skills.[86] Health Authorities were meant to listen to 'local voices' to become the 'champions of the people'.[87] However, most people did not know that their champions existed. The Patient's Charter aimed to turn citizens into consumers: individuals with a varied selection of quasi-rights rather than active, engaged, collective citizens.

After abolishing CHCs in 2003, New Labour put in place a rapid succession of complex arrangements with the appearance and disappearance of bodies such as ICAS, PALS, PPIF and CPPIH.[88] The system finally comprised Local Involvement Networks (LINks), local authority overview and scrutiny committees (OSC) and governors and members of FTs. However, these bodies were based on very different models (local 'voluntary' citizens; elected councillors; and citizens as elected members, respectively) and there is little evidence for the impact of these initiatives.[89]

Similarly, both Conservative and New Labour governments have favoured greater conditionality, linking rights and obligations.[90] This key feature of neo-republican citizenship appears to be in line with the view of many citizens that rights should be 'earned' and should be 'conditional' and that other citizens should not have 'something for nothing'.[91] The main debates are concerned with the so-called 'New Public Health' (NPH). However, clear definitions of the term remain elusive. Although most commentators view its emergence as linked with the Lalonde Report of 1974, the importance of 'lifestyle' factors is not clear. Hunter claims that the 'health field' concept has been criticized by many commentators because of its emphasis on lifestyle factors and that it lends itself to 'victim blaming'.[92]

Alan Petersen and Deborah Lupton see the NPH as an arena in which the individual is expected to take responsibility for their health, but point to the complexities and difficulties of adopting the idea of the 'healthy citizen'. They cite the WHO European Charter on Environment and Health to the effect that 'the entitlements of individuals do not exist without corresponding responsibilities', arguing that a broadening of the concept of social citizenship and an emphasis on '"rights implies duties", have profound implications'.[93] On the other hand, Robin Gauld writes that the NPH has come to the fore in the new millennium, partly in response to a pendulum swing in politics away from neoliberalism, but also due to increasing evidence showing that action is required around issues such as reducing health and other inequalities, improving housing, promoting comprehensive primary care and changing the way people live. Michael Fitzpatrick sees the aim of the new public health movement as shifting the focus of health promotion from the level of the individual to tackle the wider social determinants of ill health. He points to the 'curious combination of utopian fantasy and cynical rhetoric that characterized the new public health movement' where 'delegates to conferences in exotic international locations endorsed revolutionary declarations'.[94]

Beyond problems of definition, the policy impact of the NPH is also unclear. Fitzpatrick discusses the 'state-sponsored medical regulation of lifestyle', arguing that in the late 1970s the Labour government first took up the cause of prevention, in a series of policy initiatives which made little immediate impact. He cites Department of Health and Social Security (DHSS) documents from the 1970s which state that 'much of the responsibility for ensuring his own good health lies with the individual' and that 'much ill-health in Britain today arises from over-indulgence and unwise behaviour'. He contends that, anxious to avoid 'victim-blaming', the Conservative Secretary of State, William Waldegrave wrote that 'for too long ... the health debate has been bedevilled by two extreme claims of, on the one hand, "It's all up to individuals" and on the other hand "It's all up to Government" – we need a proper balance between individual responsibility and Government action'. Similarly, according to his successor, Virginia Bottomley, 'we must get the balance right between governments and individuals'.[95] The implications of this thesis, including financial considerations, were not made clear. For example, 'healthy' food is more expensive in some cases and the 'fitness industry', with its private gyms, makes it expensive to be healthy.

In its early years in government, New Labour broadly continued this rhetoric. According to New Labour's *Our Healthier Nation*, in the past, efforts to improve health have been too much about blame. Individuals were to blame for failing to listen to well-intentioned but misdirected health advice. Or government was blamed for failing to embrace grand plans for social engineering which would make people healthier automatically: 'Our Healthier Nation' set out a third way between the old extremes of individual victim blaming on the one hand and nanny state social engineering on the other'.[96]

David Hunter notes that the neoliberal principles stressing individual lifestyle issues in *Choosing Health* received further endorsement in July 2006 in a major speech on public health delivered by then prime minister, Tony Blair – 'our public health problems are not, strictly speaking, public health questions at all. They are questions of individual lifestyles'.[97] In rhetoric, at least, Blair presented more neoliberal citizenship credentials than the previous Conservative government.

However, speeches do not implement policy and it is difficult to determine the impact of policy rhetoric without considering policy mechanisms. While it is possible to point to individualist rhetoric such as Chief Medical Officer Liam Donaldson's Ten Tips for Better Health, the ten commandments of the European Code against Cancer and the American Institute of Public Medicine's Ten New Year Resolutions, it is more difficult to see the 'conditionality' involved.[98] While there are clear consequences in employment policy such as benefit reduction for those that the government deem not to be shouldering their 'obligations', similar consequences are far from clear in health. For example, Fitzpatrick observes that although the Conservative 'Health of the Nation' had an authoritarian character, it was not perceived as coercive by the vast majority of people.[99]

Some recent events illustrate the problem of attempting to increase responsibility and conditionality in health care. A teenager who suffered acute liver failure after drinking thirty cans of lager on a weekend was admitted to hospital, but 'still in his slippers, holding the needle of a drip in his hand and wearing his hospital name band', tried to order a pint at a bar. His father planned to launch a judicial review to try to overturn NHS guidelines which meant that his son has to be alcohol free for six months before he could get a liver transplant.[100] The former footballer, George Best, promised to give up alcohol in order to receive a liver transplant, but was drinking again, including a 'seven-day binge' within a year and died a little over two years later. Critics argued that the 'opportunity cost' of the transplant meant that a 'more deserving case' went without the transplant.[101]

Many 'Accident and Emergency' Departments are swamped by alcohol related incidents on Friday and Saturday nights, including binge-drinking 'frequent fliers' and alcohol related assaults. There have been nearly 170,000 violent incidents in English NHS hospitals each year, which have recently included several murders and rapes. Some hospital Accident and Emergency (A&E) departments have been described as 'war zones' on a typical Friday or Saturday night, with critics arguing that the Labour government's promises to tackle violence within the NHS were 'worthless'.[102]

NHS costs for treating overweight people are projected to double to £10 billion a year by the middle of the century, with the wider costs to business and other parts of society estimated to reach almost £50 billion a year. As an illustration, the world's heaviest man, at 70-stone (about 450 kilos), needs a team of carers to wash, move and feed him as well as adapted doorways, strengthened furniture and other equipment inside his house, that has cost the taxpayer hundreds of thousands of pounds over the past few years. Some people feel that obesity, like smoking and drinking, is a 'lifestyle choice' rather than an illness and therefore something for which the NHS should not pick up the bill.[103] In short, then, while there has been a great deal of rhetoric about 'responsibility', claims of 'conditional citizenship' are overstated.[104]

Conclusion

The thesis outlined in the introduction to this volume – that the definition of the citizen has shifted towards being a neo-republican citizen or an active communitarian citizen – is partial and limited in the case of the British NHS. Two main reasons can be adduced for this. First, even the 'classic' NHS was never fully compatible with Marshallian citizenship. For example, it did not treat all medical claims, patients were 'clients' rather than citizens and 'rights' were professionally determined.

Second, although some of the elements of neo-republican citizenship such as choice, consumerism, markets, the 'new public health' or 'healthism' can be found, none are fully developed and these issues change over time. For example, New Labour initially claimed to abolish the Conservatives' 'wholesale' and 'retail' market (managers made decisions collectively on behalf of patients, largely between NHS hospitals), but subsequently introduced a 'retail' and 'external' market (individual patients choose from NHS and private hospitals). Similarly, there have been documents on 'The Health of the Nation' and 'Our Healthier Nation' and policies such as healthy living campaigns and smoking bans, but their importance and consistency have varied. Although the policies of the current Coalition government may lead to radical changes in the future, at present the NHS patient is not a full neo-republican citizen.

9 STRUGGLING WITH SCIENCE AND DEMOCRACY: PUBLIC HEALTH AND CITIZENSHIP IN THE NETHERLANDS

Klasien Horstman

Public health appears to be intrinsically connected to the public domain and hence is expected to do justice to and to stimulate notions of citizenship, yet the meaning of citizenship in public health is problematic. In this chapter, I analyse the relation between public health and citizenship by drawing from political philosophy, sociology and science and technology studies. I will show that – especially the last decades in the twentieth century – relations between public health, science, politics and society have become captured in a rationalistic technocratic style. This implies that, while in society at large processes of democratization are intensified, in public health citizens are constructed more as the object than the subject of policies and interventions. As public health in the last decades of the twentieth century developed primarily as a technocratic practice, so the meaning of public health as a practice of democratic citizenship became limited.

In the introduction to this volume different ideals and practices of citizenship are distinguished, with different balances between freedom and equality, rights and duties, inclusion and exclusion, uniformity and diversity, autonomy and communion. While the nineteenth century is characterized by the editors in terms of liberal-democratic citizenship because of the strivings for political rights of the lower social classes and women, the twentieth century is characterized by the rise of social-liberal and social-democratic citizenship that combines political rights and specific welfare entitlements. At the end of the twentieth century the editors identify the rise of neo-republican citizenship, which stresses civic responsibilities and obligations. While these historical distinctions provide a fruitful lens through which to study different practices of citizenship, they do little justice to the growing importance of science and technology in modern societies and the specific influence of scientific-technological cultures in public and political life.[1]

In this chapter, I argue that the growing role of scientific disciplines like epidemiology, health education and health psychology in public health in the twentieth century brought about the transformation of the social-democratic or social-liberal notion of citizenship, not into a neo-republican ideal of citizenship, but into a *quasi*-neo-republican notion of citizenship. In the first half of the twentieth century public health became embedded in paternalistic ideals and practices, in social policies that aimed at integrating the lower social classes into society and in developing shared values about hygiene, vaccination and good parenthood. Since the 1970s, public health practices appeared to distance themselves from these paternalistic approaches as they stressed individual choice and the responsibility of citizens regarding their own health and lifestyle. At the same time, however, the developing public health sciences framed 'the healthy choice' and 'a healthy lifestyle' in such a way that responsible citizenship implied complying with the advice of public health experts. Current individualistic, evidence based public health can be considered an 'expertocracy' and as such, a liberal rhetoric notwithstanding, current Western public health practices can be understood as paternalism in disguise. To put it strongly, as post-World War II public health policies and practices have become caught in a dynamic of rationalization and scientification, public health stimulates neither social nor liberal citizenship but tends rather to destroy the political and civil character of public health.

In developing this argument, I will make use of empirical examples and illustrations from the Netherlands. Notwithstanding international differences in the interaction between science, professions, policy and citizenship – both in Europe and elsewhere – this analysis may fruitfully be used to explore the complicated relationship between public health, science and democracy in other countries.[2] Further to the analysis, I will argue for a pragmatic philosophical perspective that permits a more balanced approach to the relation between science and democracy, public health and citizenship.

Proliferating Risks, Rising Ambitions, Disappointing Results

The ideals of current public health practices are very ambitious, namely to create a society in which everyone remains fit, healthy and active for as long as possible. Health is no longer something that just happens to you or is bestowed by God, neither is it a question of luck; rather it is a project of effective risk management.[3] A century ago, the aim of public health was to prevent people from becoming ill and it was especially aimed at preventing the spread of epidemic diseases. Sewerage systems and water supply networks were constructed in order to tackle epidemics and the lower classes were taught how to run a household hygienically through the considerable efforts made by the middle and upper classes to 'civilize' them. In the twenty-first century, public health not only focuses on preventing illness but also on ensuring that people remain healthy for as long as possible and the emphasis has shifted from changing the environment towards changing people's lifestyle. While in the 1960s lifestyle still referred to the collective – 'we' had developed an unhealthy Western lifestyle – since the 1980s it increasingly came to be regarded as the choice and responsibility of individuals. In tandem with this process of individualization of responsibility for 'healthy living', the domain of public health expanded considerably. Public health now covered everything from eating, drinking and exercise to sleep, sex and work, and addressed lifestyle from before conception right into extreme old age. There is almost no domain in our lives that now escapes the ambition of the proponents of 'healthy living'.

Of course, everyday practices do not fit these ideals nicely and policymakers as well as public health experts worry about 'the obesity epidemic' and other manifestations of an unhealthy lifestyle. Sociologists and anthropologists are less surprised about the gap between policy and practice, since they acknowledge that everyday local practices have their own dynamics and rationality and cannot simply be steered by technocratic health policies.[4] Anthropology has shown that in daily life people generally do not consider health in terms of 'risk factors' but rather in terms of meanings and experiences. Further, in daily life healthy living is one of the many issues people have to deal with and individuals may give priority to working hard, solving conflicts in a marriage, adhering to family traditions and living life to the full.[5] In general, people raised in different socio-cultural settings develop different habits with respect to healthy living: while some learn a taste for vegetables, other learn that a happy family life entails alcohol and snacks. Pierre Bourdieu refers to the 'taste of distinction': by exhibiting a specific taste, people indicate their allegiance to a certain social group and distinguish themselves from others.[6] Moreover, philosophers, sociologists and anthropologists have demonstrated that human beings are made of flesh and blood, operate in specific contexts at their own rhythms and make up their own ideas about risk and safety. Even when acknowledging the specific value of scientific expertise,[7] it is naive to assume – as many public health policies and programmes do – that expert driven interventions actually result in behaviour change in everyday life on short notice.

Public health experts and public health policies nonetheless articulate an urgent need for more scientific based preventive interventions. Prevention is considered a major strategy for the control of the rising costs of health care in an era of obesity and chronic diseases. In public health we see the contours of a 'risk society', as it has been described by the German sociologist Ulrich Beck;[8] a society in which uncertainties do not arise externally but emerge from within, not as a product of nature but as a product of science and technology. In public health however, science and technology are primarily regarded as the solution to a problem, rather than as part of a problem. Beck and others who are engaged in this debate about 'risk society' like Anthony Giddens, argue that the uncertainties produced by science and technology cannot be resolved with conventional rationalistic political strategies that are guided by scientific expertise and that the failures of such rationalistic policies in that respect may undermine trust in political and scientific institutions.[9] They put forward the notion of 'new modernity' and argue that this requires new forms of reflexivity and politics. Although there is much to be said for this diagnosis, it is striking that policymakers and experts in the field of public health pay little attention to these debates.

Looking closely at current public health policies and programmes in Europe and the Netherlands, it becomes clear that specific public health issues are primarily framed as *technical problems* which have to be solved through *scientific expertise*. The fact that important 'risk groups' are 'not reached' is conceptualized as a question of effective steering tools. In other words, public health ideals and policies are characterized by a rationalistic approach that attempts to steer the behaviour of citizens by calling for more evidence about effective tools for achieving the aim of healthy behaviour. It is assumed that evidence based interventions will turn risk behaviour into healthy behaviour, thereby reducing the gap between policy ambitions and every day practices. In line with this, public health has invested in effectiveness studies. National databases of 'proven' effective interventions have been developed, in the expectation that the concept 'academic' will come to refer to technical expertise rather than to reflexive competence. At times, it seems as though ineffectiveness is also regarded as a moral issue: then the argument is that individuals who do not make the effort to stay healthy incur significant costs and are not fulfilling their duty as citizens and therefore they must pay for the consequences, for example by being excluded from health insurance and care. Yet this apparent moralization of public health problems again is framed as an issue of evidence: assigning guilt, levying penalties and imposing sanctions on unhealthy behaviour are only considered good when the effectiveness of such strategy is proven.

Current public health practices thus define themselves primarily as technocratic knowledge practices and are blind to their own unintended effects, namely the undermining of practices of citizenship – the destruction of 'the political' and 'the social' as the anchors of public health. In the twentieth century, paternalistic approaches in public health developed that contributed to social citizenship, since they pointed to mutual dependency between different social classes and called for the emancipation of the lower classes. This paternalism fitted the early twentieth-century context and cannot be maintained as a public health model for the relationship between experts and citizens in more democratized societies. The rise of a rationalistic public health in the last decades of the twentieth century at first sight appears to express an ideal of neo-republican citizenship that does fit this more democratized context, as much attention is paid to individual responsibility for risk behaviour. However, as I will show below, it is more appropriate to formulate this approach as quasi-neo-republicanism, since in this expert-driven public health the voice of citizens is not heard and little attention is paid to the (re)production of the political and social character of practices of citizenship. This point can be illustrated by three Dutch examples of public health practice: public youth care, health promotion among employees and vaccination.

The Missing Voice of Parents and Children in Public Youth Care

A society in which everyone has a duty to live by a strict health regime is portrayed in Juli Zeh's novel, *Corpus delicti: A Trial* (2009).[10] In one scene, a father is on trial on suspicion of having violated the law that states that every child has to be screened for all kinds of risks (such as cerebral risks and allergic reactions): the father is accused of negligence. This criminalization of parenthood might seem ridiculous, but in Europe as well as in the United States parents are sometimes considered as careless and abusive when they have grossly overweight children. In the Netherlands, where vending machines selling candy bars and soda cans can still be found in many schools, we already see indications that parents of overweight children are being framed in terms of abuse.[11] And public concerns about youth health are much broader than just weight: consumption of alcohol and drugs, youth crime, truancy and depression are all considered to be major problems. While the capability of parents to raise their children is questioned, professional youth care does not have a good reputation either: bureaucratic procedures, waiting lists and severe incidents like the imprisonment of autistic children attract public condemnation.

In an attempt to solve these problems, the Dutch Ministry of Youth and Family developed the *Een gezin, een plan* (One family, one plan) policy, which advocates early identification of children-at-risk and improved cooperation in the youth care chain. A great deal is expected from information technology in this regard: provincial and national electronic systems have been introduced that enable professionals such as doctors, teachers or crèche supervisors to signal a child considered as 'at risk' and to stimulate coordinated help when more than two signals about a child are put in the system. This is the so-called child index. In many municipalities, all children are registered in the electronic child index at birth, so that name and address details are immediately available the first time a child is signalled 'at risk'. Useful as these information systems may be in some respects, the way they function in practice is often contrary to their intended goals and in some senses might be called perverse. Thus in the evaluations of the index, success is measured by the entry of many signals of children at risk; when few appear it is often concluded that the system is not working well. As some authors have argued, the index system turns all children into children-at-risk and considers all parents untrustworthy.[12]

As far as policymakers are concerned, information technology is the 'magic bullet' solution to problems in the youth care chain. However, many professionals have reservations. In their experience, reporting a child is akin to labelling him or her on the basis of a somewhat arbitrary standard: should a child be reported if he or she is overweight, is withdrawn or is extremely ill-tempered? But then, what is deemed to be overweight and is a temper a problem? Does a teacher interpret these traits the same way as a general practitioner or a social worker? Further, professionals are legally obliged to inform parents if they qualify a child as 'at risk' in the index. They fear parental criticism and resistance and lack the professional confidence to meet that criticism since they themselves consider the risk-construction somewhat arbitrary. In fact, many professionals feel that reporting children in this way hampers the provision of adequate help as parents become afraid to ask for fear of being put 'in the system'. Some professionals have severe doubts about the information system model. They consider that, despite the many privacy protocols in place, trust between professionals and parents is a fragile construct that is threatened by the index system.[13]

Many explanations are given for the problems of public youth care, but almost all frame them technocratically: instruments to steer professionals as well as parents in the right direction are lacking, so investment in science and technology should do the job. So, policymakers as well as experts call for more scientific research to design and support interventions in youth care. 'The evidence beast', as the Dutch pedagogy professor Mischa De Winter called it, is running riot in the youth care system.[14] It is, for example, considered that improved scientific insights into children-at-risk will resolve the uncertainty with regard to determining when a child is to be considered at risk and the degree of urgency level to be assigned to the problem. It is expected that if children could be monitored on a large scale, data would be produced to provide a basis for categorizing at-risk children more effectively and for improving the criteria for determining whether a child is at low, medium or high risk. Furthermore, it is expected that this kind of evidence will facilitate making adequate definitions, enabling professionals from different disciplines to work together more efficiently.[15] Scientific evidence, so it is assumed, will reduce uncertainty among professionals and will give rise to a more effective youth care system. Yet this focus on producing more expertise does not address the relationship between professionals, parents and children. The voice of parents and children in the endeavour to improve the quality of youth care is lacking, their experiences are not heard and their possible distrust not acknowledged. The Dutch website Parents on line (*Ouders-on-line*) that gathers experiences of parents with youth care is not popular with professionals. Tense relations between this website and youth care professionals symbolize the difficulty in addressing the issues at hand in ways other than as a lack of scientific expertise. Policymakers and professionals are trapped in a rationalistic paradigm which prevents them from noticing the one sidedness of the rationalistic focus on science and technology.

The Missing Voice of Employees in Health Promotion at the Work Place

The workplace has recently been seized upon as providing an excellent opportunity to promote health. In the Netherlands a process of privatization of sick-leave costs, the new Zorgverzekeringswet (Care Insurance Act) and a shrinking employment market due to demographic change, form the backdrop for new initiatives in the field of occupational health. While occupational health in the past focused on structural working conditions like chemical substances and safety, such concerns are now being replaced by attention to the individual lifestyle of employees. Occupational health services, coaching agencies, psychologists, fitness centres and insurers all offer a range of services to employers with the aim of promoting the health, vitality and working capacity of employees. The idea is that employees must stay fit, enthusiastic and motivated into old age. The focus is therefore not on people who are ill (sickness absence in the Netherlands is at a historic low of 4 per cent) but on people who are still healthy but might become ill in future. After all, they could be even fitter, healthier and more motivated. In other words, just as all children in the Netherlands are framed as being at-risk, all workers are framed as being at-risk workers. Thus fitness studios are introduced in the workplace, yoga courses are offered, canteens are changing their menus to healthy food and the occupational health physician performs regular health checks, while the whole team begins training for a half-marathon.[16] Recently it has been proposed that people who are frequently absent due to illness or who demonstrate an unhealthy lifestyle or are overweight should be dismissed.

Yet just as the effectiveness of the child index has become an issue, so the effectiveness of these health promotion activities has become a concern. There are indications that while slim white-collar workers may welcome fitness initiatives in the workplace, overweight truck drivers will not change their habits. They will not refrain from stopping at their customary stopping points because the food there is too fatty – they enjoy the place and the food. Sports facilities may create greater loyalty to the employer, but there are reasons to suspect that health promotion in the workplace increases socio-economic differences in health. In his excellent study on the nature of the psychoanalytic setting, Dutch sociologist Abram de Swaan has shown that the intake procedure for psychotherapy is not a neutral way of identifying a client's problem; rather, it is a means of distinguishing who is and who is not suited for psychotherapeutic treatment.[17] Those individuals who are not inclined to reflect on their behaviour, who do not find it easy to talk about themselves, who are not already familiar with the language game of psychotherapy, are not suited for therapy and are excluded. The therapy session therefore is a test in 'proto-professionalization', that has to be passed. Something similar goes for health promotion: those who do not already define their lifestyle in terms of health risks and are not already in the habit of 'healthy living' will not receive the help that they might need. By not tuning health promotion to social and cultural differences, social and cultural inequalities may increase. Apart from issues of effectiveness, there are also privacy concerns with respect to health promotion in the work place. When employers require healthy behaviour, non-smoking, weight loss and good sleep, the classic divide between work and private life is threatened. We may wonder to what extent the requirements of the workplace should be allowed to discipline private lives.

As with youth care, doubts and concerns regarding health promotion in the workplace are primarily defined as technical issues: as issues of effectiveness and thus of expertise. Public justification of new developments in workplace health promotion is sought through a rationalistic strategy. Knowledge institutions such as universities and the Netherlands Organization for Applied Scientific Research (TNO) have designed evidence-based programmes to assist smoking cessation, tools to measure fatigue and questionnaires to monitor workers who are at increased risk of exhaustion. For example, TNO offers companies a service by which it charts problems of poor exercise levels and employees' lifestyles and subsequently indicates the most effective solutions. TNO's promotional material reads as follows:

> Enthusiastic employees, work that inspires and work that those employees can be proud of. These are things that employees, managers, organizations and clients can all benefit from. Enthusiasm, that is what it is all about and it is increasingly an area of focus as it reduces the likelihood of health problems and has an effect on the quality of service provision ... What does TNO offer? TNO analyses the bottlenecks that exist in work processes and the factors at work that promote enthusiasm, or indeed hamper it. The analysis is based on an employee questionnaire ... In the analysis, TNO focuses on both those elements that workers enjoy and that inspire them and the bottlenecks that hamper job satisfaction ... If you would like your workers to be enthusiastic and healthy, then get in touch with us.[18]

Maastricht University similarly has developed the *Balansmeter* questionnaire, which can be used to map the risk of individual workers being absent in the future:

> We use this unique questionnaire to identify 'at-risk' employees and we prevent absence from work by providing targeted support. The Balansmeter is a scientifically-tested tool that we use in close collaboration with Maastricht University[19] ... A tool [in other words, a questionnaire] that can predict which office staff members are more likely to be absent for an extended period due to illness. A follow-up study also showed that early intervention could reduce absence rates in this group by 35%.[20]

These knowledge institutions, which are to a certain degree themselves dependent on the growing commercial market for health promotion at the work place, determine to a significant extent what is meant by 'risks' in the domain of health and work. Moreover, they lend an element of 'scientific justification' to the health promotion programmes so developed, through the rhetoric of 'measuring is knowing' that they employ. In the quest for 'effective steering and control' and for 'evidence of effectiveness', troublesome issues regarding the objectives and resources of the current 'health mission' at the workplace are pushed into the background. Moreover, organizations like trade unions do not actively address these issues. Their experience is in classic regulatory issues like dealing with toxic substances. They do not feel capable of dealing with the growing attention to the individualistic responsibility of employees and as a result their attitude is somewhat defensive. Thus while health promotion in the workplace is becoming big business and much is invested in a rationalistic justification of the programmes, the voice of employees – the subjects of these programmes – is neither heard in occupational public health nor organized to critique it.

The Missing Voice of Citizens in Vaccination Programmes

Although it was long believed that infectious diseases were on the verge of eradication, we have been startled by the rise of new epidemics in recent decades. The AIDS epidemic of the 1980s soon became associated with promiscuity, homosexuality and Africa and allowed most Western citizens to carry on believing they were rather safe.[21] However, prosperity, international travel, close proximity of humans and animals, the limitations of preventive virology and the rise of antibiotic-resistance have created conditions in which a whole range of familiar and unfamiliar disease agents may become problematic. New infections are constantly emerging, as the examples of AIDS, SARS and West Nile virus indicate and how significant such infections may become is largely unknown. Dealing with infectious disease is likely to pose many new challenges for public health in the future.

As far as prevention of the classic infectious diseases such as polio and diphtheria among children is concerned, loyal attendance at vaccination programmes could be counted on in the Netherlands for decades, except in some rather strict orthodox Protestant regions. Vaccination rates in the Netherlands were and still are high, at over 95 per cent. But the introduction of new immunization programmes is not unproblematic.[22] Turnout for the first Dutch Human Papiloma Virus (HPV) vaccination programme in 2009, designed to protect teenage girls against the HPV virus which can cause cervical cancer, was unexpectedly low. The vaccination programme raised many questions among girls and parents, but also among experts.[23] On the internet and the Dutch social networking site Hyves, parents and girls discussed issues of safety and risk of the vaccine in the long term and whether or not the vaccination programme effectively stigmatized girls as being sexually active at a very young age. In the case of vaccination against Mexican swine flu in 2009, there was also far more public discussion than had been expected and even many health care professionals refused to be vaccinated.

In both debates, attention was drawn to the potential financial interests of the pharmaceutical industry and the independence of the medical experts involved was questioned.

Reactions to these discussions varied. While some experts viewed members of the public as irrational and criticized the use of social media and internet, others argued that the communication strategy of the public health authorities had not been effective enough.[24] Both types of reactions assume, however, that the objectives of the vaccination programmes could be achieved by an instrumental technocratic strategy of steering and control; more scientific research into the effectiveness of vaccination as well as into the effectiveness of communication should point the way to public compliance. In line with this, in the attempt to ensure that more citizens are loyal to the national vaccination programme, public health institutions have stressed the need for more scientific research into how the public deals with risk information about vaccination and into how risks can better be communicated to the public. It is striking that public health policymakers and experts tried to solve the tension between experts and citizens by calling for more scientific expertise. The perspectives and experiences of citizens are not taken seriously as such, but are addressed by calling for a more evidence based communication strategy which is more oriented to steering citizens in the right direction than to understanding the perspectives, ambiguities, fears and convictions of citizens in their own right.

Questioning a Rationalistic Strategy in Public Health

To the categories of at-risk children, exhausted employees and unfamiliar viruses, we can add unhealthy neighbourhoods and risky pregnancies. The fact that citizens do not identify with the ideals of public health and do not respond to public health initiatives and interventions as expected, is regarded by public health experts primarily as a technical problem that can be resolved with increased scientific-technical evidence with respect to the effectiveness of interventions. Since the 1980s, there has, of course, been a critical counter discourse in public health: sociologists, political scientists and anthropologists realized the complexity of the public health endeavour which requires the cooperation of 'the target group'; the route from every day experiences to statistics and from statistical evidence towards effective control is mediated by citizens and by communities.[25] Sociologists, political scientists and anthropologists have argued that 'the social', 'the political' or 'the cultural' cannot simply be controlled and engineered, since they have their own dynamics. The work of philosophers like Jürgen Habermas, Paul Karl Feierabend and Michel Foucault have inspired health promotion scientists and professionals to advocate and develop bottom–up approaches, dialogue with the public, community participation and practice-based evidence.[26] Following movements like the WHO Healthy Cities initiative, critical public health researchers have reflected on the role of politics and policy processes in public health. They have called for innovations in policy processes in the direction of developing network approaches that will engage citizens and other stakeholders.[27] David Buchanan has argued that public health has embraced 'the medical model' of 'intervening' and has become blind to the notion that health promotion should involve careful learning and experimenting rather than intervening.[28] However, the impact of these initiatives has been limited and they have difficulty in escaping – in Wittgenstein's terms – the rationalistic language game of 'steering and control'. In current rationalistic political cultures the justification of dialogue and community participation ultimately lies in the effective reduction of risky behaviour, otherwise a dialogue will be regarded as a waste of scarce means. In other words, even while approaches have been developed that move beyond a technocratic discourse of steering and control, it appears to be difficult to enact these approaches in a sustainable way.

In newly emerging technological sciences – such as genomics and nanotechnology – there is an increasing awareness that knowledge of whether a technology 'works' does not ensure that these new technologies can be successfully introduced in every day practice and that interaction with civil society is of crucial importance to make the new technologies socially valid and useful. The ELSA programme (Ethical, Legal, Social Aspects) associated with the Human Genome Project set a standard. Since then, dealing with the social dimension of newly emerging technologies has become an obligatory passage point in the development of new technologies.[29] In fields like science and technology studies and innovation studies the interrelatedness of science, technology, politics and society has been studied thoroughly over the last three decades, which has resulted in new ideas about 'democratization of technology design', 'science-society interaction' and 'socially responsible and sustainable innovation'.[30] In the practice of public health sciences, however, such reflexivity is largely missing. Public health, by transforming from a social political enterprise that engaged with citizens in a social-paternalistic way into a technocratic expertocracy that focuses on steering and controlling citizens, has increasingly turned away from politics and from society. How can this development be understood?

Rationalization as a Product of Democratization

The rise of public health as an expertocracy must, of course, be considered an unplanned, unintended outcome of specific social and political processes. Public health scientists could not foresee how their work – unintentionally – contributed to the creation of expertocracy. To understand this development historians of science, sociologists and researchers in science and technology studies have pointed to the interrelatedness of processes of rationalization of professional interventions 'in the social' on the one hand and processes of democratization on the other.

The historian Theodore Porter for instance distinguishes between disciplinary and mechanical objectivity to characterize how in the twentieth century the expertise of professionals changed in relation to the growing public quest for accountability.[31] In the first half of the twentieth century, in the context of shared moral values between professionals and citizens, the paternalistic approach was a typical feature of public health. Relationships between politicians, professionals and the general public could be characterized in terms of trust. Professionals were trusted because of the specific training and experience that granted them wisdom and authority. Moreover, they represented a social elite and 'trust in professionals', as expressed in compliance to hygiene instructions, offered the lower social classes an opportunity to climb the social ladder. Government did not interfere much in the professional domain and professionals did not need to prove the value of their expertise, since professionalism was accepted by definition. In Porter's terms, professional insights and experiences were accepted because of disciplinary objectivity: in a political culture of trust, expertise was discussed among professionals but was not contested in the social and political domain. However, in the final decades of the twentieth century, relationships between politicians, professionals, experts and the public were increasingly modelled in terms of distrust. Democratization, increasing pluralism and the emancipation of citizens gave rise to greater pressure for social policies to be accountable to the public. In developing welfare states the social rights of citizens increased but growing controversies over the spending of scarce public money and increasing disputes about claims and entitlements stimulated a 'quest for accountability' and in line with that a quest for steering and control.[32] In order to justify social policies, politicians did not appeal to collective moral principles such as professional integrity and social trust, which in fact were disappearing, but rather to the authority of objective scientific knowledge. Scientific expertise came to act as a referee in the pluralistic political arena, since scientific knowledge was associated with objectivity and empirical evidence. In other words, the social sciences achieved an instrumental and technical role in democratic welfare states and became more and more interwoven with the 'bureaucratic machinery' of the state.

The growing political role of social sciences engaged with the welfare state did not leave the character of these sciences untouched. As Porter demonstrates, because of the quest for accountability in a democratic political culture, the ideal of objectivity in the social sciences and the professions involved was transformed from the disciplinary to the mechanical. In response to the quest for public accountability this expertise was becoming increasingly formalized and rationalized. Porter shows that in this formalization process one specific ideal of expertise became dominant, namely the ideal of quantitative, statistical knowledge. In modern democratic welfare states policies are increasingly backed up and accounted for and evaluated in terms of 'hard' statistical data. Thus, after the Second World War, institutions for large scale statistical research were established and the technical infrastructures for data production and data traffic continuously improved. The digital revolution in particular contributed to the flourishing of statistical research practices. In relation to processes of democratization, statistics, developed into a technology of 'trust in numbers'. In public health this development is expressed in, for instance, the dominance – in journals as well as funding bodies – of statistical research designs that aim to measure the success of public health interventions in controlled settings. As this statistical ideal of 'knowledge' is considered the basis of 'scientific evidence', reflection on this knowledge practice in public health is lacking.

Intriguingly, with the development of a rationalistic style in public health, a public health ethics has developed that criticized the older paternalistic style and that stressed the importance of autonomy, thereby defining autonomy as an informed free choice for citizens. Although this may sound like a genuine liberal-democratic approach, the actual options available to citizens were not that great. While in the past civic freedom was limited by moral values and the authority of professionals, it has now become limited by scientific, statistical risk assessments and evidence-based preventive strategies. Whether the issue be one of bringing up children, smoking, diet, exercise or pre-natal screening, public health experts feel that people should be guided by their expertise to make 'the right' – or the 'healthy' – choices. Of course, citizens have an 'exit' option, namely the unhealthy option, but in current public health formulations this is not regarded as a real option but rather as irrational behaviour. Thus the field of public health appears to be stuck between an expert-driven rationalistic approach to public health on the one hand and an ethics that stresses the importance of autonomous choice on the other.

Lacking Evidence or Lacking Social Practices of Citizenship?

The rationalization of professional practices may have paradoxical effects, however. Initially, these processes resulted in greater authority of experts such as epidemiologists and health scientists since they possessed something that the general public does not, namely databases, statistics and an 'ideology of evidence'. Experts developed the power to determine risks and the gap between experts and the lay public grew. However, as Porter argues, such processes of rationalization are sooner or later followed by a process in which trust in experts and professionals is replaced by trust in the ability of their tools – statistics, standards and explicit methodological rules – to identify and calculate risks. And when statistics, formal procedures and methods constitute how public services are provided, the clients of these public services – the average child, the average worker, the average citizen – will be homogenized and made in to objects of control, but experts and professionals become mutually homogenous, measurable, controllable and exchangeable as well. The increasing pressure of accountability in the public domain leads to a situation in which scientific and professional experts are increasingly required to 'prove' by 'objective' indicators and standards that the work they do is valuable. With the advent of the 'audit society',[33] public health practices are caught between performance indicators and a critical public on the one hand and a one-size-fits-all approach and customized preventive strategies on the other and the authority of experts is increasingly contested by both politics and the public.

This analysis leads to the conclusion that the current problems in public health should not be diagnosed in terms of lack of scientific expertise but in terms of neglect of democracy, pluralism and active citizenship. Paradoxically, democratization results in the rationalization of politics, which in turn results, unintentionally, in the democratization of expertise. If experts become engaged in policy and politics, their claims become increasingly infected by political pluralism and as such are held up to democratic transparency, scrutiny and debate. In this context, the current cry for more evidence-based interventions in response to failure to discipline people into a healthy lifestyle misses the point. The presumed authority of experts to guide the life choices of citizens fails in a political culture that appears to fit the rationalistic approach to public health really well, in the sense that it has become characterized by a striving for rationality and science-based policymaking. The reason for this is not that scientific expertise is not valuable, but that too much is expected from it in a pluralist democratic society.

In the context of a historical reconstruction of the changing relations between policy, experts, professionals and citizens, it is more appropriate to diagnose the gap between public health ambitions and results in terms of a clash of 'experts' and 'citizens' claims and values rather than in terms of lack of evidence about effective management of citizens' risk behaviour. Citizens may doubt that vaccination is safe or they have other concerns and priorities in life than dieting and quitting smoking, even when they think it would be wise to do so. These 'facts of social life' cannot simply be overruled by the provision of more risk information and the design of more effective interventions. Any such attempt would further exacerbate the vicious circle of distrust between state, experts and citizens. Historical analysis can teach us that to resolve the misfit between policy and practice in public health, experts should not focus on the question of which instruments, methods and technologies are required to make non-compliant citizens compliant, but should reflect on the relationship between science, politics and society in shaping public health as a democratic practice of citizenship. In this respect, a pragmatic approach might be helpful.

A Pragmatic View

A pragmatic view of public health does not characterize relationships between politicians, scientists, professionals and the public in terms of blind trust in the authority and integrity of professionals – in other words, traditional paternalism. Nor does it define these relationships in terms of trust in objective knowledge and statistical evidence, steering and control. It defines these relations in terms of experimentation and public learning.[34] From a pragmatic perspective, public health should be considered a practice of democratic citizenship in the sense that, by taking citizen perspectives seriously and by actively organizing dialogue and deliberation, it continuously frames, shapes and enables citizen voice, autonomy and responsibility. In this formulation, people are regarded not as individuals but as citizens who work together with experts, professionals and policymakers to shape public health and the risks and relations that make up public health. But, it may be asked, why is it necessary to replace the language of steering (and control) by a language of learning?

According to philosophers, science and technology researchers and sociologists such as Herman van Gunsteren, Zygmunt Bauman, Ulrich Beck and Michel Callon, present-day global and technologically-advanced risk cultures and their most important institutions can be characterized as in principle – epistemological as well as political – uncertain, unpredictable and unknowable, although more knowledge and information is available than ever before.[35] There is no central Archimedean point from which to develop an objective view on reality: all knowledge is partial and temporary. Political institutions as well as economic markets have proved to be more unstable than we assumed and neither the Pope nor the Cochrane database can offer definitive guidance.[36] In order to boost the resilience of such an 'unknowable' society, it is important when it comes to controversial issues that we do not focus solely on steering by technical knowledge, but instead organize public learning processes that mobilize and reproduce pluralism and diversity. Herman van Gunsteren considers dealing with plurality as one of the most important capacities of citizenship in an 'unknown society', because plurality is a main stimulus for public learning processes. Without differences, these learning processes would be blocked. For example, issues relating to the introduction of genetic knowledge and technology into society have not only been framed as problems of effectiveness to be dealt with by genetic experts, but also as public, moral and political issues. By exploring facets of these issues through public debate and deliberation, new 'experimental' genetic practices have been developed in which ideas about the use of genetic knowledge and technology are technically and socially tested.[37] Considering the current state of public health as diagnosed above and considering the tension between expertocracy and democracy as it developed in the twentieth century, public health might also be considered in need of public learning processes and new practices of citizenship. Instead of stressing that smokers, fat people, irresponsible parents and vaccination refuters should learn from experts about individual behaviour change, the question should rather be how to learn from the daily life experiences of smokers and fat people and to reflect how interaction and dialogue between policymakers, experts, professionals and citizens might help to co-shape public health as a societal practice. To be sure, from a pragmatic perspective citizens are not considered as individual actors, but as embedded by social relations. Instead of celebrating a quasi-neo-republican ideal of citizenship, public health needs to explore how it actually might create a real republican ideal of citizenship and how it can contribute to a social world in which this kind of citizenship might flourish.

In order to be able to learn from controversial issues and the unintentional consequences of public health practices, these issues need to be articulated as public issues.[38] The problem of public health, however, is that controversial issues are poorly identified and do not find a place on the public agenda. By focussing on evidence rather than on controversial issues, policymakers, experts and professionals do not stimulate public reflection and do not contribute to 'making' public issues, which also implies that they neither actively engage 'a public'. Parents, children, employees, target vaccination groups – these are not mobilized as participants in the public sphere, as citizens. In the curative care sector, the patient's perspective has gradually been taken more seriously over the last twenty years, expressed in a legal discourse of patients' rights as well as a growing importance of clients in the governance of health care organizations and more client-centred care. In Dutch mental health care institutions 'lay experts' have been appointed to facilitate professional learning from the lay knowledge and experience of being psychotic or schizophrenic, or of being placed in isolation. Public health as a provider of collective care and as contributor to the public good, might be expected to engage its public, yet in reality it does not allow the public a voice. Because of the mechanisms described above and even more through competition with curative medicine to acquire social standing as a disciplinary field, public health has developed a rationalistic style and has turned its back on its main 'client' – society or the public. The tragedy of modern public health is that by breaking away from 'the public', it has become disconnected from its main object as well as from a source of public learning. The rationalistic strategy of guidance through knowledge has turned overweight women, powerless parents and fatigued men into objects and denies their capacity to generate knowledge and provide interpretations, as well as to contribute towards defining public health. The work of the philosopher Herman van Gunsteren suggests that a refusal to learn from differences constitutes a threat to the resilience of public health and society.[39] The work of science and technology scholar Sheila Jasanoff indicates that a rationalistic strategy should be considered as a 'technology of hubris' that embodies a risk to socially-robust knowledge as it will result in a growing distrust in the authority of expertise.[40] The ethicist Miranda Fricker's concept of epistemic injustice makes clear that it can be a kind of injustice to refuse to take seriously the experiences, ideas and interpretations of 'the object' of public health.[41]

A pragmatic approach that fosters and promotes plurality does not signal the end of public accountability, but a broadening of it: such an approach requires that experts and professionals test their ideas about prevention strategies much more rigorously. Testing should occur not only in the (quasi-)controlled setting of scientific study, but also in the uncontrolled social environment of parents, employees and other groups involved in public health – in deliberative democracy. Precisely because the success of public health policies and interventions cannot be guaranteed, because these are fundamentally uncertain practices, because the standard for success can be called into doubt and because multiple and competing ideals exist with regard to what constitutes healthy living, the public must not be regarded as an object to be dealt with but as the co-constructor of public health. To that end, controversies over knowledge and values must not be avoided but encouraged. As society is the core business of public health, it must therefore be taken seriously, not as a collection of individual citizens who have a choice to live healthy, but as citizenry constituted in socially embedded practises. A change in perspective, from a rationalistic to a pragmatic approach, has many implications. Concepts such as professional responsibility, change, implementation, intervention, evaluation and quality, as well as methodical strategies, must be reconsidered and practices reorganized. However, this is the only way for researchers and professionals to regain authority and trust in a society in which they are no longer automatically placed on a pedestal.

Conclusion

The introduction to this book argued that today we see the shift from social-liberal or social-democratic ideals of citizenship into a neo-republican ideal of citizenship, which stresses individual rights as well as responsibilities. In my reconstruction of the development of the interrelations between policy, science, professions and citizenship in public health, the Netherlands serves as the case study. I have argued that despite a neo-republican rhetoric of autonomous choice and individual responsibility, neo-republican ideals are not practised in public health and that it is better to speak of a *quasi*-neo-republican notion of citizenship. There is no structural engagement with social practices of citizenship – on local, national or international levels – and there is too little awareness of the social embeddings of citizenship. This diagnosis explicitly takes into account the changing role of public health sciences and public health professions in the context of processes of democratization. The focus on the interrelationship between policy, science, professionals and citizens demonstrates how a somewhat paradoxical trend of both democratization and rationalization puts a limit to the development of neo-republican citizenship. However, public health may not be a special case. Paying more attention to how science and technology may affect citizenship in curative health, mental health and other domains of health, will provide further insight into whether the hypothesis of the rise of neo-republican citizenship in the field of illness and health will hold.

10 UNDERWRITING CITIZENSHIP: THE INTRODUCTION OF PREDICTIVE MEDICINE IN PRIVATE INSURANCE

Ine Van Hoyweghen

> The fear, amongst some, that medical examinations in insurance may create some imperfection cult, in line with the propaganda of the rights of the imperfect to have their place under the economic sun and that it will be difficult for the imperfect to sustain themselves economically due to insurance medical examinations, is in general unfounded.[1]

During the expansion of the private insurance business at the end of the nineteenth century, the practice of medical underwriting in private insurance became a subject of public debate.[2] Since then, the issue has virtually disappeared from the public agenda. Medical risk selection has been accepted as a routine step in the application procedure for private life insurance, while medicine's gatekeeper role in insurance has rarely been criticized. The legitimacy of this practice rests in the scientific medico-actuarial dealing with risks via the development of actuarial science, mortality tables, medical expertise and technologies. The rise of predictive medicine, however, has prompted new debates on the issue of medical selection in private insurance, bringing the relationship between medicine and insurance back into the foreground.

Over the past decade the potential of genetics for understanding health and disease in radically new ways has been widely discussed. Genetic researchers anticipate that it will be possible to test for a variety of susceptibility genes and consider appropriate prevention strategies. Others view this attention to genetics as part of an existing transformation from a clinical, complaints-bound medicine to a predictive, risk-oriented medicine. Since the 1970s, new disciplines have taken shape within public health and prenatal care that have contributed to a framework in which problems of health and disease have become problems of health *risks*, shifting the focus from symptoms and treatment to pre-symptomatic diagnosis and preventive intervention. Where once health was defined as the 'present absence of disease', it might now be better understood as the 'absence of an increased statistical chance of future disease'. New intermediate or in-between health categories have emerged where individuals are identified as 'risk carriers', derived from risk probabilities and statistical correlations. People identified as being at high risk for, say, breast cancer, inhabit an intermediate disease state as neither necessarily healthy nor ill, they are neither 'already diseased' nor are they 'disease free'. The introduction of predictive medicine, then, is likely to change our definitions of health and disease. On a broader level, this shift towards a predictive style in medicine may redistribute responsibilities of individuals, health care institutions and the state concerning both public and personal health.

Given medicine's gatekeeper role in private insurance, it is not surprising that the issue of predictive medicine is intriguing in the context of insurance because assessing people's health forms the very criterion for access to private life insurance. Predictive medicine is to be expected to play a prominent role in the design of insurance risk profiles and risk categorization of high and low risk applicants. In this chapter, I will reflect on the introduction of predictive medicine in private life insurance. I will demonstrate how private insurance, in applying the new definitions of health and disease of predictive medicine, contributes to new conceptualizations and ideals of citizenship. In doing so, I will connect with broader sociologies on risk society, neo-liberal governmentality and the individualization of responsibility for health.[3] For, as we will see, the framing of predictive medicine in insurance is consonant with contemporary neo-republican emphases on individual responsibility for health, self-governance and a prudential approach to controlling and transforming one's future.

In this way, the chapter will outline the role of private insurance as an important producer of ideals and competencies linked up with health and citizenship. Drawing on contributions from sociology of insurance, insurance institutions do not simply or passively reflect wider social and cultural visions on health and citizenship. Rather, in creating risk categories and selecting risk profiles, insurance actively *produces* a range of moral duties, civic virtues and cultural values, for example on what counts as a 'suitable life' in insurance.[4] Private insurance is a method of organizing mutual aid by deciding which citizens qualify or disqualify as members. As a 'normative technology',[5] it defines the criteria and norms to be eligible in insurance, contributing to the development of the ideals and competencies linked to ideals of citizenship. As D. Stone has argued: 'Insurance is a social institution that helps define norms and values in political culture and ultimately shapes how citizens think about issues of membership, community, responsibility and moral obligation'.[6] This role of insurance as a 'norm-giver' is articulated in the insurers' management of moral attitudes – towards savings, welfare, health, life and death.[7] But above all, it is expressed in the management of moral hazard of insurance applicants in the process of underwriting.

While insurers have always been concerned with the control of moral hazard, I argue that the introduction of predictive medicine enables the insurance industry to control the 'immoral' in a medically and technically mediated way. New predictive technologies allow insurers to evaluate our behaviour towards our health, or our capacity to control our health. Moreover, these developments create the possibility of tightening the norms for 'suitable lives' in insurance, increasing the conditions to be fulfilled as part of the insurance group. In playing a gatekeeper role in insurance, predictive medicine therefore performs an important part in creating the ideals and competencies linked to current ideals of neo-republican citizenship.

The material presented here is part of a research project on the construction of risk in private life insurance.[8] Research included ethnographic fieldwork in Belgian insurance companies (2001–4) and in international reinsurance companies (2005–6), analysis of national and international primary written insurance sources on medical underwriting, interviews with key persons in the European life insurance market and an analysis of secondary historical sources on medical underwriting in private insurance. The central focus has been on life insurers' assemblage work in performing medical underwriting and the heterogeneous considerations, tools and ingredients involved in transforming insurance applicants into insurance risks. One major strategy relied on was following an insurance risk 'trajectory',[9] from the initial application to the final risk assessment, with particular attention to the different 'inscription devices' used by medical underwriters,[10] like reinsurance manuals, guidelines, computer programmes, statistics and forms (medical questionnaires, protocols) that frame the underwriting process. The material has been analysed using the software program Nvivo.

Managing Moral Hazard in Insurance: Insurers as Producers of Ideals of Citizenship

The development of the private insurance industry is commonly traced back to the opening of Edward Lloyd's coffee house in Tower Street, London, in 1687.[11] Many of the insurance principles for coping with the vagaries of seventeenth-century maritime trade continue to underpin today's life and health insurance industry. While insurers provide for the pooling of risks and mutual aid among policyholders, at the same time, they also select their policyholders in advance, group them and price them according to market considerations. To this end, they rely on the principle of risk classification. It holds that premium rates should be differentiated so that each person will pay in accordance with his or her 'risk quality'.[12] Underwriting is the method to assess this 'risk quality' and to classify people according to their risk profile into 'standard', 'substandard' or 'excluded' risks. According to insurance logic, underwriting is essential to the workings of private insurance because the insurance relationship takes the form of a private contract and, as such, it fulfils the requirement regarding the validity of consent. Insurance contracts must be made *uberrima fides* – in the utmost good faith – with full disclosure from the applicant. This is particularly important because the insurance applicants' knowledge regarding their risk status may also affect their insurance behaviour. In insurance terms, this is the principle of moral hazard. Moral hazard arises when insurance applicants misrepresent information while applying for insurance, resulting in increased costs (claims) for the insurance company (or other policyholders).

A central concern for any insurance company is therefore determining which applicants they can accept and which ones they cannot. The idea was (and continues to be) that there are certain types of individuals whose characteristics or morals lead them to be less cautious, or worse, to cause losses in search of payments. For example, the immoral homeowner might try to burn his home down for the insurance money. Or the malingerer might try to defraud the insurance company for accident insurance coverage. The whole underwriting process is exactly the *raison d'être* in insurance for predicting and controlling this moral hazard. Several detection tools trace where dishonesty and non-performance are likely to occur, refusing insurance in some instances ('excluded risk') and adjusting premiums in others ('substandard risks'). Whenever moral hazard is identified, individual financial responsibility is claimed by refusing cover or having to pay a substandard rate. In other words, making the 'morally hazardous' share *a priori* the cost burden of risk – by paying higher premiums or excluding them – encourages citizens to act in a responsible manner. To be 'beyond insurance' is therefore often seen as a moral assessment that a person is imprudent or even irresponsible.

In producing the conditions and criteria for eligibility for insurance, insurance therefore contributes to the development of ideals and competencies linked up with citizenship. In this respect, private insurance is a form of discipline or social control, of inculcating norms, supervising behaviours and enforcing compliance.[13] Private insurers' attempts to manage moral hazard reflect and reinforce moral duties and cultural values on people's 'trustworthiness'. So private insurers do not just manage or spread risks. In producing risk categories, they also regulate behaviour, by excluding some and mandating the conditions of inclusion for others. As Stone puts it: 'Insurance underwriting, far from being a dry statistical exercise, is a political exercise in drawing the boundaries of community membership'.[14] By defining criteria on 'suitable lives' (as a way of preventing moral hazard), insurers put boundaries between those who are 'Accepted' members of society and those who form the 'Other'.[15] Like certification societies, standard-setting bodies and credit inspectors, insurers make evaluations of who is worthy or not, while other organizations rely on these risk assessments by insurance companies. In this way, private insurance has always been an important producer of reigning ideals and competencies linked up with citizenship.

At the beginning of the industry, life insurers had carefully to select what were called 'quality lives' in order to keep the 'immoral' at bay.[16] In preventing this moral hazard, insurers gradually resorted to the profession of medicine with the medical examination of the insurance candidate's life. Yet assessing the general health of an individual was a challenge. It was usually sufficient for the applicant to submit a signed declaration of health, denying experiences of serious diseases such as smallpox or cowpox and to include references by third parties, including friends, particularly regarding 'habits' like intemperance. Medical examiners had to rely heavily on the applicant's word and on oral or written testimonies, which were scarcely adequate. As T. M. Porter notes, these 'quality of life' assessments were 'rather like admitting someone to a gentleman's club. The company had to be satisfied that the applicant was honourable and trustworthy'.[17] In this regard, medical knowledge was subordinate to a general assessment of dignity and morality, in terms of (particularly middle-class) values and civic virtues, such as prudence and moderation, personal responsibility and self-help.[18] Underwriting standards in the nineteenth century were thus informed as much by the medical examiner's judgements of membership in society, as by qualities relating to the actual health of the applicant. In defining the criteria of health and insurability in line with the reigning norms of membership to society, insurance companies contributed to ideals and norms linked to *liberal citizenship*. At the beginning of the twentieth century, the insurance industry increasingly met with criticism and distrust. The public saw medical examinations as suspect because they were dependent on the medical advisor's judgement. Moreover, the public increasingly demanded the insurability of people who did not meet the insurance business's standards for insurability but who still had a very low risk of early death. A notion of equality of opportunity within the market for life insurance had become evident. The insured life was considered no longer exclusive to the 'healthy, wealthy', but there was growing demand that lower middle-class and even working-class applicants should be entitled to life insurance, as a means of social citizenship. Insurers, for their part, shared this interest in marketing towards 'the great mass of people' for profit reasons. They began to speculate on the development of a whole new enterprise of insuring 'lesser', 'half' or 'unsuitable' lives, that would extend their market. The insurance industry began to develop a more *objective* approach of medicine, by resorting to an extended assortment of medical measurements. This resulted in the establishment of a specific classification scheme in insurance, called the numerical rating system.[19] The idea of judging an applicant was replaced by mathematically justified matrices and objective measuring tools that rate individuals according to their risk and charge them an appropriate premium. The development of this system, including the extensive mortality investigations prompted by it, facilitated a vast expansion of 'substandard' underwriting, expanding the insurance business's potential clientele. With the insuring of the unhealthy, private insurance interests in up-scaling of markets reflected a more general social and political process of democratization (towards modern mass-society). In liberalizing the conditions for insurability and in expanding insurance cover to more people, private insurance, with the aid of medicine, was contributing to the then reigning ideals of *social citizenship* – with an emphasis on entitlement to income-guarantees for the working class, fostering self-control and social responsibility and binding claimants into a system of solidarity and mutual obligation.[20] In this way, medical expertise and testing instruments played an important role in re-establishing public trust in insurance, reconciling the economic interests of the insurance industry with societal interests while articulating the *public* role of medicine and insurance.

In the past decades, the insurance industry has introduced more medical test instruments and, recently, it seems that the relevance of these technologies has only increased.[21] What these new technologies most of all reveal is that they are *predictive*, enhancing the detection of predictive markers in the body and, as such, affecting the applicant's insurability. Moreover, these technologies are capable of 'quantifying' lifestyle behaviour. Thanks to the new predictive technologies, insurers are able to 'measure' our individual health behaviour and our individual responsibility towards health. In the next sections, I will discuss in more detail private insurers' control of moral hazard through predictive medicine (lifestyle and genetic predictive health information) and reflect on the consequences this has for the production of current ideals and competencies of citizenship.

Lifestyle as Predictive Health Information in Private Insurance

If we take a look at private insurers' current medical underwriting, 'lifestyle underwriting' is a trend that is increasingly being deployed by insurance companies. As this website of an international reinsurance company for example states:

> Lifestyle indicators such as sports, diet, stress, weight and smoking are becoming more and more important for lifelong health conditions. They have a substantial impact on life expectancy. Future underwriting systems will be based to a vast extent on these indicators.[22]

In the course of fieldwork it became clear that the underwriters paid much attention to lifestyle characteristics. Invariably, when tracing medical information from applicants, they alluded to notions of 'lifestyle risks':

> We are most of all presented with things like depression. And also diseases arising from high affluence like increased liver values, high blood pressure and so. Or increase of blood sugar levels. So these are all matters, well, that deal with stress and bad life habits. Really things one can do something about, in my opinion. So that usually happens most of the time.[23]

In the same way, the instruments and forms used to assess the insurance applicant's health reflect this attention to lifestyle. The medical questionnaire, for example, entails an exclusive section dedicated to questions about weight, alcohol use, smoking and drug use. The section was headed 'Important Information', with the lifestyle questions highlighted in grey to attract extra attention. The same attention to lifestyle is again seen in the statistics constituting the risk calculations. A recent internal company actuarial study, documented the following 'pre-existent conditions' with an excess mortality: under and overweight, alcoholism, hypertension, smoking, depression and cardiac abnormalities. Based on the study, the company's management decided to increase the premium for these characteristics. Originally, however, they were somewhat hesitant about selecting insurance applicants on the basis of health-behaviour characteristics alone. They acknowledged that, if this information was only derived from the medical questionnaire, it could give rise to fraud by insurance applicants. To overcome this, the decision was made that an extra premium would be charged only in those cases where this information could be corroborated by more 'objective' instruments, like blood analysis, liver tests, lung radiography or a codeine test. Thanks to these technologies, lifestyle characteristics thus can be *objectified* and *quantified* and, as such, considered as a legitimate base to charge extra premiums.

The guidelines from reinsurance companies on cholesterol level and overweight further underline the relevance of lifestyle characteristics. While these risk factors statistically indicate an increased chance of developing a possible future disease, they are constructed in insurance as *primary* mortality risks, as the *independent* basis for excess mortality and thus for charging extra premiums. That is, they are conceived in a qualitatively similar way to 'pre-existent conditions', defined as 'past illness and current health status',[24] as the example of increased cholesterol level illustrates. A high cholesterol level indicates a greater risk of arterial congestion or other cardiovascular abnormalities. For insurers, a high cholesterol level is taken directly as synonymous with extra mortality risk. The same logic is manifest in the calculation of those who are overweight. There is thus a tendency in insurance underwriting to *reify* predictive lifestyle risk factors as independent mortality risks.[25] Accordingly, these lifestyle characteristics are considered as already 'pre-existent conditions', or as 'pre-existent impairments' or 'abnormalities'. Insurers thus transform epidemiological risks (defined as probabilities for future disease) into pre-existent conditions or abnormalities. Probabilistic risk factors become physical abnormalities or impairments requiring exclusion or an increased premium. Moreover, by constructing these lifestyle risk factors as 'impairments', intervention and prevention are highlighted, stressing individual responsibility for health. So people with some lifestyle risk factors are seen by insurers as already ill and what is more, as people responsible for causing their own illness and therefore deserving of an extra premium.

In addition to the use of lifestyle risk factors as primary mortality risks, lifestyle characteristics also appear to be relevant in rating applicants already suffering from (other) impairments. As such, the manuals indicate that lifestyle is used to *adjust* the statistically average substandard premium for a particular disorder. By asking extra information, via the applicant's GP or the medical expert's examination, lifestyle characteristics are revealed concerning the circumstances of the disorder. These are used as positive or negative prognosis determining factors in the individual risk assessment. In that way, personalized clinical information, including the time of onset, periods of relapse, course of the disorder, reactions to treatment and causes can be traced to influence the final risk assessment. For example, in the case of high cholesterol level, underwriters can ask multiple test values with time intervals as a way to assess whether the person takes his or her medication regularly to stabilize the cholesterol level:

> Here is the GP letter with the examinations of the last two years and you see [points to section in the letter]: these blood values are continuously fine. So I think this man is following his treatment with pills quite well, there are no excesses in these values you see? He's holding his disease under control. So I'll accept him now at a better rate.[26]

In other words, the issue of compliant behaviour now comes to the fore. Not only is the medical risk a subject of assessment but also the moral risk, the patient's reliability and disease management. Applicants are charged with responsibility for their own health. If they are good patients, they are rewarded with a reduced premium. If instead they are disobedient, they will be charged extra rates.

Above all, the insurers' smoking policy is an indication that lifestyle is assuming an ever more prominent role in insurance underwriting. Currently, smoking is used as a risk-classification factor and smokers are charged a substandard premium.[27] The statistical studies of life insurance companies all seem to target smokers as a relevant risk group. For example, one study notes that 'smoking up to now has been significantly under-rated, both in itself and in combination with other impairments'.[28] In addition, smoking has also recently been introduced into the calculation of the standard premium. Whereas the standard premium usually is calculated according to non-medical characteristics, like age, capital sum assured and sex, the smoking factor is now also included. In practice, this means that, at the start of the medical underwriting, the standard rate is calculated on the basis of smoking. If afterwards it turns out that the applicant is in fact a non-smoker, he can get a reduced standard rate. On the other hand, in the case of a smoker, the person will have to pay the increased smoking 'standard' rate. Yet, if it concerns a heavy smoker (that is defined in the guidelines as: 'smoking more than 2 packets a day'), the person will have to pay an additional extra premium above the standard smoking rate. This further illustrates how normative views around individual responsibility for health are embedded in underwriting. By calculating the standard premium based on 'smoking', the non-smokers are rewarded. In explaining this strategy, the management claimed they wished to make their clients responsible for their health. But besides penalizing the unhealthy smokers, this strategy was also a means of attracting the healthy clients:

> Instead of the usual option of charging the unhealthy people, we took the option to reduce the standard premium in case of non-smoking. In doing so, we wanted to give a sign to our applicants, that their lifestyle really matters. So when they don't smoke, the company remunerates them by giving them a reduced standard rate. And of course, we find it more positive if an applicant is originally charged at the smoking standard rate and if he turns out to be a non-smoker that we can charge him less, then in reverse, if he declares to be a non-smoker and then afterwards the codeine test shows he is a smoker and he has to pay more. The first strategy is more customer-friendly, isn't it?[29]

Consequently, the new smoking policy reinforces the difference between a healthy and unhealthy lifestyle.

Making the Normal Deviant

The introduction of predictive lifestyle information in private insurance raises questions about the meaning of the standard rate in insurance. After all, the use of predictive lifestyle risk factors contributes to the idea of the 'worried well', the idea that we are neither yet ill, nor completely healthy. But, for insurers, as I have demonstrated, if your health behaviour is considered risky, you are considered 'already ill'. In that way, more and more conditions are stipulated in order to be able to receive insurance at a standard rate. In this situation, the margin for being normal is actually quite small and the scope for deviation relatively wide. Predictive medicine eliminates more and more risk factors from the standard rate in insurance, eroding the standard rate to some extent, which results in a far more restricted meaning of what counts as 'healthy' or 'normal' in life and health insurance. Normality (as conceived in the assessment of 'standard risk') in insurance has been transformed from a state of health as the *absence of past and current illness* to a state of health defined as *risk resistant*. Predictive medicine thus 'immunizes' the standard rate in insurance against risk, by deploying a new definition of health as 'risk resistance', that way widening the indicators of excess mortality risks and making the conditions of insurability more stringent.

As we have seen, at the beginning of the twentieth century, medical knowledge and technologies were specifically devised in insurance to allow 'unsuitable' or 'half' lives to participate in the insurance group, with the creation of 'substandard risks' in insurance. By establishing mortality statistics for particular disorders and tools for assessing excess mortality risk, these people, instead of being declined, have been integrated into the insurance risk pool, as a way to *normalize* them. Today however, the new knowledge of predictive medicine is increasingly restricting the conditions for access to the insurance risk pool. To some extent, this suggests that people are increasingly being *made abnormal* in insurance. Ironically, while our average life expectancy increases, the norm to be accepted at standard rate in insurance narrows. The *norm* for 'standard risk' in insurance thus becomes more detached from the *average* health status.

This tendency is also underpinned by current insurance market trends towards the marketing of products to 'preferred lives', where individuals are subjected to medical underwriting in return for a *reduction* in the standard premium. Is the 'standard rate' in insurance more accurately expressed then as a 'more-than-standard' rate? Or do these tendencies mean that our social and cultural norms and ideals of health have changed to a more stringent definition of health? As an insurer comments on preferred underwriting in the American market:

> When did 'standard' become rated? As preferred products have evolved, we've encountered a further stratifying of the standard class, with ever increasing variations in the criteria used to classify these risks. In many respects, standard has been recast as preferred and we've created additional substandard categories ... Now everything but preferred is considered a rated class ... A word is no more than a symbol of a concept. Healthy individuals once were labelled standard, now we're calling them preferred.[30]

In increasing the range of risk factors by the use of predictive medicine in insurance, potentially fewer insurance applicants are assessed into the standard category, prompting the question who may still fulfil the conditions to be rated as 'standard risk' or as 'suitable life' in the future? A reinsurance spokesman discusses the preferred life policy approach thus:

> The initial intention was certainly a valid one, i.e. to apply more efficiently the principles of risk classification and charge policyholders more accurately for the cost of their cover, thereby emphasizing a healthy lifestyle. The practical result of such an approach, however, is that for an increasing number of people, i.e. those which do not qualify as Preferred Lives or those belonging to segments of the population which do not retain the interest of product development units, insurance may become more and more expensive, possibly unaffordable, or even unavailable![31]

The above tendencies can be considered as a continuation of the medical underwriting workings in insurance. Insurers have always been concerned with the management of moral hazard through underwriting. But clearly, the involvement of increasing predictive lifestyle technologies represents a precedent in insurance practice. Predictive medicine in private insurance may promote a dynamic of health standards that excludes more and more people who cannot meet them. By broadening its scope to the detection and prognosis of illness in the future, predictive medicine may lead to increasing exclusion from insurance, 'undoing' the democratization process in insurance which since the twentieth century has been linked to ideals of *social citizenship*, while bringing increasingly more people in danger of being marginalized as second-class citizens.

'Behave': Assessing the Capacity to Self-Control

Predictive medicine brings to the fore not only our medical characteristics, but also our moral behaviour in relation to our health. By stressing the relevance of lifestyle to financial incentives or penalties, insurers focus on individual self-control over health risks, or our body maintenance. In expanding the definition of health in insurance towards self-control over health, present-day insurance contributes to new ideals and competencies linked up with citizenship. The individual responsibility for preventing illness is part of a broader public morality in which one is expected to be as little a nuisance to others as possible, avoid social dependency and display a sense of autonomy. In this ideal of neo-republican citizenship, the balance is shifted from rights and entitlements to responsibilities and obligations, with an emphasis on the idea that individual behaviour should be in the interest of personal health, or else demonstrates lack of self-control. The concept of health, as deployed by predictive medicine in insurance, frames the insurance applicant as active and self-conscious, ultimately responsible for the assessment and avoidance of risk and his/her own health and well-being. In this way, health becomes associated with the older republican ideals of 'virtuousness' and managing one's relation to health has currently become an important means by which individuals can express their ethical selves, fulfilling their obligations as neo-republican citizens.

Insurers can trace to what extent an applicant is capable of controlling his health through the measurement of lifestyle characteristics. If you are showing responsibility for your health, you will get your insurance at standard rate but if you display *irresponsible* behaviour you must pay an appropriate rate. Accordingly, normality in insurance expresses a morally embedded (neo-)republican civic notion of control over health. By ascribing these moral claims to applicants, insurers contribute to the construction of the *voluntary* character of lifestyle risks. Identifying fault and blame is the basis for penalization. Where the disease is not your fault, you will be considered a *victim*.

> We are increasingly confronted with obesity, high blood pressure, diabetes. These are the main disorders for the moment. And the heavy smokers of course, let's not forget them. Besides that, you have their 'anti-poles', like the cancers. Those are the legitimate victims, really.[32]

Requesting extra premiums from people who exhibit bad lifestyles forms the basis of an *own-fault* approach in insurance; those who demonstrate 'good manners' to their own health will be rewarded, and those who fail to do so must face the consequences (that is: paying extra premium). So we see here a form of 'healthism' in insurance, where insurance applicants are expected to be active in keeping and optimizing their health by adopting a good lifestyle, thereby appealing to and producing a neo-republican ideal of citizenship stressing the reflexive, competent and entrepreneurial self.

Measuring Trustworthiness

The use of predictive lifestyle factors in insurance not only emphasizes responsible health behaviour but also fabricates the trustworthiness of applicants. As we have seen, this positioning of people in a trustworthiness continuum in insurance is again not new, quite the reverse. Insurance institutions have always been concerned with the management of moral hazard. The argument here is that the emergence of predictive lifestyle risk assessment has taken shape within these historical continuities in insurance. By increasing the scope of lifestyle predictive risk factors in epidemiology and predictive medico-actuarial techniques, insurers are able to take into account moral characteristics in a new way. Nineteenth-century assessments of moral judgement of applicants (for example, 'the total abstainers') have undergone important shifts, notably a quantification and objectification of lifestyle behaviour through predictive medicine. Moral judgements on the applicant's moral hazard have been translated into the morally *neutral* considered medical devices of predictive technologies. Lifestyle behaviour can be traced in insurance through the objective expert risk assessment of lifestyle predictive technologies and testing instruments, lifestyle statistics, insurance manuals and guidelines. Objective predictive measures have thus become the basis on which the moral duty of insurance applicants is currently taking shape.

And yet there are also some discontinuities here. The increasing availability of predictive technologies further enhances or takes beyond its limits the idea of the controllability of death in insurance.[33] From the fatalism of an inevitable death we are now enmeshed in a view of mortality that is *individually* controllable. The introduction of predictive medicine comes with an individual 'duty to prevent', indicating a shift from collective responsibility for the consequences of illness to individual responsibility for the prevention of illness. Where once managing moral hazard may have been the primary responsibility of insurers (via risk selection), it is increasingly that of individuals, mediated through predictive technologies. From a *collective* risk management (via insurance risk selection), a shift moves towards an *a priori*, *individualized* risk management. By stressing individual responsibility for health as a condition for insurability, insurers are, to some extent, requesting that applicants institute 'safety measures' as preconditions for insurance coverage – as, for example, would be the case in buildings insurance where a policy may be offered only where fire and theft prevention devices have been installed. Predictive technologies increasingly play a similar role, especially as financial inducements for people to alter their health behaviour. A good lifestyle as a sign of individual responsibility for health has become decisive in offering insurance cover and at what cost. And of course, this is likely to play an important role in reshaping the wider public and cultural dynamics of accountability for health.

The Involuntary Character of Genetic Risks in Private Insurance

How did Belgian insurers deal with predictive *genetic* information? This issue has been, to a large extent, confined to and regulated by the Belgian Insurance Law.[34] In fact, Belgium has been one of the first European countries introducing a legal prohibition on the use of genetic data by insurance companies. In practice, however, Belgian underwriters are exceptionally confronted with genetic test results or genetic information (such as with Down syndrome, cystic fibrosis and Huntington). In these cases, the general rule was to refer the risk to the reinsurance company. Moreover, Belgian law does not prohibit *to the letter* the use of family history. All insurance companies analysed in the study asked for family history in the medical questionnaire or requested this type of information from GP or specialists' reports.

The underwriting policies were, however, fairly reticent about the use of family medical history in their risk assessment. First of all, when receiving incomplete answers to the family history question, the questionnaire would not necessarily be returned to the applicant. Further, in the underwriting guidelines, this information only played a denying or confirming role in regard to disorders an applicant might already suffer from. As in the case of a person with cardiovascular problems:

> If the person himself shows some symptoms related to cardiovascular diseases, then family history comes into the picture. In that case, if there are also family members with some cardiovascular problems we have to charge more seriously. Yet, if a person declares that his father was a heart sufferer, but he himself is in good health at the moment, then we won't charge him (case 1, underwriter E).

Current pathology is thus ultimately qualifying whether family history is important or not. A *messy* family history may in these circumstances raise the statistically average extra premium for a particular disorder (for example, to 60 per cent instead of 50 per cent). As an underwriter explains in regard to familiar hypercholesterolaemia (FH):

> If the applicant declares a family history of FH, but he himself doesn't suffer from a high LDL cholesterol level, then he will be accepted at standard rate. However, if he indeed suffers from high cholesterol and we can also see that in the family there are some aggravating circumstances, then everything will be added and he will pay some higher than average extra premium. And if he declares nothing about family history and he suffers from high cholesterol, then we will charge him the average extra premium (case 1, underwriter P).

Although family history thus plays a role in underwriting, it is of less relevance if compared to lifestyle risk information. So the insurance companies did not distinguish between applicants with a good and a bad family record *per se*, nor penalized them on the basis of family history alone. Unlike lifestyle, predictive family history risk factors are thus not reified as main, decisive mortality risks. A family history of illness does not yet make that person ill. The underwriters also raised normative objections to the use of family history as a decisive risk factor:

> We can't afford to rate on the basis of family history alone. We can't tell our clients they have to pay more because their father had heart problems. That doesn't sound customer-friendly, you see? If someone declares in full honesty that he suffers from nothing and the examinations confirm that there's nothing wrong, well, then a decision to charge him an extra premium would be very hard to defend, wouldn't it? (case 1, underwriter K)

Again we see that moral judgements are embedded in the risk assessment process. Charging somebody because of his genes or family's health condition alone is considered unjustifiable. Family history or 'bad genes' are considered not to be a matter of own choice or control. In other words, that way, the *involuntary* character of genetic risks is constructed.

Risk Carriers and Risk Takers

If we compare the underwriters' approaches to predictive medicine, lifestyle risks are far more pressing in the risk assessment than genetic risks. In the first case, the risk pool will not subsidize the applicant: he must bear his own risk. In the latter case, insurance companies are willing to take the risk. Consequently, insurers construct the voluntary or involuntary character of, respectively, lifestyle and genetic risk factors.

Moral judgements involved in predictive medicine create on the one hand 'at risk people' – that is, people with risks which are perceived as completely out of individual control – and, on the other hand, 'risky selves': or people whose risk derives from their ignorance or lack of self-control. The same tendency seems to occur in the Belgian insurance practice: lifestyle *risk takers* are treated differently from the genetic *risk carriers*. This results in a fault/no fault approach in underwriting: Risks are differently assessed according to whether they are a result of the applicant's own fault or not. In the first case, the applicant is made a culprit, in the latter, considered a victim. Implicitly then, insurers disseminate moral judgements on responsibility for health. Although lifestyle, genetics and family history are all predictors of individual future health status, insurers have introduced a ranking of them – with lifestyle risks considered as the most 'decisive' risk factors for assigning premiums.

This prompts questions not so much about the emergence of these judgements but what they *imply*. That is, by stressing the difference between lifestyle and genetic risks, we see how quite distinct moralities are attributed to applicants and, consequently, different (financial) responsibilities as well. Other sociological work has argued that genetic knowledge production is associated with new forms of determinism, a 'geneticization' or 'genetic essentialism' in which genes are allocated an over deterministic role.[35] This encourages the tendency to differentiate people according to genetic characteristics and to categorize diseases into genetic and non-genetic, with the result that different responsibilities are attributed to genetic and non-genetic diseases: where genes are linked to fatalism or lack of control, lifestyle is associated to individual control or responsibility. The same approach occurs in Belgian legislative and insurance practices. Where genetic risks are seen as 'fate', as 'involuntary' or 'uncontrollable', lifestyle risks are considered as self-induced, voluntary and 'own responsibility'. The outcome is a collective financial responsibility for the genetic *risk carriers* – the collective risk pool is prepared to pay for them – and individual financial responsibility for lifestyle *risk takers* – they have to pay themselves for their risk via extra premiums. While we consider solidarity for the genetic risks, lifestyle risks have to bear their own responsibility.[36]

However, the question of which health characteristics ought to be considered controllable is an open one.[37] What does it mean to 'have control' over one's health? In this regard, the developments in genomics may create some interesting surprises. In the light of genetic risks, there may be an even greater ascription of individual responsibility for lifestyle risks. Consider for example current developments in behavioural genetics research. The former suggests that genetic factors may account, at least partly, for many behavioural traits and psychiatric disorders. If one accepts that genetic factors contribute to conditions such as alcoholism[38] and nicotine addiction,[39] are smokers or problem drinkers still responsible for the health consequences of their behaviour? This possibility is particularly ironic in light of the fact that smoking and alcohol are currently taken as *the* examples of bad lifestyles. Yet this could also be turned around: as the breadth of the genetically *at risk* broadens, notions of self-inflicted lifestyle and individual responsibility may intensify. Take for example the case of a genetic mutation for smoking. Studies are underway to examine the genetic factors contributing to smoking, nicotine dependence and inability to quit. The involuntary smoker, the genetic carrier, is considered a victim. But doesn't this imply that for the non-genetic carrier, who still smokes, the individual responsibility will be additionally stressed? In other words, compared to the smoking-genetic-carrier, the smoker's freedom to influence his own fate is even more emphasized. In the light of genetics, the contrast will be deepened.

Paradoxically, the most important consequence of the genetics discovery might be that it is individual *lifestyle* that will be given an ever-increasing importance. This is further applicable given that most diseases are multi-factorial, meaning that a complex mix of lifestyle, environment and genes contributes to the possible development of a condition. Conditions with a genetic component can be primarily triggered by a particular health behaviour. Instead of a 'genetic determinism', it seems more plausible that we are all subject to different levels of susceptibility. As a consequence, if society discovers a genetic mutation for some disease, the individual's lifestyle habits, preventive initiatives and compliant behaviour in relation to these susceptibilities will be stressed even more. The explicit withdrawal of responsibility in the case of genetic risks is the other side of the coin of an increasing ascription of responsibility for lifestyle risks. In 'the genetic era', we will be confronted with a radicalized appeal to individual responsibility and accountability towards health and prevention of illness.[40]

Conclusion

In this chapter, I have reflected on the introduction of predictive medicine in private insurance and its consequences for the construction of ideals of citizenship. I argue that these developments in insurance underwriting practice can be understood as both continuous with traditional underwriting and yet discontinuous. Even with the introduction of highly sophisticated medical technologies, insurance companies to the present day still accept and refuse coverage on the basis of the insurance applicant's morality, as a way to prevent moral hazard. In time, however, this moral judgement has found *objective* expression in medical predictive knowledge. In other words, the control of moral hazard is now medically and technically mediated. So while the concepts of character and morality still inform insurers' underwriting decisions, they are now veiled in the language of the medico-actuarial soundness of the rating classes and expert risk assessment tools. The introduction of predictive medicine enables insurers to trace the insurance applicants' moral hazard along with their lifestyle risk factors, or their self-capacity to control health. Predictive medicine thus functions as a *new* technology in applying the same *old* principles of underwriting, that is, in ascribing morality to applicants in the distribution of responsibility for risks in insurance.

I have also demonstrated some important discontinuities in present-day insurance, more particularly in the shift from a collective risk management to a more individual risk management. Predictive medicine, with its early detection of risk factors, encourages people *individually* to manage their health risks. Individual responsibility for managing one's health becomes the gold standard for assessing one's *fitness* for membership to the insurance pool. This shift from a collective to an individual risk management goes together with the introduction of market-based trends in insurance, such as Preferred Underwriting and excessive stratification, indicating a transformation of insurance from care arrangement to private insurance institutions. In this alignment of predictive medicine and risk stratification underwriting strategies, private insurers contribute to new norms and ideals of citizenship, in the form of a neo-republican citizenship. There is a potential for those seen to be in 'at risk' categories, who do not take preventive action, to be seen as failing in their duties of citizenship.

These developments present society with some important challenges. Do we agree risk selection to be based on our individual responsibility for health or our capacity to self-control? Moreover, by applying predictive technologies, a form of economically imposed solidarity between those included in large risk groups may disappear. In that way, insurance contributes to an increasing differentiation between people. These developments create the possibility of tightening the norms of 'suitable lives' in insurance. This might contribute to the classification of increasing numbers of individuals as uninsurable or substandard in insurance. While the standards for citizenship in a regime of predictive medicine thus become more stringent (monitoring of health risks), there is a possibility that fewer people will receive access to the infrastructure they need for developing the competencies for this ideal of citizenship. On the basis of predictive risks, they may be excluded – both formally and informally – from insurance and other routes that lead to concrete social and economic independence or that contribute to a sense of self-respect. In this regard, predictive medicine may undermine the democratic principles of equity and solidarity, which are the foundations of civil and social rights. Present-day insurance thus produces and articulates a shift away from ideals of social citizenship to a neo-republican citizenship, resulting in a more restrictive notion of inclusion, as a form of 'conditional citizenship'.

Further, it is also doubtful whether it will be ever possible to assess individual control or individual responsibility over health. Where are fate, blame and bad luck in this regard? The American debate around the risk classification of domestically-abused women may highlight this.[41] The victims of domestic violence were 'substandard risks' from the perspective of the insurer. The public, however, argued that charging them increased premiums was unfair because the increased risk was beyond their control. One suggestion then was that victims of domestic violence should be insured at standard rate but that the difference between the standard and the actuarially accurate substandard premium should be sought from the abuser. In other words, financial accountability was redistributed here to the 'cause' of the 'uncontrollable' risk. It is of little surprise, then, that penetrating socio-political issues will arise about who should and who should not carry the burden of blame for health risks with the advent of predictive medicine.

The above discussion prompts questions concerning medicine's present role in insurance and, more broadly, in society. As we have seen, at the end of the nineteenth century, the profession of medicine was deployed in insurance as a way to establish public trust in insurance, articulating the *public* role of medicine and insurance. Medical underwriting thus served as an instrument that allowed for a seamless connection of economic and societal interests. Current developments in predictive medicine, however, point to a potential discrepancy of these interests in insurance. They suggest a tendency where market-based concerns, such as profit margins achieved through differentiation and risk segmentation, may prevail over societal concerns. It can be asked therefore whether predictive medicine is a vehicle for the destruction of public trust in insurance and to dispute the public role of present-day medicine. When a growing number of basically healthy individuals who have no particular health complaints are assessed as 'unhealthy risks' in insurance, will medicine indeed contribute to an 'imperfection cult' in society? As I have demonstrated in this chapter, in being insurance's gatekeeper, medicine contributes to the development of the ideals and competencies linked to citizenship. In this role of *underwriting* citizenship, medicine is tasked with deciding which conditions people have to fulfil to be part of society. Implicit within these decisions are important re-workings of collective and individual responsibility for health. Predictive medicine constitutes new ground in old debates about individual control, responsibility and blame for health. This goes to the heart of producing the ideals and competencies linked to citizenship and how this articulates with membership in – or, if you wish, exclusion from – the insurance pool.

NOTES

Oosterhuis and Huisman, 'The Politics of Health and Citizenship: Historical and Contemporary Perspectives'

1. *Constitution of the World Health Organization, signed at the International Health Conference, New York, 1946* (Geneva: WHO, 1946).
2. Cited by M. B. Dembour, 'Medical Care as Human Right: The Negation of Law, Citizenship and Power?', in T. Kohn and R. McKechnie (eds), *Extending the Boundaries of Care: Medical Ethics and Caring Practises* (Oxford and New York: Berg, 1999), pp. 89–106, on p. 91.
3. For a compelling overview of the post-World War II development of medicine, see J. Le Fanu, *The Rise and Fall of Modern Medicine* (London: Little, Brown and Company, 1999).
4. Cf. R. A. Stevens, C. E. Rosenberg and L. R. Burns (eds), *History and Health Policy in the United States: Putting the Past Back in* (New Brunswick, NJ and London: Rutgers University Press, 2006); V. Berridge, 'History Matters? History's Role in Health Policy Making', *Medical History*, 52:3 (2008), pp. 311–26.
5. See for example H. Sigerist, *Civilization and Disease* (Ithaca, NY: Cornell University Press, 1943) and G. Rosen, *A History of Public Health* (Cambridge, MA: Harvard University Press, 1958).
6. M. Foucault, *Naissance de la clinique: Une archéologie du regard médical* (Paris: PUF, 1963); M. Foucault, 'La politique de la santé au XVIIIe siècle', in M. Foucault et al., *Les machines à guérir: Aux origines de l'hôpital moderne* (Brussels: Pierre Mardaga, 1979), pp. 7–18 ; D. Armstrong, 'The Rise of Surveillance Medicine', *Sociology of Health and Illness: A Journal of Medical Sociology*, 17:3 (1995), pp. 393–404; C. Jones and R. Porter (eds), *Reassessing Foucault: Power, Medicine and the Body* (London: Routledge, 1994); J. Rolies (ed.), *De gezonde burger: Gezondheid als norm* (Nijmegen: SUN, 1988); B. S. Turner, *Medical Power and Social Knowledge* (London: Sage, 1995); A. Petersen and R. Bunton (eds), *Foucault, Health and Medicine* (London and New York: Routledge, 1997).
7. E. Freidson, *Profession of Medicine: A Study of the Sociology of Applied Knowledge* (New York: Harper & Row, 1970); E. Freidson, *Professionalism: The Third Logic* (Chicago, IL: University of Chicago Press, 2001); I. Zola, 'Medicine as an Institution of Social Control', *Sociological Review*, 20 (1972), pp. 487–504; I. Zola, 'In the Name of Health and Illness: On Some Socio-Political Consequences of Medical Influence', *Social Science and Medicine*, 9 (1975), pp. 83–7.
8. N. Elias, *Über den Prozess der Zivilisation* (Bern: Francke, 1969); J. Goudsblom, 'Openbare gezondheidszorg en het civilisatieproces', in J. Goudsblom, *De sociologie van Norbert Elias* (Amsterdam: Meulenhoff Informatief, 1987), pp. 183–210; A. Labisch, *Homo*

Hygienicus: Geschichte und Medizin in der Neuzeit (Frankfurt: Campus, 1992); A. de Swaan, *In Care of the State: Health Care, Education and Welfare in Europe and the USA in the Modern Era* (Cambridge: Polity Press, 1988).

9. A. de Swaan, *De mens is de mens een zorg* (Amsterdam: Meulenhof, 1983); De Swaan, *In Care of the State*; D. Porter (ed.), *The History of Public Health and the Modern State* (Amsterdam and Atlanta: Rodopi, 1994), pp. 1–44; H. Oosterhuis, *Stepchildren of Nature: Krafft-Ebing, Psychiatry, and the Making of Sexual Identity* (Chicago, IL and London: University of Chicago Press, 2000); L. Nys et al. (eds), *De zieke natie: over de medicalisering van de samenleving 1860–1914* (Groningen: Historische Uitgeverij, 2002).

10. Cited by M. Pijnenburg, 'Verdelingsproblemen in de gezondheidszorg', in Rolies (ed.), *De gezonde burger*, pp. 175–207, here p. 180.

11. M. Foucault, *The History of Sexuality. Volume 1: An Introduction* (New York: Random House, 1978), pp. 122–7; G. Göckenjan, *Kurieren und Staat machen. Gesundheit und Medizin in der bürgerlichen Welt* (Frankfurt am Main: Suhrkamp, 1985); Rolies (ed.), *De gezonde burger*; E. S. Houwaart, *De hygiënisten. Artsen, staat & volksgezondheid in Nederland 1840–1890* (Groningen: Historische Uitgeverij Groningen, 1991), pp. 50–5; P. Weindling, 'Bourgeois Values, Doctors and the State: The Professionalization of Medicine in Germany 1848–1933', in D. Blackbourn and R. J. Evans (eds), *The German Bourgeoisie: Essays on the Social History of the German Middle Class from the Late Eighteenth to the Early Twentieth Century* (London and New York: Routledge, 1991), pp. 198–223; Labisch, *Homo Hygienicus*; M. Frey, *Der reinliche Bürger: Entstehung und Verbreitung bürgerlicher Tugenden in Deutschland, 1760–1860* (Göttingen: Vandenhoeck & Ruprecht, 1997).

12. G. Manenschijn, 'Gezondheid in de burgerlijke filosofie: de onderwerping van het lichaam', in Rolies (ed.), *De gezonde burger*, pp. 31–49.

13. K. Danziger, 'The Historical Formation of Selves', in R. D. Ashmore and L. Jussim (eds), *Self and Identity: Fundamental Issues* (New York and Oxford: University Press, 1997), pp. 137–59.

14. B. S. Turner, 'Postmodern Culture/Modern Citizens', in B. van Steenbergen (ed.), *The Condition of Citizenship* (London, Thousand Oaks and New Delhi: Sage Publications, 1994), pp. 153–68, on p. 159.

15. For the historical conceptualization of citizenship we rely on: M. Walzer, 'Citizenship', in T. Ball and J. Farr (eds), *Political Innovation and Conceptual Change* (Cambridge: Cambridge University Press, 1989), pp. 211–19; B. S. Turner, 'Outline of a Theory of Citizenship', *Sociology*, 24 (1989), pp. 189–217; J. B. D. Simonis, A. C. Hemerijck and P. B. Lehning (eds), *De staat van de burger: Beschouwingen over hedendaags burgerschap* (Meppel: Boom, 1992); H. R. van Gunsteren (ed.), *Eigentijds burgerschap* (The Hague: Sdu, 1992); Van Steenbergen (ed.), *The Condition of Citizenship*; R. Beiner (ed.), *Theorizing Citizenship* (Albany, NY: State University of New York Press, 1995); K. Faulks, *Citizenship* (London and New York: Routledge, 2000).

16. T. H. Marshall, *Citizenship and Social Class* (Cambridge: Cambridge University Press, 1950); cf. T. H. Marshall, *Class, Citizenship, and Social Development* (New York: Anchor, 1965).

17. Recently an extension of Marshall's model has been proposed: after the development of civil, political and social citizenship, Western democracies now would also require cultural citizenship to guarantee an egalitarian pattern of cultural participation and the competence to deal with cultural and ethnic diversity. Van Gunsteren (ed.), *Eigentijds burgerschap*; Turner, 'Postmodern Culture/Modern Citizens'.

18. N. Fraser and L. Gordon, 'Civil Citizenship against Social Citizenship? On the Ideology of Contract-Versus-Charity', in Van Steenbergen (ed.), *The Condition of Citizenship*, pp. 90–107, on pp. 101–5.

19. F. Manuel, *Freedom from History and Other Untimely Essays* (New York: New York University Press, 1972), pp. 221–41; J. O'Neill, *Five Bodies: The Human Shape of Modern Society* (Ithaca, NY and London: Cornell University Press, 1985), pp. 67–90; G. Jahoda, *Crossroads between Culture and Mind: Continuities and Change in Theories of Human Nature* (New York: Harvester/Wheatsheaf, 1992); T. R. Schatzki and W. Natter, *The Social and Political Body* (New York and London: Guilford Press, 1996), pp. 1–25.

20. Foucault, *The History of Sexuality*, pp. 133–59; M. Foucault, 'Governmentality', *Ideology and Consciousness*, 6 (1979), pp. 5–21.

21. G. Rosen, 'Cameralism and the Concept of Medical Police', *Bulletin of the History of Medicine*, 27 (1953), pp. 21–42; G. Rosen, *From Medical Police to Social Medicine: Essays on the History of Health Care* (New York: Science History Publications, 1974), pp. 142–58.

22. C. Fox, R. Porter and R. Wokler (eds), *Inventing Human Science: Eighteenth-Century Domains* (Berkeley, Los Angeles, CA and London: University of California Press, 1995) pp. 1–30, 88–111, 53–87; R. Porter, *The Greatest Benefit to Mankind: A Medical History of Humanity from Antiquity to the Present* (London: Harper Collins Publishers, 1997), pp. 245–303.

23. D. B. Weiner, *The Citizen-Patient in Revolutionary and Imperial Paris* (Baltimore, MD: Johns Hopkins University Press), p. 3.

24. Weiner, *The Citizen-Patient*, pp. 3–11, 316–19; Rosen, *From Medical Police to Social Medicine*, pp. 220–45; E. A. Williams, *The Physical and the Moral: Anthropology, Physiology, and Philosophical Medicine in France, 1750–1850* (Cambridge: Cambridge University Press, 1994), p. 17.

25. E. H. Ackerknecht, *Medicine at the Paris Hospital, 1794–1848* (Baltimore, MD and London: Johns Hopkins University Press, 1967); Foucault, *Naissance de la clinique*; J. Goldstein, *Console and Classify: The French Psychiatric Profession in the Nineteenth Century* (Cambridge: Cambridge University Press, 1990); W. F. Bynum, *Science and the Practice of Medicine in the Nineteenth Century* (Cambridge, New York and Melbourne: Cambridge University Press, 1994), pp. 25–46.

26. G. Rosen, 'The Philosophy of Ideology and the Emergence of Modern Medicine in France', *Bulletin of the History of Medicine* 20 (1946), pp. 328–39; M. S. Staum, *Cabanis: Enlightenment and Medical Philosophy in the French Revolution* (Princeton, NJ: Princeton University Press, 1980); S. Moravia, *Beobachtende Vernunf: Philosophie und Anthropologie in der Aufkläring* (Frankfurt am Main, Berlin and Vienna: Ullstein, 1977), pp. 40–50, 50–8, 58–64, 64–9, 82–8; Williams, *The Physical and the Moral*.

27. Rosen, *From Medical Police to Social Medicine*, pp. 246–58.

28. H. A. M. J. ten Have, *Geneeskunde en filosofie: De invloed van Jeremy Bentham op het medisch denken en handelen* (Lochem: Uitgeversmaatschappij de Tijdstroom, 1983); H. A. M. J. ten Have, *Jeremy Bentham. Een quantumtheorie van de ethiek* (Kampen: Kok Agora, 1986); J. Semple, 'Bentham's Utilitarianism and the Provision of Medical Care', in D. Porter and R. Porter (eds), *Doctors, Politics and Society: Historical Essays* (Amsterdam and Atlanta: Rodopi, 1993), pp. 30–45.

29. M. Foucault, *Surveiller et punir: Naissance de la prison* (Paris: Gallimard, 1975).

30. Porter, *The Greatest Benefit*, pp. 397–427, 628–67; Porter (ed.), *The History of Public Health*; D. Porter, *Health, Civilization and the State: A History of Public Health from*

Ancient to Modern Times (London and New York: Routledge, 1999); Bynum, *Science and the Practice of Medicine*, pp. 55–91; E. Fee and D. Porter, 'Public Health, Preventive Medicine and Professionalization: England and America in the Nineteenth Century', in A. Wear (ed.), *Medicine in Society: Historical Essays* (Cambridge: Cambridge University Press, 1992), pp. 249–75; P. Weindling, 'Hygienepolitik als sozialintegrative Strategie im späten Deutschen Kaiserreich', in A. Labisch and R. Spree (eds), *Medizinische Deutungsmacht im sozialen Wandel* (Bonn: Psychiatrie-Verlag, 1989), pp. 37–55; U. Frevert, *Krankheit als politiches Problem 1770–1880: Soziale Unterschichten in Preussen zwischen medizinischer Polizei und staatlicher Sozialversicherung* (Göttingen: Vandenhoeck & Ruprecht, 1984); W. Coleman, *Death is a Social Disease: Public Health and Political Economy in Early Industrial France* (Wisconsin and London: University of Wisconsin Press, 1982); Houwaart, *De hygiënisten*; M. Berg and G. Cocks (eds), *Medicine and Modernity. Public Health and Medical Care in Nineteenth- and Twentieth-Century Germany* (Cambridge: Cambridge University Press, 1997); Nys et al. (eds), *De zieke natie*.

31. B. Haines, 'The Inter-Relations between Social, Biological and Medical Thought, 1750–1850: Saint-Simon and Comte', *British Journal for the History of Science*, 11 (1978), pp. 19–35; J. V. Pickstone, 'Bureaucracy, Liberalism and the Body in Post-Revolutionary France: Bichat's Physiology and the Paris School of Medicine', *History of Science*, 19 (1981), pp. 115–42.

32. Cited by Houwaart, *De hygiënisten*, p. 105; cf. K. Figlio and P. Weindling, 'Was Social Medicine Revolutionary? Rudolf Virchow and the Revolutions of 1848', *Bulletin of the Society for the Social History of Medicine*, 34 (1984), pp. 10–18.

33. Cited by Houwaart, *De hygiënisten*, p. 104.

34. E. Mendelsohn, 'Revolution and Reduction. The Sociology of Methodological and Philosophical Concerns in Nineteenth Century Biology', in Y. Elkana (ed.), *The Interaction between Science and Philosophy* (Atlantic Highlands: Humanities Press, 1974), pp. 407–26; T. Lenoir, *Instituting Science: The Cultural Production of Scientific Disciplines* (Stanford, CA: Stanford University Press, 1997), pp. 75–95.

35. Porter, *The Greatest Benefit*, p. 331.

36. Houwaart, *De hygiënisten*; L. Nys, 'Nationale plagen: hygiënisten over het maatschappelijk lichaam', in Nys et al. (eds), *De zieke natie*, pp. 220–41; R. Schepers, 'Een wereld van belangen: artsen en de ontwikkeling van de openbare gezondheidszorg', in Nys et al. (eds), *De zieke natie*, pp. 200–18.

37. Bynum, *Science and the Practice of Medicine*, p. 86; Porter and Porter (eds), *Doctors, Politics and Society*, pp. 6, 12; Porter (ed.), *The History of Public Health*, p. 10.

38. M. Durey, 'Medical Elites, the General Practitioner and Patient Power in Britain during the Cholera Epidemic of 1831–2', in I. Inkster and J. Morrell (eds), *Metropolis and Province: Science in British Culture, 1780–1850* (Philadelphia, PA: University of Pennsylvania Press, 1983), pp. 257–78; Porter, *The Greatest Benefit*, pp. 348, 358; Schepers, 'Een wereld van belangen'; W. de Blecourt, F. Huisman and H. van der Velden (eds), 'De medische markt in Nederland, 1850–1950', *Tijdschrift voor sociale geschiedenis*, special issue, 25 (1999).

39. W. Conze and J. Kocka, *Bildungsbürgertum im 19. Jahrhundert: Bildungssystem und Professionalisierung in internationalen Vergleichen* (Stuttgart: Klett-Cotta, 1985); C. Huerkamp, *Der Aufstieg der Ärzte im 19. Jahrhundert: Vom gelehrten Stand zum professionellen Experten. Das Beispiel Preussens* (Göttingen: Vandenhoeck & Ruprecht, 1985); C. E. McClelland, *The German Experience of Professionalization: Modern Learned*

Professions and their Organizations from the Early Nineteenth Century to the Hitler Era (Cambridge: Cambridge University Press, 1991); Weindling, 'Bourgeois Values'.

40. Fee and Porter, 'Public Health', pp. 249–58, 265–7, 270–3; Houwaart, *De hygiënisten*, pp. 105–7, 136; Porter and Porter, *Doctors, Politics and Society*, p. 16.

41. T. Osborne, 'On Liberalism, Neoliberalism and the "Liberal Profession" of Medicine', *Economy and Society*, 22:3 (1993), pp. 345–56; T. Osborne, 'Of Health and Statecraft', in Petersen and Bunton (eds), *Foucault, Health and Medicine*, pp. 173–88; G. Burdell, C. Gordon and P. Miller (eds), *The Foucault Effect: Studies in Governmentality* (London: Harvester/Wheatsheaf, 1991); A. Barry, T. Osborne and N. Rose (eds), *Foucault and Political Reason: Liberalism, Neo-Liberalism, and Rationalities of Government* (London: University College London Press, 1996); M. Dean, *Governmentality: Power and Rule in Modern Society* (London, Thousand Oaks and New Delhi: Sage Publications, 1999); G. Eghigian, A. Killen and C. Leuenberger (eds), *The Self as Scientific and Political Project*, Osiris series (Chicago, IL: University of Chicago Press, 2007), pp. 1–25; P. Miller and N. Rose, *Governing the Present: Administering Economic, Social and Personal Life* (Cambridge and Malden: Polity Press, 2008).

42. S. L. Gilman and E. Chamberlain (eds), *Degeneration: The Dark Side of Progress* (New York: Columbia University Press, 1985); D. Pick, *Faces of Degeneration: A European Disorder 1848–1918* (Cambridge: Cambridge University Press, 1989); M. Hawkins, *Social Darwinism in European and American thought, 1860–1945* (Cambridge, New York and Melbourne: Cambridge University Press, 1997).

43. R. A. Nye, *Crime, Madness, and Politics in Modern France: The Medical Concept of National Decline* (Princeton, NJ: Princeton University Press, 1984); R. Smith, *The Fontana History of the Human Sciences* (London: Fontana.Smith, 1997), pp. 392–433.

44. D. J. Kevles, *In the Name of Eugenics: Genetics and the Uses of Human Heredity* (Berkeley, CA: University of California Press; Cambridge, MA: Harvard University Press, 1985); M. B. Adams (ed.), *The Wellborn Science: Eugenics in Germany, France, Brazil, and Russia* (New York and Oxford: Oxford University Press, 1990); G. Broberg and N. Roll-Hansen, *Eugenics and the Welfare State: Sterilization Policy in Denmark, Sweden, Norway, and Finland* (East Lansing, MI: Michigan State University Press, 1996); M. A. Hasian, *The Rhetoric of Eugenics in Anglo-American Thought* (Athens, GA: University of Georgia Press, 1996); I. R. Dowbiggin, *Keeping America Sane: Psychiatry and Eugenics in the United States and Canada, 1880–1940* (Ithaca, NY and London: Cornell University Press, 1997); D. Porter, 'Eugenics and the Sterilization Debate in Sweden and Britain before World War II', *Scandinavian Journal of History*, 24 (1999), pp. 145–62.

45. S. Faith Weiss, *Race, Hygiene and National Efficiency: The Eugenics of Wilhelm Schallmeyer* (Chicago, IL: University of Chicago Press, 1987); P. Weindling, *Health, Race and German Politics between National Unification and Nazism, 1870–1945* (Cambridge: Cambridge University Press, 1989); P. Weingart, J. Kroll and K. Bayertz, *Rasse, Blut, und Gene: Geschichte der Eugenik und Rassenhygiene in Deutschland* (Frankfurt am Main: Suhrkamp, 1992).

46. R. J. Lifton, *The Nazi Doctors: Medical Killing and the Psychology of Genocide* (New York: Basic Books, 1986); R. N. Proctor, *Racial Hygiene: Medicine Under the Nazis* (Cambridge, MA and London: Harvard University Press, 1988); M. Burleigh, *Death and Deliverance: 'Euthanasia' in Germany c. 1900–1945* (Cambridge, New York and Melbourne: Cambridge University Press, 1994); M. Burleigh and W. Wippermann, *The Racial State: Germany 1933–1945* (Cambridge, New York and Melbourne: Cambridge

University Press, 1998); A. Götz, *Cleansing the Fatherland: Nazi Medicine and Racial Hygiene* (Baltimore, MD: Johns Hopkins University Press, 1994).

47. J. Donzelot, *The Policing of Families* (New York: Pantheon, 1979).
48. De Swaan, *In Care of the State*.
49. Weindling, 'Hygienepolitik'; Weindling, 'Bourgeois Values'; K. Horstman, *Public Bodies, Private Lives: The Historical Construction of Life Insurance, Health Risks, and Citizenship in the Netherlands 1880–1920* (Rotterdam: Erasmus Publishing, 2001).
50. C. Hamlin, 'State Medicine in Great Britain', in Porter (ed.), *The History of Public Health*, pp. 132–64; M. Ramsey, 'Public Health in France', in Porter (ed.), *The History of Public Health*, pp. 45–118; P. Weindling, 'Public Health in Germany', in Porter (ed.), *The History of Public Health*, pp. 119–31; R. van Daalen, 'Honderd jaar vrouwen en gezondheidsdeskundigen', in R. van Daalen and M. Gijswijt-Hofstra (eds), *Gezond en wel: Vrouwen en de zorg voor gezondheid in de twintigste eeuw* (Amsterdam: Amsterdam University Press, 1998), pp. 15–29; M. Daru, 'Hygiënisering en moralisering van de gezondheidszorg', in Van Daalen and Gijswijt-Hofstra (eds), *Gezond en wel*, pp. 30–51; L. Frohman, 'Prevention, Welfare, and Citizenship: The War on Tuberculosis and Infant Mortality in Germany, 1900–1930', *Central European History*, 39 (2006), pp. 431–81.
51. Frevert, *Krankheit als politiches Problem*, pp. 185–330; Huerkamp, *Der Aufstieg der Ärzte*; McClelland, *The German Experience of Professionalization*, pp. 82–6, 236–9; Ramsey, 'Public Health in France'.
52. D. J. Rothman, *Beginnings Count: The Technological Imperative in American Health Care* (New York and Oxford: Oxford University Press, 1997).
53. Pijnenburg, 'Verdelingsproblemen'; Ramsey, 'Public Health in France', 97; E. Fee, 'Public Health and the State: The United States', in Porter (ed.), *The History of Public Health*, pp. 224–75, on pp. 248–52; D. van der Meer, 'Marktwerking in de gezondheidszorg: kostenbeheersing?', in L. Aarts et al. (eds), *Het bedrijf van de verzorgingsstaat: Naar nieuwe verhoudingen tussen staat, markt en burger* (Amsterdam and Meppel: Boom), pp. 117–33; Porter, *The Greatest Benefit*, pp. 642–54.
54. Freidson, *Professionalism*; cf. J. W. Duyvendak, T. Knijn and M. Kremer (eds), *Policy, People, and the New Professional: De-professionalization and Re-professionalization in Care and Welfare* (Amsterdam: Amsterdam University Press, 2006); G. van der Laan, 'Vraagsturing, professionaliteit en burgerschap', *Sociale Interventie*, 11:2 (2002), pp. 44–51.
55. A. Giddens, *The Consequences of Modernity* (Cambridge: Polity, 1990); A. Giddens, *Modernity and Self-Identity: Self and Society in the Late Modern Age* (Cambridge: Polity, 1991); R. Castel, 'From Dangerousness to Risk', in Burchell, Gordon and Miller (eds), *The Foucault Effect*, pp. 281–98; U. Beck, *Risk Society: Towards a New Modernity* (London: Sage, 1992); D. Lupton, *The Imperative of Health: Public Health and the Regulated Body* (London: Sage, 1995); R. Bunton, S. Nettleton and R. Burrows (eds), *The Sociology of Health Promotion: Critical Analyses of Consumption, Lifestyle and Risk* (London: Routledge, 1995); A. R. Petersen and D. Lupton, *The New Public Health: Health and Self in the Age of Risk* (Sydney: Allen and Unwin; London: Sage, 1996); Petersen and Bunton (eds), *Foucault, Health and Medicine*; K. Horstman, G. H. de Vries and O. Haveman, *Gezondheidspolitiek in een risicocultuur: Burgerschap in het tijdperk van de voorspellende geneeskunde* (The Hague: Rathenau Instituut, 1999).
56. Kohn and McKechie (eds), *Extending the Boundaries of Care*, pp. 1–13; 181–201.
57. See D. Nelkin and L. Tancredi, *Dangerous Diagnostics: The Social Power of Biological Information* (New York: Basic Books, 1989); Horstman, De Vries and Haveman, *Gezondheidspolitiek*; F. Fukuyama, *Our Posthuman Future: Consequences of the Biotech-*

nology Revolution (London: Profile Books, 2002); J. Habermas, *The Future of Human Nature* (Cambridge: Polity Press, 2003).

58. J. van Steenbergen and C. Th. Bakker (eds), *Het leeft onder de bevolking: Maatschappelijke aspecten van infectieziektebestrijding vroeger en nu* (Alphen aan den Rijn: Van Zuiden Communications, 2010); K. Horstman and R. Houtepen, *Worstelen met gezond leven: Ethiek in de preventie van hart- en vaatziekten* (Amsterdam: Het Spinhuis, 2005); K. Horstman, *Dikke kinderen, uitgebluste werknemers en vreemde virussen: Filosofie van de publieke gezondheidszorg in de 21ᵉ eeuw* (Maastricht: Maastricht University, 2010).

59. K. Horstman, 'Experts en hun publiek: over vertrouwen, achterdocht en dialoog', in Van Steenbergen and Bakker (eds), *Het leeft*, pp. 83–93.

1 Ramsey, 'Before *l'État-Providence*: Health and Liberal Citizenship in Revolutionary and Post-Revolutionary France'

1. Universal Declaration of Human Rights, http://www.un.org/en/documents/udhr, art. 25 [accessed 27 September 2013]; emphasis added.

2. Law no. 99–641, 27 July 1999, http://www.legifrance.gouv.fr/affichTexte.do;jsessionid=0B21021CD5BED4BEE549A3611CFD4201.tpdjo05v_3?cidTexte=JORFTEXT000000198392&categorieLien=id, art. 1 [accessed 27 September 2013]. Unless otherwise indicated, all translations are by the author.

3. Charter of Fundamental Rights of the European Union (2000/C 364/01), http://www.europarl.europa.eu/charter/pdf/text_en.pdf, art. 35 [accessed 27 September 2013]. On the question of principle versus right, see C. Rapoport, 'L'opposabilité des "droits-créances" constitutionnels en droit public français', http://www.droitconstitutionnel.org/congresParis/comC8/RapoportTXT.pdf, p. 3 [accessed 27 September 2013].

4. On citizenship and rights in the French context, see D. Schnapper, *Qu'est-ce que la citoyenneté?* (Paris: Gallimard, 2000).

5. For a detailed analysis of the legislation, see P. H. Douglas, 'The French Social Insurance Act', *Annals of the American Academy of Political and Social Science*, 164 (1932), pp. 211–48.

6. A useful overview of the French health care system in the twentieth century can be found in P. V. Dutton, *Differential Diagnoses: A Comparative History of Health Care Problems and Solutions in the US and France* (Ithaca, NY: Cornell University Press, 2007). On the legislation of 1930 in the context of the broader history of French institutions of social welfare before 1945, see T. B. Smith, *Creating the Welfare State in France, 1880–1940* (Montreal: McGill-Queen's University Press, 2003) and P. V. Dutton, *Origins of the French Welfare State: The Struggle for Social Reform in France, 1914–1947* (Cambridge: Cambridge University Press, 2002). On the debates over policies and institutions, see H. Hatzfeld, *Du paupérisme à la Sécurité sociale, 1850–1940: Essai sur les origines de la Sécurité sociale en France* (Nancy: Presses Universitaires de Nancy, 1989).

7. On social and economic rights, see L. Pech, 'France', in M. Langford (ed.), *Socio-Economic Rights Jurisprudence: Emerging Trends in Comparative and International Law* (Cambridge: Cambridge University Press, 2008), pp. 267–75.

8. Schnapper, *Qu'est-ce que la citoyenneté?*, pp. 104–5.

9. Préambule de la Constitution du 27 Octobre 1946, http://www.legifrance.gouv.fr/Droit-francais/Constitution/Preambule-de-la-Constitution-du-27-octobre-1946, arts 10–11 [accessed 27 September 2013].

10. See, for example, Pech, 'France', pp. 266, 269; Rapoport, 'L'opposabilité', pp. 3, 8, 9; and F. Rangeon, 'Droits-libertés et droits-créances: les contradictions du préambule de la Constitution de 1946', in G. Koubi et al., *Le Préambule de la Constitution de 1946: Antinomies juridiques et contradictions politiques* (Paris: Presses Universitaires de France,1996), pp. 169–86 (p. 169 on the right to health).

11. Charte de l'environnement de 2004, http://www.legifrance.gouv.fr/Droit-francais/Constitution/Charte-de-l-environnement-de-2004, art. 1 [accessed 25 June 2013].

12. T. H. Marshall, *Class, Citizenship, and Social Development* (Garden City, NY: Doubleday & Company, Inc., 1964), ch. 4, 'Citizenship and Social Class', pp. 70–4, on p. 70.

13. On 'contradictions' in the preamble of 1946, see Rangeon, 'Droits-libertés et droits-créances'.

14. J. Rivero and H. Moutouh, *Libertés publiques*, 2 vols (Paris: Presses Universitaires de France, 2003), vol. 1, p. 8. See also Pech, 'France'.

15. Rapoport, 'L'opposabilité'.

16. Pech, 'France', pp. 268–9.

17. Marshall, 'Citizenship and Social Class', pp. 104–5.

18. I. Berlin, *Two Concepts of Liberty: An Inaugural Lecture Delivered Before the University of Oxford on 31 October 1958* (Oxford: Clarendon Press, 1958).

19. 'Lecture on Liberal Legislation and Freedom of Contract', in *Works of Thomas Hill Green*, 3 vols (Longmans, Green & Co.: London, 1906–1908), vol. 3, p. 379.

20. J. S. Mill, *On Liberty*, ed. G. Alexander (Peterborough, ON: Broadview Press, 1999), p. 42; quotation from W. von Humboldt, *The Sphere and Duties of Government (Ideen zu einem Versuch die Grenzen der Wirksamkeit des Staats zu bestimmen)*, trans. J. Cailthard (London: Champman, 1854), p. 65.

21. Dutton, *Differential Diagnoses*, p. 3.

22. P. L. R. Higonnet, *Sister Republics: The Origins of French and American Republicanism* (Cambridge, MA: Harvard University Press, 1988), cited in Dutton, *Differential Diagnoses*, p. 223, n. 2.

23. Higonnet, *Class, Ideology, and the Rights of Nobles during the French Revolution* (Oxford: Clarendon Press, 1981) and *Goodness Beyond Virtue: Jacobins during the French Revolution* (Cambridge, MA: Harvard University Press, 1998).

24. Higonnet, *Sister Republics*, pp. 6–7, 218, 271.

25. Higonnet, *Class, Ideology and the Rights of Nobles*, p. 23.

26. E. J. Sieyès, *Qu'est-ce que le tiers état?* (n.p., 1789).

27. For an overview of this question, see M. P. Fitzsimmons, *The Night the Old Regime Ended* (University Park, PA: Pennsylvania State University Press, 2003), pp. 178–212.

28. M. Foucault, *The Birth of the Clinic: An Archaeology of Medical Perception*, trans. A. M. Sheridan (New York: Pantheon Books, 1973), p. 46.

29. M. Ramsey, 'The Politics of Professional Monopoly in Nineteenth-Century Medicine: The French Model and Its Rivals', in G. L. Geison (ed.), *Professions and the French State, 1700–1900* (Philadelphia, PA: University of Pennsylvania Press, 1984), pp. 225–305. On Raspail, see D. B. Weiner, *Raspail: Scientist and Reformer* (New York: Columbia University Press, 1968).

30. M. Ramsey, 'France', in D. Porter (ed.), *The History of Public Health and the Modern State* (Amsterdam: Rodopi, 1994), pp. 45–118. See also G. Jorland, *Une société à soigner: hygiène et salubrité publiques en France au XIXᵉ siècle* (Paris: Gallimard, 2010).

31. D. B. Weiner, 'Le droit de l'homme a la santé: Une belle idée devant l'Assemblée constituante, 1790–1791', *Clio Medica*, 5 (1970), pp. 208–23.

32. *Nouveau plan de constitution pour la médecine en France, présenté à l'assemblée nationale par la Société royale de médecine, 1790* (n.p., 1790), pp. 68–73, on p. 73.

33. Weiner, 'Le droit de l'homme', p. 209; A. R. J. Turgot, 'Fondation', in D. Diderot and J. le Rond D'Alembert (eds), *Encyclopédie ou Dictionnaire raisonné des sciences, des arts et des métiers*, 17 vols (Paris, 1761–5), vol. 7, p. 73.

34. Weiner, 'Le droit de l'homme', p. 210. Liancourt, 'Quatrième rapport du Comité de mendicité: Secours à donner à la classe indigente dans les différents âges et dans les différentes circonstances de la vie', in C. Bloch and A. Tuetey (eds), *Procès-verbaux et rapports du Comité de mendicité de la Constituante, 1790–1791* (Paris: Imprimerie nationale, 1991), p. 391.

35. On the terminology, see C. Jones, *Charity and Bienfaisance: The Treatment of the Poor in the Montpellier Region, 1740–1815* (Cambridge: Cambridge University Press, 1982), pp. 1–8.

36. Two older works are still useful: C. Bloch, *L'Assistance et l'État en France à la veille de la Révolution* (Paris : A. Picard et fils, 1908), ch. 5 (on the Comité de Mendicité) and H. Ingrand, *Le Comité de salubrité de l'Assemblée nationale constituante (1790–1791)* (Paris: M. Vigné, 1934).

37. D. B. Weiner, *The Citizen-Patient in Revolutionary and Imperial Paris* (Baltimore, MD: Johns Hopkins University Press, 1993), pp. 3, 21, 84, 311, 318.

38. One recent example is a study of the spinning workshops set up during the Revolution to employ needy women, which draws on Weiner for its interpretive framework: L. DiCaprio, *The Origins of the Welfare State: Women, Work, and the French Revolution* (Urbana, IL: University of Illinois Press, 2007), pp. ix, 37.

39. E. J. Sieyès, 'Reconnaissance et exposition raisonné des droits de l'homme et du citoyen, 20 et 21 juillet 1789', arts 24 and 25', in F. Furet and R. Halévi (eds), *Orateurs de la Révolution française*, vol. 1 : *Les Constituants* (Paris: Gallimard, 1989), pp. 1005–18, on pp. 1012, 1018.

40. *Plan de travail du Comité pour l'extinction de la mendicité, présenté à l'Assemblée nationale...*, in Bloch and Tuetey (eds), *Procès-verbaux et rapports*, p. 310.

41. *Premier rapport du Comité de mendicité: exposé des principes généraux qui ont dirigé son travail...*, in Bloch and Tuetey (eds), *Procès-verbaux et rapports*, pp. 327–8.

42. *Troisième rapport du Comité de mendicité: bases constitutionnelles du système général de la législation et de l'administration des secours...*, 21 January 1791, in Bloch and Tuetey (eds), *Procès-verbaux et rapports*, pp. 369, 378–9; *Troisième Rapport du Comité de mendicité sur les bases de répartition des secours dans les différens Départemens, Districts et Municipalités, de leur administration et du système général qui lie cette branche de la Législation et d'Administration à la Constitution*, 15 July 1790 (Paris: Imprimerie nationale, 1790), p. 29 (art. 16). On the two versions of the report, see Bloch and Tuetey (eds), *Procès-verbaux et rapports*, pp. 355–6.

43. *Quatrième rapport*, p. 384.

44. B. d'Airy, *Rapport sur l'organisation générale des secours publics, et sur la destruction de la mendicité, présenté a l'Assemblée nationale, au nom du Comité des secours publics, le 13 juin 1792* (Paris: Imprimerie nationale, 1792), pp. 7, 9, 83, 108.

45. J. Locke, *Two Treatises of Government* (London: Awnsham Churchill, 1690), pp. 52–3, 222, 305.

46. 'Déclaration des droits de l'homme et du citoyen', http://www.conseil-constitutionnel. fr/conseil-constitutionnel/francais/la-constitution/la-constitution-du-4-octobre-1958/ declaration-des-droits-de-l-homme-et-du-citoyen-de-1789.5076.html, art. 4 [accessed 27 September 2013].

47. M. de Robespierre, 'Sur les subsistances', 2 December 1792, in M. de Robespierre, *Discours et rapports à la Convention* (Paris: Union Générale des Éditions, 1965), pp. 53–4.

48. M. de Robespierre, 'Sur la nouvelle déclaration des droits', 24 April 1793, arts 2, 7, 11, 12, in Robespierre, *Discours et rapports*, pp. 123–4.

49. France, Constitution de 1791, title 1, http://www.conseil-constitutionnel.fr/conseil -constitutionnel/francais/la-constitution/les-constitutions-de-la-france/constitution- de-1791.5082.html [accessed 25 June 2013].

50. On the development of public assistance under the Revolution, see I. Woloch, *The New Regime: Transformations of the French Civic Order, 1789–1820s* (New York: W. W. Norton & Company, 1994), ch. 8, 'The Rise and Fall of Revolutionary *Bienfaisance*', and, for a regional perspective, Jones, *Charity and Bienfaisance*, chs 8, 'Towards a "Welfare State", 1789–c. 1795' and 9, 'Retreat from the "Welfare State", c. 1795–c 1800'. On the Revolution's impact on the hospitals and nursing orders, see D. B. Weiner, 'The French Revolution, Napoleon, and the Nursing Profession', *Bulletin of the History of Medicine* 46:3 (1972), pp. 274–305 and J. C. Sournia, *La Médecine révolutionnaire, 1789–1799* (Paris: Payot, 1989), ch. 2, 'L'Institution hospitalière menacée'.

51. See, for example, M. L. Kennedy, *The Jacobin Clubs in the French Revolution, 1793–1795* (Oxford: Berghahn Books, 2000), p. 141.

52. The complex story is well told in I. Woloch, 'From Charity to Welfare in Revolutionary Paris', *Journal of Modern History*, 58:4 (1986), pp. 780–812.

53. 'Décret concernant la nouvelle organisation des secours publics', 19 March 1793, arts 11–12, in A. de Watteville (ed.), *Législation charitable, ou Recueil des lois ... qui régissent les établissements de bienfaisance*, 2nd edn (Paris: Librairie de Jurisprudence de Cotillon, 1847), p. 18.

54. 'Décret qui ordonne la formation d'un Livre de la bienfaisance nationale', title IV, in Watteville (ed.), *Législation charitable,* pp. 30–1.

55. C. Duprat, *Le Temps des philanthropes: la philanthropie parisienne des Lumières à la monarchie de Juillet* (Paris: Éditions du CTHS, 1993), pt 2, ch. 4.

56. On welfare policy and the role of the state in the post-revolutionary period, see P. Rosanvallon, *L'État en France, de 1789 à nos jours* (Paris: Éditions du Seuil, 1990), pt 3, chs 1–2.

57. J.-B. Say, *Traité d'économie politique*, 6th edn (Paris: Guillaumin, 1841), pp. 493–7, on p. 493.

58. A. Thiers, *De l'assistance et de la prévoyance publiques* (Brussels: veuve Wouters, 1850), pp. 10–11, 15, 21–2.

59. J. M. de Gérando, *De la Bienfaisance publique*, 4 vols (Paris: J. Renouard, 1839) and J. M. de Gérando, *Le Visiteur du pauvre* (Paris: L. Colas, 1820).

60. Gérando, *Le Visiteur*, pp. 5, 11–12.

61. Gérando, *Bienfaisance*, vol. 1, pp. lxxvi, 74, 205, 471, 486; vol. 4, pp. 247–53 (on medical assistance).

62. Considerant, *Le Socialisme devant le vieux monde ou le vivant devant les morts* (Paris: Librairie Phalanstérienne, 1848), pp. 138–42.

63. Considerant, *Exposition abrégée du système phalanstérien de Fourier*, 3rd edn (Paris: Librairie Phalanstérienne, 1848), pp. 47–8.

64. É. Cabet, *Voyage en Icarie*, 5th edn (Paris: Bureau du *Populaire*, 1848), 'Santé-Médecins-Hospices', pp. 111–23, on pp. 112–13, 121.

65. F. V. Raspail, *Histoire naturelle de la santé et de la maladie chez les végétaux et chez les animaux en général, et en particulier chez l'homme; suivie du formulaire pour la nouvelle méthode de traitement hygiénique et curatif*, 3rd edn, 3 vols (Paris: chez l'éditeur des ouvrages de M. Raspail, 1860), vol. 1, pp. liv–lv, quoting from the first edition. See D. B.

Weiner, 'François-Vincent Raspail: Doctor and Champion of the Poor', *French Historical Studies*, 1:2 (1959), pp. 141–71.

66. On the development of medical assistance, see O. Faure, 'La Médecine gratuite au XIXe siècle: de la charité à l'assistance', *Histoire, économie et société*, 3 (1984), pp. 593–610.

67. G. D. Sussman, 'Enlightened Health Reform, Professional Medicine and Traditional Society: The Cantonal Physicians of the Bas-Rhin, 1810–1870', *Bulletin of the History of Medicine*, 51:4 (1977), pp. 565–84.

68. See E. Ackerman, 'Medical Care in the Countryside near Paris, 1800–1914', *Annals of the New York Academy of Sciences*, 412 (1983), pp. 1–18.

69. G. Weisz, 'The Politics of Medical Professionalization in France, 1845–1848', *Journal of Social History*, 12 (1978–1979), pp. 3–30.

70. J. Guérin, 'La Médecine sociale et la médecine politique', *Gazette médicale de Paris*, 25 March 1848, and 'La Médecine sociale et la médecine socialiste', *Gazette médicale de Paris*, 18 March 1848.

71. Constitution of 4 November 1848, preamble, art. 8, http://www.conseil-constitutionnel.fr/conseil-constitutionnel/francais/la-constitution/les-constitutions-de-la-france/constitution-de-1848-iie-republique.5106.html [accessed 25 June 2013].

72. J. D. Ellis, *The Physician-Legislators of France: Medicine and Politics in the Early Third Republic, 1870–1914* (Cambridge: Cambridge University Press, 1990), p. 9.

73. J. Gaillard, 'Une expérience de médecine gratuite au XIXe siècle: l'arrêté d'Haussmann du 20 avril 1853', *Actes du 103e Congrès National des Sociétés Savantes, Nancy, 1978: Colloque sur l'histoire de la sécurité sociale, problèmes et méthodes* (Paris: Association pour l'Étude de l'Histoire la Sécurité Sociale, 1978), pp. 61–73.

74. On welfare policy, see P. Nord, 'The Welfare State in France, 1870–1914', *French Historical Studies*, 18 (1983), pp. 821–38. For a broader discussion of the changing role of the state, see Rosanvallon, *L'État en France*, pt 3, ch. 3.

75. See J. E. S. Hayward, '"Solidarity" and the Reformist Sociology of Alfred Fouillée', *American Journal of Economics and Sociology*, 22:1 (1963), pp. 205–22, 303–12.

76. A useful overview can be found in T. Zeldin, *France 1848–1945*, 2 vols (Oxford: Clarendon Press, 1973–7), vol. 1: *Ambition, Love, and Politics*, ch. 21, 'Solidarism'.

77. France, Constitution du 5 Fructidor An III, arts 2, 4 and 9, http://www.conseil-constitutionnel.fr/conseil-constitutionnel/francais/la-constitution/les-constitutions-de-la-france/constitution-du-5-fructidor-an-iii.5086.html [accessed 25 June 2013].

78. L. Bourgeois, *Solidarité*, 3rd edn (Paris: Librairie Armand Colin, 1902), pp. 19, 21, 55–6, 94, 101–2, 138, 141, 152.

79. N. and A. J. Arnaud, 'Une doctrine de l'État tranquillisante: le solidarisme juridique', *Archives de philosophie du droit* 21 (1976), pp. 131–5; pp. 146–7 on the idea of an enforceable right.

80. See A. Mitchell, *The Divided Path: The German Influence on Social Reform in France After 1870* (Chapel Hill, NC: University of North Carolina Press, 1991); pp. 278–9 on the Belgian model.

81. On the medical profession in parliament, see Ellis, *Physician-Legislators*; pp. 223–5 deal with the law of 1893.

82. The text of the law can be found in *Bulletin des lois de la République française*, 12th series, vol. 47 (Paris: Imprimerie Nationale, 1894), bulletin no. 1583, law no. 27052, pp. 841–9; quotation from art. 1.

83. M. L. Hildreth, 'Medical Rivalries and Medical Politics in France: The Physicians' Union Movement and the Medical Assistance Law of 1893', *Journal of the History of Medicine*,

42 (1987), pp. 5–29. M. L. Hildreth, *Doctors, Bureaucrats, and Public Health in France, 1888–1902* (New York and London: Garland Publishing, Inc., 1987), chs 4–5.

84. On the complexities of French socialism in the late nineteenth century, see Zeldin, *France*, vol. 1, ch. 23.

85. R. C. Stuart, *Marxism at Work: Ideology, Class, and French Socialism during the Third Republic* (Cambridge: Cambridge University Press, 1992), p. 333 and passim. On the debate over pensions, see B. Dumons and G. Pollet, 'Les Socialistes français et la question des retraites (1880–1914)', *Vingtième Siècle: Revue d'histoire*, 38:38 (1993), pp. 34–46.

86. D. Stafford, *From Anarchism to Reformism: A Study of the Political Activities of Paul Brousse within the First International and the French Socialist Movement 1870–90* (Toronto: University of Toronto Press, 1971).

87. The standard biography remains H. Goldberg, *The Life of Jean Jaurès* (Madison: University of Wisconsin Press, 1962).

88. J. Jaurès, 'Sa profession de foi aux élections législatives de 1906', http://www.assemblee-nationale.fr/histoire/jaures/prof-foi.asp [accessed 25 June 2013].

89. *Compte rendu du 7ᵉ congrès national du Parti socialiste (SFIO)*, Nîmes, 6–9 February 1910 (Paris: l'Émancipatrice, n.d.), p. 377, quoted by Dumont and Pollet, 'Les Socialistes français', pp. 43–4.

90. On the post-war Social Security system, see Rosanvallon, *L'État en France*, pt 3, ch. 4.

2 Hardy, 'An Oyster Odyssey: Science, State and Commerce in England, 1895–1905'

1. D. Porter, *Health, Civilization and the State: A History of Public Health from Ancient to Modern Times* (London and New York: Routledge, 1999), p. 97.

2. For a briefer account of this episode, and for French responses to a similar situation at this period, see R. Neild, *The English, the French and the Oyster* (London: Quiller, 1995), ch. 8. For an account of American responses to the oyster problem, see A. Hardy, 'Scientific Strategy Versus ad hoc Response: The Problem of Typhoid in England and America, c 1910–1950', *Journal of the History of Medicine and Allied Sciences*, pre-published online, April 2012; R. V. Tauxe and E. J. Esteban, 'Advances in Food Safety to Prevent Foodborne Diseases in the United States', in J. W. Ward and C. Warren, *Silent Victories: The History and Practice of Public Health in Twentieth-century America* (Oxford and New York, 2007), pp. 18–43, on p. 20; M. Kurlansky, *The Big Oyster: History on the Half Shell* (New York: Random House, 2006), pp. 259–65. Issues of citizenship do not feature in these accounts.

3. Editorial, 'Typhoid and Oysters', *British Medical Journal*, 1 (1894), p. 41. For the Christmas trade in oysters, see A. Hardy, 'Exorcising Molly Malone: Typhoid and Shellfish Consumption in Urban Britain, 1850–1960', *History Workshop Journal*, 55 (2003), pp. 73–90.

4. Sir W. Broadbent, 'A Note on the Transmission of the Infection of Typhoid Fever by Oysters', *British Medical Journal*, 1 (1895), p. 61.

5. Editorial, 'Typhoid Fever and Oyster Eating', *British Medical Journal*, 1 (12 January 1895), pp. 92–3.

6. 'Copy of a Report on an Outbreak of Typhoid Fever at Wesleyan University by Professor H. W. Conn', British Parliamentary Papers, 1896, xxxvii, Appendix 3, pp. 274–89, on p. 274. Note that the bound volume of parliamentary papers was printed in the year following the original report.

7. Ibid., p. 285.
8. J. G. Bertram, *The Harvest of the Sea* (London: John Murray, 1865), p. 374.
9. Correspondence, 'Typhoid Fever and Oysters', *British Medical Journal*, 1 (1895), p. 217.
10. Anon., 'Oh, those Medical Papers', *Fish Trades Gazette*, 12 January 1895, p. 8.
11. Medical Officer's Annual Report, Local Government Board, BPP, 1896, xxxvii, 'Supplement to the Medical Officer's twenty-fourth annual report, on Oyster Culture in Relation to Disease' (hereafter 'Oyster culture'), p. 30.
12. H. J. Lewis-Johnston, 'The Possible Conveyance of certain Water Borne Diseases, especially Typhoid Fever, by Oysters and other Molluscs', *British Medical Journal*, 1 (1895), p. 559.
13. H. Timbrell Bulstrode, 'Report on an Inquiry into the Conditions under which Oysters ... are Cultivated and Stored along the Coast of England and Wales', BPP 1896, xxxvii, Appendix no 1, pp. 29–198.
14. Editorial, 'Oysters and Disease', *British Medical Journal*, 2 (1896), p. 1663.
15. Anon., 'Pathogenic Organisms and Sea Water', *British Medical Journal*, 2 (1895), p. 390.
16. See G. E. Cartwright Wood, 'Special Report to the *British Medical Journal* on the Circumstances under which Infectious Diseases may be Conveyed by Shellfish with Special Reference to Oysters', *British Medical Journal*, 2 (1896), pp. 664–6, 759–64, 759.
17. C. Hamlin, *A Science of Impurity: Water Analysis in Nineteenth-Century England* (Bristol: Hilger, 1990).
18. Wood, 'Special Report', p. 759
19. R. Thorne, 'Introduction', Supplement to the 24th Annual Report of the Local Government Board, PP, 1896, xxxvii, p. 26
20. Ibid.
21. J. M. Tabor, 'The Position of the Oyster Industry in Great Britain', *F.T.G.*, 9 September 1899, p. 57.
22. Editorial, 'Oysters and Typhoid Fever', *British Medical Journal*, 2 (1896), p. 1736.
23. 'Our Trawl Net', *F.T.G.*, 12 January 1895, pp. 10–11. Analytical chemists were employed by the local authorities in relation to food adulteration regulations. They were known as public analysts.
24. Ibid.
25. Editorial, 'The Oyster Report II. Dr Klein as Balaam', *F.T.G.*, 19 December 1896, pp. 8–9.
26. Ibid.
27. Annotation, *Lancet*, 2 (1896), p. 1695.
28. Editorial, 'Oysters and Typhoid Fever', *British Medical Journal*, 2 (1896), p. 1736.
29. Editorial, 'The Oyster Report III', *F.T.G.*, 26 December 1896, pp. 8–9.
30. Sir William Abbott Herdman (1858–1924), *DNB*. The Sea Fisheries Committees were officially committees of the county or borough authorities, singly or in combination, with additional members representing the fishery interests of the district. The number of fishery trade members on any given committee was not to be less than that of the local authority members.
31. Editorial, 'Oysters and 'rrors', *F.T.G.*, 4 April 1896, p. 8.
32. W. A. Herdman and R. Boyce, *Oysters and Disease*, Lancashire Sea Fisheries Memoir no 1 (1899), p. 38.
33. Editorial, 'Oysters For Ever', *F.T.G.*, 13 February 1897, p. 8.
34. Editorial, 'The Oyster Question', *F.T.G.*, 10 September 1898, p. 14.
35. Editorial, 'A Word to Medical Officers', *F.T.G.*, 6 January 1900, p. 8.
36. Annotation, 'Oysters and Disease', *British Medical Journal*, 1 (1900), p. 338.

37.	Since the Oyster Bill did not make it to the statute book, it appears not to have been recorded.
38.	Editorial, 'The Government's Oyster Bill', *F.T.G.*, 20 May 1899, p. 12.
39.	Editorial, 'The Oyster Bill', *F.T.G.*, 27 May 1899, p. 14; Editorial, 'The Oysters Bill – Objections from Essex', *F.T.G.*, 17 June 1899, p. 18.
40.	'Our Trawl Net', *F.T.G.*, 24 June 1899, p. 13.
41.	Editorial, 'Fish Trades in Parliament', *F.T.G.*, 5 August 1899, p. 9.
42.	Editorial, 'The Abandoned Oysters Bill', *British Medical Journal*, 2 (1899), p. 422.
43.	Editorial, 'The Oyster Trade', *F.T.G.* 15 December 1900, p. 23; Editorial, *F.T.G.*, 29 December 1900, p. 17.
44.	Editorial, 'The Oyster Trade', *F.T.G.*, 9 February 1901, p. 27.
45.	Editorial, 'The Oyster Trade', *F.T.G.*, 7 September 1901, p. 15.
46.	Editorial, 'The Oyster Trade', *F.T.G.*, 1 April 1901, p. 27.
47.	'Our Trawl Net – Oyster Merchants in a New Profession', *F.T.G.*, 9 January 1904, p. 18.
48.	'Our Trawl Net', *F.T.G.*, 19 December 1896, p. 9.
49.	Ibid., *F.T.G.*, 18 September 1897, p. 9.
50.	Editorial, 'Oyster Report III', *F.T.G.*, 26 December 1896, pp. 8–9.
51.	'Our Trawl Net', *F.T.G.*, 2 May 1896, p. 9.
52.	'Our Trawl Net', *F.T.G.*, 26 December 1896, p. 10. 'The Oyster Trade', *F.T.G.*, 17 November 1900, p. 17.
53.	Editorial, 'The Oyster Trade', *F.T.G.*, 17 November 1900, p. 17.
54.	Ibid.
55.	P. Quant, 'Fish Snacks', *F.T.G.*, 6 November 1897, p. 10.
56.	Editorial, 'The Oyster Trade', *F.T.G.*, 15 December 1900, p. 23.
57.	Editorial, 'The Oyster Trade', *F.T.G.*, 10 August 1901, p. 35.
58.	Editorial, 'Shellfish Trade at Billingsgate', *F.T.G.*, 8 February 1902, pp. 28–9.
59.	Editorial, 'Shellfish Trade at Billingsgate', *F.T.G.*, 23 August 1902, p. 29; *F.T.G.*, 18 October 1902, p. 29.
60.	Editorial, 'Shellfish Trade at Billingsgate', *F.T.G.*, 23 August 1902, p. 29.
61.	H. Timbrell Bulstrode, 'Report Upon Alleged Oyster-borne Enteric Fever and Other Illness following on the Mayoral Banquets at Winchester and Southampton', BPP 1904, xxvi, Appendix A no 9, pp. 129–89.
62.	'Our Trawl Net', *F.T.G.*, 20 December 1902, p. 19; Editorial, 'The Oyster Trade', *F.T.G.*, p. 27 December 1902, p. 16; Editorial, 'Oysters for London', *F.T.G.*, 3 January 1903, p. 23.
63.	Editorial, 'Oysters for London', *F.T.G.*, 3 January 1903, p. 23.
64.	'Our Trawl Net: Opening of the Oyster Season', *F.T.G.*, 8 August 1903, pp. 16–17.
65.	'Cleethorpes Again', *F.T.G.*, 26 September 1903, p. 19.
66.	Editorial, 'Gann's Princesses', *F.T.G.*, 2 January 1904, p. 20.
67.	Ibid.
68.	Ibid. See also Bulstrode, 'Report upon Alleged Oyster-borne Enteric Fever', p. 152.
69.	'Our Trawl Net – Royal Commission on Sewage Report', *F.T.G.*, 9 January 1904, p. 18.
70.	Editorial, 'Dr A. A. Kanthack and B. Coli Communis', *F.T.G.*, 9 January 1904, p. 19.
71.	'Our Trawl Net – Oyster Merchants and a New Profession', *F.T.G.*, 9 January 1904, p. 18.
72.	Editorial, 'Sewage and Shell-fish', *F.T.G.*, 16 January 1904, p. 19.
73.	Royal Commission on Sewage Disposal, Fourth Report, BPP, 1904, xxxvii, pp. 32–3.
74.	'Our Trawl Net', *F.T.G.*, 23 January 1904, p. 21.
75.	E. Klein, *Report of Experiments and Observations on the Vitality of the Bacillus of Typhoid and of Sewage Micrtobes in Oysters and Other Fish* (London, 1905).

76. Editorial, 'Dr Klein's Report', *F.T.G.*, 29 July 1905, p. 16.
77. Ibid.
78. Editoial, 'B.coli Communis', *F.T.G.*, 5 August 1905, p. 16.
79. J. H. Eyre, *Bacteriological Techniques*, 3rd edn (London: Balliere, Tindall and Cox, 1930), p. 560.
80. Ibid., p. 559.
81. Royal Commission on Sewage Disposal, Fourth Report, p. 22.
82. J. H. Eyre, 'The Control and Marketing of Shellfish', *Journal of the Royal Sanitary Institute*, 49 (1928–9), pp. 275–82.
83. Ibid., p. 282.

3 Huisman, 'Monopoly or Freedom of Healing? The Role of Medicine in a Modernizing Society'

1. Nationaal Archief Den Haag (NA), archief van de Tweede Kamer der Staten-Generaal, 1815–1945 (2.02.22), inv.nr. 1252. The petition was registered as number 39 by the Committee for Petitions: *Handelingen van de Tweede Kamer* 1913/1914, 78. In the same period, a very similar petition was submitted by the Comité (later on: Nationale Vereeniging) tot Propaganda voor Wijziging der Wetten betreffende de Uitoefening der Geneeskunst: NA, archief Tweede Kamer 1815–1945, inv.nr. 1252 (72 en 210) and 1253 (348).
2. For a first batch of adhesions to the petition nr. 39, see NA, archief Tweede Kamer 1815–1945, inv.nr. 1254, 1255 and 1518.
3. Cf. R. O. van Holthe tot Echten, *De vrije uitoefening der geneeskunst of het artsenmonopolie?* (Den Haag, 1913) and 'Het Nederlandsche tijdschrift voor geneeskunde over het artsenmonopolie en de geneesvrijheid', *Het toekomstig leven*, 18 (1914), pp. 301–8, 321–6, 337–43 351–7; J. A. van Hamel (pro) and E. C. van Leersum (contra), *Vrije uitoefening van de geneeskunde*, published in the series *Pro en contra betreffende vraagstukken van algemeen belang* (Baarn, 1914).
4. See, for example, *Weekblad van het recht*, 48 (1886), 5304.1; 73 (1911), 9240.3. In most cases, it proved impossible to collect the evidence, because former patients refused to testify, or because the law was not clear.
5. Van Holthe tot Echten: 'Why should the State protect *my* health, *my* life, when my health and my life are in danger only due *to my own will and my own doing? De vrije uitoefening*, p 49 [original italics] Van Hamel argued that current legislation was lacking in fairness, responsibility and freedom: *Pro en contra vrije uitoefening van de geneeskunde*, p. 20.
6. *Handelingen Tweede Kamer 1913/14*, pp. 1450–1, 1454, 1464, 1472–3; bijlage A, hfst. 5, par. 12, 3e afd., 6; par. 13, 3e afd., p. 37.
7. J. T. Minderaa, 'Pacificatie en democratisering in Nederland rond 1918', in R. A. Koole (ed.), *Van Bastille tot Binnenhof: De Franse revolutie en haar invloed op de Nederlandse politieke partijen* (Houten, 1989), pp. 49–65, on p. 59.
8. 'Adults should not be kept from submission to treatment by someone of their own choosing. And that the man who cures him should be prosecuted for it is a second folly in our legislation', *Handelingen Tweede Kamer 1913/14* (1464). De Savornin Lohman was greatly interested in the topic, about which he collected much documentation: NA, archief De Savornin Lohman (2.21.148), inv.nrs. 614–19.

9. NA, Ministerie van BiZa, Volksgezondheid en Armwezen 1910–1918, inv.nr. 417, 23 December 1916. The report is attached as Supplement I to the *Verslag van de [juridische] Staatscommissie benoemd bij K.B. van 31 juli 1917 no. 39* (z.p. z.j.).
10. NA, Afdeling Volksgezondheid en Armwezen van het Ministerie van Binnenlandse Zaken, 1910–1918 (2.04.54) inv.nr. 417. Apart from the three H's members included: Jhr Mr J. W. M. Bosch van Oud-Amelisweerd, President of the District Court of Utrecht and a member of the Senate; Mr D. Simons, Professor of criminal law in Utrecht and Mr B. Edersheim, attorney in The Hague.
11. *Verslag van de [juridische] Staatscommissie benoemd bij K.B. van 31 juli 1917 no. 39* (z.p. z.j.).
12. J. F. Selhorst, 'Het meervoudig juristenmonopolie en zijn consequenties voor den staat I', *Vox medicorum*, 31 October 1917.
13. The Health committee of Gorinchem was an exception to this. Having realized the potential threat from the beginning, it submitted a counter petition to Parliament in November 1913, in which it urged not to take the petition by Van Houten c.s. in consideration: NA, archief Tweede Kamer 1815–1945, inv.nr. 1252 (138). The Health committees of Oldenzaal and Franeker pledged their adhesion: inv.nr. 1518.
14. *Nederlandsch tijdschrift voor geneeskunde*, 58 (1914) IB, pp. 1846–2044 (30 May). All further reference to the *NTvG* are to this special issue, unless otherwise stated.
15. J. Slingenberg, 'Het artsen-monopolie in andere landen', *NTvG*, pp. 1859–1885.
16. Ibid., p. 1870.
17. See, for example, C. Lawrence, 'Incommunicable Knowledge: Science, Technology and the Clinical Art in Britain 1850–1914', *Journal of Contemporary History*, 20 (1985), pp. 503–20; J. H. Warner, 'Science in Medicine', *Osiris*, 2nd series 1 (1985), pp. 37–58.
18. Van Rijnberk, 'Een woord', p. 1848.
19. W. Nolen, 'De toekomst der geneeskunde', *NTvG*, pp. 2013–22 on p. 2018.
20. See also P. van der Wielen on the herbal practitioners of his days: 'Van de kruiden, die genazen', *NTvG*, pp. 1961–9, on p. 1962.
21. P. Muntendam, 'De gevaren van z.g. populaire boeken over geneeskunde', *NTvG*, pp. 1929–33.
22. E. C. van Leersum, 'Over de waardeering van oude en volks-geneesmiddelen', *NTvG*, pp. 1952–60.
23. *Rapport van de [medische] Staatscommissie benoemd bij K.B. 31 juli 1917* (Den Haag z.j.). Members of the committee included: Prof. C. A. Pekelharing (chair), Storm van Leeuwen (secretary), Prof. A. A. Hijmans v. d. Bergh, Prof. Laméris, Dr L. Polak Daniels, Dr D. Schermers, Dr Schuurmans Stekhoven, Dr M. P. van Spanje, prof. Treub, Prof. J. Wertheim Salomonson, Prof. C. Winkler and Prof. W. P. C. Zeeman.
24. Ibid., p. 33.
25. See, for example, *Vox medicorum*, 2 April and 28 May 1919.
26. R. O. van Holthe tot Echten, 'Het Nederlandsche tijdschrift voor geneeskunde over het artsenmonopolie en de geneesvrijheid', *Het toekomstig leven*, 18 (1914), pp. 301–8, 321–6, 337–43, 351–7.
27. Van Holthe tot Echten, 'Het Nederlandsche tijdschrift voor geneeskunde', p. 326.
28. Ibid., p. 324.
29. 'Het adres van de drie Meesters' and 'Het meervoudig juristenmonopolie en zijn consequenties voor den staat'. Both series were published in *Vox medicorum;* the first one in the editions of 11 and 25 July 1917, the second one in those of 31 October, 14 and 28 November, 12 and 26 December 1917 en 9 and 23 January 1918.

30. *Vox medicorum*, 14 November 1917. It would seem that Selhorst was writing on behalf of many of his colleagues; see the opening address to the general meeting of the NMG in 1906 held by the chair, M. W. Pijnappel: *NTvG*, 50 (1906) IIB, pp. 81–9.

31. *Vox medicorum*, 23 January 1918.

32. R. O. van Holthe tot Echten, *Het goed recht van het zoogenaamde menschelijke magnetisme als geneeskracht* (Den Haag, 1911), p. 39.

33. Cf. Van Holthe tot Echten, 'Het NTvG', 302 and 356. His faith in reincarnation becomes clear in *Reincarnatie: Historische, ethische, wijsgeerige en wetenschappelijke beschouwing* (Bussum, 1921).

34. See, for example, *Nieuwe Rotterdamsche Courant*, 27 September 1913; *De Telegraaf*, 11 October 1913; Hector Treub, 'Vrije uitoefening der geneeskunst', *Vragen des tijds*, 39:1 (1913) pp. 155–72; A. W. van Renterghem, 'De vrije uitoefening der geneeskunst in Nederland', *De Gids*, 78:2 (1914), pp. 482–513 and 78:3, pp. 74–103.

35. G. van Rijnberk, 'Hedendaagsch mirakelgeloof', p. 5. 'Over somnambulisme', *NTvG*, pp. 1969–73 on p. 1973; *Vox medicorum*, 12 March 1913; H. Pinkhof, in *Pro en contra natuurgeneeswijze* (Baarn, 1917), p. 29. Although there was general support for the petition, the number of notables is striking.

36. *Handelingen Tweede Kamer 1913/14*, p. 1464.

37. B. Willink, *De tweede Gouden Eeuw: Nederland en de Nobelprijzen voor natuurwetenschappen 1870–1940* (Amsterdam: Bakker, 1998).

38. H. Pinkhof, 'De homoeopathie', *NTvG*, pp. 1981–9 on p. 1982. For his sharp response to the appointing of the State Committee, see H. Pinkhof, 'De vrucht van de monopoliebeweging', *NTvG*, 61 (1917) IIA, pp. 507–9.

39. *Vox medicorum*, 5 November 1913.

40. Ibid., 8 October 1913; Pinkhof in *Pro en contra natuurgeneeswijze*, 16 (original).

41. This trend was observed by contemporaries as well. See, for example, B. H. C. K. van der Wijck, 'De wetenschappen', in Smissaert (ed.), *Nederland*, pp. 261–98 on p. 264; *Vox medicorum*, 31 October 1917.

42. To name but a few examples: the Gouda physician A. C. A. Hoffman advocated homeopathy and miraculous healing in Lourdes, while his Amsterdam colleague W. van Renterghem did the same for hypnosis. Their colleague G. Luchtmans was an ardent anti-vivisectionist.

43. J. Bank and M. van Buuren, *1900. Hoogtij van burgerlijke cultuur* (Den Haag, 2000), p. 230.

44. Van Leersum, *Pro en contra vrije uitoefening van de geneeskunde*, p. 21.

45. In his *Op het breukvlak van twee eeuwen: De westerse wereld rond 1900* (Amsterdam, 1976), Jan Romein labelled all these systems and movements as 'the small religions' (ch. 33). For a reassessment of the 'medical' small religions, see F. Huisman and H. te Velde (eds), *De 'medische' kleine geloven rond 1900*. Special issue of *De negentiende eeuw*, 25 (2001).

46. *Pro en contra natuurgeneeswijze*. Beijlevelt knew and supported the petition of the three H's: Ibid., p. 15.

47. *Pro en contra vivisectie* (Baarn, 1905). On Ortt, see André de Raaij, 'Felix Ortts pneumat-energetisch monisme: Een filosofie van het christen-anarchisme', *Geschiedenis van de wijsbegeerte in Nederland*, 8 (1997), pp. 93–102.

48. For example in *Pro en contra dierlijk magnetisme* (Baarn, 1911).

49. See also H. N. de Frémery, *De gave der gezondmaking* Bussum, 1911).

50. *Pro en contra spiritisme* (Baarn, 1906).

51. Ibid., p. 21.

52. *Pro en contra Christian Science* (Baarn, 1915).
53. For the citations, see ibid., pp. 6, 11 (emphasis added).
54. See also R. Cooter (ed.), *Studies in the History of Alternative Medicine* (New York, 1988); W. de Blecourt, *Het Amazonenleger. Irreguliere genezeressen in Nederland 1850–1930* (Amsterdam, 1999).
55. See, for example, H. G. Thieme, *Open brief aan de heeren S. van Houten, R. O. Van Holthe tot Echten en J. A. van Hamel inzake het artsen-monopolie* (Zutphen z.j., [1916]).
56. See also Van Holthe tot Echten, *Het goed recht*, pp. 16–18, 22. To Van Holthe tot Echten, the attraction of magnetism was the fact that it bridged the gap between body and mind. The fluidum mediated between the soul and the material organism: *De vrije uitoefening*, p. 30.
57. *Verslag van de [juridische] Staatscommissie*, 5 (supplement I).
58. Cf. an observation made by Van Holthe tot Echten: 'The matter cannot be solved using purely medical arguments; rather, what we need are legal and political arguments: *NTvG*, p. 303.
59. See J. Talsma, *Het recht van petitie, verzoekschriften aan de Tweede Kamer en het ombudsvraagstuk. Nederland, 1795–1983* (Arnhem, 1989), esp. p. 189. The petition of the Nationale Vereeniging tot Propaganda voor Wijziging der Wetten betreffende de Uitoefening der Geneeskunst was almost ignored, probably because the chief petitioner (the Amsterdam policeman G. Bruijn) was of much more humble status than Van Houten.
60. On Van Houten, see G. M. Bos, *Mr. S. van Houten. Analyse van zijn denkbeelden, voorafgegaan door een schets van zijn leven* (Purmerend, 1952); Stuurman, *Wacht op onze daden*, ch. 5.
61. S. van Houten, *Staatkundige brieven*, 28 November 1913. For the same reasons, he was opposed to forced vaccination: NA, papieren van S. van Houten (2.21.026.06), inv.nr. 38.
62. On Cort van der Linden, see A. O. Minderaa, 'Pacificatie'; Henk te Velde, *Gemeenschapszin en plichtsbesef: Liberalisme en nationalisme in Nederland, 1870–1918* (Den Haag, 1992), pp. 243–8; S. Dudink, *Deugdzaam liberalisme: Sociaal-liberalisme in Nederland 1870–1901* (Amsterdam, 1997), esp. ch. 6.
63. Dudink, *Deugdzaam liberalisme*, pp. 161–2. On the distinction between 'male' and 'female' politics, see A. Kluveld, *Reis door de hel der onschuldigen: De expressieve politiek van de Nederlandse anti-vivisectionisten, 1890–1940* (Amsterdam, 2000), pp. 16–21.
64. Like Cort van der Linden, Dutch Parliament had suggested to include non-academics and advocates of irregular healing methods in the committee, in an attempt to counterbalance the hostile attitude of Dutch medical faculties towards magnetism and clairvoyance: *Handelingen Tweede Kamer 1913/14*, pp. 1454 and 1464. From an internal note by Cort to his secretary-general, it becomes clear that he was sceptical of the open-mindedness of the medical committee: NA, Ministerie BiZa, Volksgezondheid en Armwezen 1910–1918, inv.nr. 417, 23 June 1917.
65. NA, Ministerie BiZa, Volksgezondheid en Armwezen 1910–1918, inv.nr. 417, 25 March 1918 (Cort) and 26 March 1918 (Van Houten and Pekelharing).
66. M. J. L. A. Stassen, *Charles Ruys de Beerenbrouck. Edelman-staatsman 1873–1936* (Maastricht, 2000).
67. Stassen, *Charles Ruys de Beerenbrouck*, pp. 51–9. Ruys, who would be the leader of three cabinets between 1918 and 1933, is characterized by his political biographer as 'the promoter of the social state': ibid., p. 197. With regard to the organization of the Dutch health care system, Henk van der Velden points to a transformation from a 'local and liberal' system to a 'central-confessional one': 'Groot of klein: de opbouw van het Nederlandse ziekenhuiswezen, 1890–1950', *Tijdschrift voor sociale geschiedenis*, 25 (1999), pp. 406–24, on pp. 408–14.

4 Peeters and Wils, 'Ambivalences of Liberal Health Policy: *Lebensreform* and Self-help Medicine in Belgium, 1890–1914'

1. A. De Swaan, *In Care of the State: Health Care, Education and Welfare in Europe and the USA in the Modern Era* (Cambridge: Polity, 1988).

2. E. Witte, 'The Battle for Monasteries, Cemeteries and Schools: Belgium', in C. Clark and W. Kaiser, *Culture Wars: Secular-Catholic Conflict in Nineteenth-Century Europe* (Cambridge: Cambridge University Press, 2003), pp. 102–28.

3. J. Deferme, *Uit de ketens van de vrijheid: het debat over de sociale politiek in België 1886–1914* (Leuven: Universitaire Pers Leuven, 2007).

4. On the place of the layman in *fin-de-siècle* health reform in Germany, see for example, C. Huerkamp, 'Medizinische Lebensreform im späten 19. Jahrhundert: Die Naturheilbewegung in Deutschland als Protest gegen die naturwissenschaftlichen Universitätsmedizin', *Vierteljahresschrift für Sozial- und Wirtschaftsgeschichte*, 73 (1986), pp. 158–82; C. Regin, *Selbsthilfe und Gesundheitspolitik. Die Naturheilbewegung im Kaiserreich, 1889 bis 1914*, Medizin, Gesellschaft und Geschichte 4 (Stuttgart: Franz Steiner Verlag, 1995); R. Jütte, *Geschichte der alternativen Medizin. Von der Volksmedizin zu den unkonventionellen Therapien von heute* (Munich: C. H. Beck, 1996) and T. Faltin, *Heil und Heilung. Geschichte der Laienheilkundigen und Struktur antimodernistischer Weltanschauungen in Kaiserreich und Weimarer Republik am Beispiel von Eugen Wenz (1856–1945)*, Medizin, Gesellschaft und Geschichte. Beihefte 15 (Stuttgart: Franz Steiner Verlag, 2000).

5. See for example, R. Cooter, 'Alternative Medicine, Alternative Cosmology', in R. Cooter (ed.), *Studies in the History of Alternative Medicine* (London: Macmillan, 1988), pp. 63–78.

6. K. Velle, 'De centrale gezondheidsadministratie in België vóór de oprichting van het eerste Ministerie van Volksgezondheid (1849–1936)', *Belgisch Tijdschrift voor Nieuwste Geschiedenis*, 21 (1990), pp. 162–210.

7. R. Schepers, *De opkomst van het medisch beroep in België. De evolutie van de wetgeving en de beroepsorganisaties in de 19de eeuw* (Amsterdam: Amsterdam University Press, 1989), pp. 515–16; M. Ramsey, 'Alternative Medicine in Modern France', *Medical History*, 43 (1999), pp. 386–422; Jütte, *Geschichte der alternativen Medizin*, pp. 20, 36.

8. G. Willems, 'De maatschappelijke rol van de Académie Royale de Médecine de Belgique (1841–1914)' (MA thesis, University of Leuven, 2003).

9. K. Velle, 'De centrale gezondheidsadministratie'; 'De overheid en de zorg voor de volksgezondheid', in J. de Maeyer et al. (eds), *Er is leven na de dood. Tweehonderd jaar gezondheidszorg in Vlaanderen* (Kapellen: Pelckmans, 1998), pp. 130–50.

10. K. Velle, 'Statistiek en sociale politiek: De medische statistiek en het gezondheidsbeleid in België in de 19de eeuw', *Belgisch Tijdschrift voor Nieuwste Geschiedenis*, 26 (1985), pp. 213–42.

11. K. Wils, *De omweg van de wetenschap: Het positivisme en de Belgische en Nederlandse intellectuele cultuur, 1845–1914* (Amsterdam: Amsterdam University Press, 2005), pp. 161–76, 306–26.

12. J. Vandendriessche, 'Medische expertise en politieke strijd: De dienst medisch schooltoezicht in Antwerpen, 1860–1900', *Stadsgeschiedenis*, 6 (2011), pp. 113–28.

13. L. Nys, 'Nationale plagen: Hygiënisten over het maatschappelijk lichaam', in L. Nys, H. de Smaele, J. Tollebeek and K. Wils (eds), *De zieke natie. Over de medicalisering van de samenleving, 1860–1914* (Groningen: Historische Uitgeverij, 2002), pp. 220–41; A. Morelli, 'Les médecins parlementaires belges (19ᵉ–20ᵉ siècles)', in *L'engagement social et politique des médecins. Belgique et Canada, Xixe et Xxe siècles. Actes du colloque tenu à l'U.L.B. les 5 et 6 février 1993*, special issue of *Socialisme* (Brussels, 1993), pp. 9–18.

14. Schepers, *De opkomst van het medisch beroep in België*, pp. 153–63, 169–77, 387–406.
15. Nys, 'Nationale plagen', pp. 220–41; Morelli, 'Les médecins parlementaires belges', J. D. Ellis, *The Physician-Legislators of France: Medicine and Politics in the Early Third Republic, 1870–1914* (Cambridge: Cambridge University Press, 1990); J. Deferme, 'Geen woorden maar daden. Politieke cultuur en sociale verantwoordelijkheid in het België van 1886', *Belgisch Tijdschrift voor Nieuwste Geschiedenis* (2000), pp. 131–71.
16. K. Velle, 'De geneeskunde en de Rooms Katholieke Kerk (1830–1940): een moeilijke verhouding?', *Trajecta. Tijdschrift voor de geschiedenis van het katholiek leven in de Nederlanden*, 4 (1995), pp. 1–21.
17. M. Stolberg, 'Homöopathie und Klerus. Zur Geschichte einer besonderen Beziehung', *Medizin, Gesellschaft und Geschichte*, 17 (1998), pp. 131–48; M. Gijswijt-Hofstra, 'Homeopathie rond 1900: een 'klein geloof'?', *De Negentiende Eeuw*, 25 (2001), p. 177.
18. A. H. Van Baal, *In Search of a Cure: The Patients of the Ghent Homoeopathic Physician Gustave A. van den Berghe (1837–1902)* (Amsterdam: Amsterdam University Press, 2004), pp. 123–6.
19. W. Van Praet, 'De receptie van de homeopathie in België: 1874–1914', *Belgisch Tijdschrift voor Nieuwste Geschiedenis*, 20 (1989), pp. 107–35.
20. Van Baal, *In Search of a Cure*, pp. 44 and 47–136.
21. For biographical details on Van den Broeck, see the commemorative series published by his pupil Aloïs van Son: A. van Son, 'Beknopte levensschets van F. J. van den Broeck I, II en III', *Maandschrift van het Hygiënisch Gesticht Van den Broeck. Natuurgeneeskundig tijdschrift*, 1:10 (1923–4), pp. 149–59; 1:11 (1923–4), pp. 165–70 and 1:12 (1923–4), pp. 191–4. See also A. van Son, 'Beknopte levensschets van F. J. van den Broeck IV', *Terug ter orde*, 2:1, 2, 5 (1924–5), pp. 207–11; 219–22; 65–70, respectively.
22. On natural healers in Belgium, see E. Peeters, 'Questioning the Medical Fringe. The "Cultural Doxy" of Catholic Hydropathy in Belgium, 1890–1914', *Bulletin of the History of Medicine*, 84 (2010), pp. 92–119.
23. On the position of the Kneipp movement: M. Hau, *The Cult of Health and Beauty in Germany: A Social History 1890–1930* (Chicago, IL: Chicago University Press, 2003), p. 232.
24. P. Van Waver, *De l'art de guérir, avec ou sans diplôme. Réponse à un membre de l'Académie* (Brussels, 1899).
25. J. Van den Broeck, *De natuurlijke behandeling. Hare beschuldigers gedaagd voor het gezond verstand* (Norderwijck: Van den Broeck, 1896); J. Van den Broeck, *Het Levensproblema en de natuurlijke behandeling der zieken* (Brecht: Van den Broeck, 1904).
26. Van den Broeck, *De natuurlijke behandeling* and *Het Levensproblema*.
27. J. Magnus, 'Over kwakzalverij en wat daarbij te pas komt', *Het Voorlichtingsblad. Tijdschrift ter Bevordering der Wetenschappelijke Natuurgeneeskunde*, 2 (1937–1938), pp. 49–56; A. Van Son, 'Kwakzalverij en … kwakzalverij', *Terug ter Orde. Vlaams Natuurgeneeskundig Tijdschrift van het Hygiënisch Gesticht Van den Broeck*, 13 (1938–9), pp. 1–19.
28. P. Van Waver, *De l'art de guérir, avec ou sans diplôme. Réponse à un membre de l'Académie* (Brussels : Van Waver, 1899), pp. 8, 23, 80, 82, 116.
29. L. Dejace, 'L'excercice de l'art de guérir sans diplôme', *Le Scalpel : Journal hebdomodaire. Organe des intérêts scientifiques et professionels de la médecine, de la pharmacie et de l'art vétérinaire*, 43:49 (1890–1), pp. 337–8.
30. A. Ruyssen, 'Echos de Wörishofen', *Kneipp Journal*, 6:4 (1897), p. 60.
31. A. Van Son, 'Een "Orde der Geneesheeren" of de Geneesheren tot de Orde?', *Terug ter Orde. Vlaams Natuurgeneeskundig Tijdschrift van het Hygiënisch Gesticht Van den Broeck*, 4 (1926–7), p. 769.

32. A. Van Son, 'Volksgeneeskundige doktersvoorlichting', *Terug ter Orde. Vlaams Natuurgeneeskundig Tijdschrift van het Hygiënisch Gesticht Van den Broeck*, 4 (1926–7), p. 778.

33. J. M. Romein, *Op het breukvlak van twee eeuwen* (Amsterdam: Querido, 1976), pp. 632, 644, 650.

34. On the vaccination debate, see K. Velle, *De nieuwe biechtvaders. De sociale geschiedenis van de arts in België* (Leuven: Kritak, 1991), pp. 44–58.

35. See for example, A. Van Son, 'Het bankroet der vaccinatie', *Terug ter Orde. Vlaams Natuurgeneeskundig Tijdschrift van het Hygiënisch Gesticht Van den Broeck*, 4 (1926–7), pp. 4–7.

36. R. Schepers, 'The Belgian Medical Profession, the Order of Physicians and the Sickness Funds (1900–1940)', *Sociology of Health and Illness*, 15 (1993), pp. 386–7.

37. Dr Danjou, 'L'action combinée des sociétés végétariennes de France, de Belgique et de Catalogne, au premier Congrès Espagnol International de la Tuberculose (Barcelone, 1910)', *La Réforme Alimentaire*, 14 (1910), p. 264.

38. L. Nys, 'Moderation as a Medical Moral: The Invention of the Hygienic Body in Belgium c. 1840–1914', unpublished paper presented at the Anglo-Dutch-German Workshop: Patients' Body Perceptions, 11–13 July 2003, pp. 2–3. For the quotation, see also K. Velle, *Lichaam en hygiëne. Naar de wortels van de huidige gezondheidskultuur* (Ghent / Leuven: Kritak, 1984), p. 50.

39. L. Nys, 'De ruiters van de apocalyps. 'Alcoholisme, tuberculose, syfilis en degeneratie in medische kringen, 1870–1940', in J. Tollebeek, G. Vanpaemel and K. Wils (eds), *Degeneratie in België 1860–1940. Een geschiedenis van ideeën en praktijken* (Leuven: Universitaire Pers, 2003), p. 230.

40. The Belgian hydrotherapist Nicolas Neuens seems to have been the only person within the Belgian *Lebensreform* movement who was in favour of a general prohibition of alcohol: N. Neuens, *Médication interne de M. L'abbé Kneipp, curé de Woerishogen. Régime, hygiène alimentaire et plantes médicinales* (Paris, 1893), p. 36. See also N. Neuens, 'La peste de l'eau de vie en Belgique', *Kneipp Journal*, 1 (1892), p. 349; G. A., 'La peste de l'alcool en Belgique', *Kneipp Journal*, 4 (1895), p. 71.

41. G. Viaud, 'L'empoisonnement du protoplasma', *La Réforme Alimentaire*, 6 (1902), pp. 21–8; Em. Nyssens-Piron, 'La lutte contre l'alcoolisme. Modération ou abstinence', *La Réforme Alimentaire*, 12 (1908), pp. 309–14; F. Kubiczek, 'Guerre au démon de l'alcool', *Kneipp Journal*, 1(1892), pp. 23–4.

42. Nys, 'De ruiters van de apocalyps', p. 13.

43. Dr A. R., 'Valeur hygiénique des promenades à pied', *Kneipp Journal*, 10 (1901), p. 156. See also Dr Danjou, 'Pourquoi et comment respirer', *La Réforme Alimentaire*, 14 (1910), p. 97, E. Nyssens, 'Un nouveau traitement des arbres fruitiers', *La Réforme Alimentaire*, 14 (1910), p. 207; N. Neuens, *Traité de médecine naturelle scientifique* (Tournai, 1901), vol. 1, pp. 360–3.

44. A. De Swarte, 'Nervosisme moderne', *La Réforme Alimentaire*, 6 (1902), pp. 14–15.

5 Frohman, 'The Right to Health and Social Citizenship in Germany, 1848–1918'

1. I have found Jane Jenson's notion of citizenship regimes to be useful in thinking about these issues. See J. Jenson, 'Making Sense of Contagion: Citizenship Regimes and Public Health in Victorian England', in P. Hall and M. Lamont (eds), *Successful Societies: How Institutions and Culture Affect Health* (Cambridge: Cambridge University Press, 2009),

pp. 201–25. For guides to the literature on the entangled topics of social medicine and the social right to health, see F. Schulz, *Das 'Recht auf Gesundheit': seine wirtschafts- und sozialpolitischen Voraussetzungen in der Geschichte der sozialmedizinischen Lehrmeinungen* (Regensburg: Transfer-Verlag, 1987) and the literature cited in note 19 below.

2. *Health, Race and German Politics between National Unification and Nazism, 1870–1945* (Cambridge: Cambridge University Press, 1989).

3. *Poor Relief and Welfare in Germany from the Reformation to World War I* (Cambridge: Cambridge University Press, 2008) and 'Prevention, Welfare and Citizenship: The War on Tuberculosis and Infant Mortality in Germany, 1900–1930', *Central European History*, 39:3 (September 2006), pp. 431–81.

4. C. Hamlin, *Public Health and Social Justice in the Age of Chadwick: Britain, 1800–1854* (Cambridge: Cambridge University Press, 1998).

5. Neumann, *Die öffentliche Gesundheitspflege und das Eigenthum* (1847), partly reprinted in K.-H. Karbe, *Salomon Neumann 1819–1908. Wegbereiter sozialmedizinischen Denkens und Handelns* (Leipzig, 1983), citation pp. 100–1.

6. Virchow, 'Report on the Typhus Epidemic in Upper Silesia', in *Collected Essays on Public Health and Epidemiology* (New York: Watson Publishing, 1985), pp. 204–319, on p. 316. For Virchow's views on the rights to health and education, see his essays from *Medicinische Reform* Nr. 5 & 7 (August 4 & 18, 1848), reprinted in ibid., pp. 14–21. On the medical reform movement, see E. Ackerknecht, *Beiträge zur Geschichte der Medizinalreform von 1848*, 25 (1932), pp. 61–183.

7. Oesterlen, *Der Mensch und seine physische Erhaltung* (Leipzig, 1859), pp. 465–6.

8. Stein, *Das Gesundheitswesen* (=*Verwaltungslehre*, Teil 3, 2. Aufl., 1887), p. 20 and F. Schulz, 'Die Lehre vom öffentlichen Gesundheitswesen bei Lorenz von Stein', *Der Staat*, 27 (1988), pp. 110–28.

9. Stein, *Das Gesundheitswesen*, pp. 128–34, on p. 294.

10. On the sanitary reform movement, see A. I. Hardy, *Ärzte, Ingenieure und städtische Gesundheit. Medizinische Theorien in der Hygienebewegung des 19. Jahrhunderts* (Frankfurt: Campus Verlag, 2005), J. Rodriguez-Lores, 'Stadthygiene und Städtebau. Zur Dialektik von Ordnung und Unordnung in den Auseinandersetzungen des Deutschen Vereins für öffentliche Gesundheitspflege 1868–1901', in Rodriguez-Lores and G. Fehl (eds), *Städtebaureform 1865–1900: Von Licht, Luft und Ordnung in der Stadt der Gründerzeit* (Hamburg, 1985), pp. 19–58, M. Rodenstein, *'Mehr Licht, Mehr Luft'. Gesundheitskonzepte im Städtebau seit 1750* (Frankfurt: Campus Verlag, 1988), B. Ladd, *Urban Planning and Civic Order in Germany, 1860–1914* (Cambridge, MA: Harvard University Press, 1990) and R. Evans, *Death in Hamburg. Society and Politics in the Cholera Years, 1830–1910* (Oxford: Oxford University Press, 1987).

11. Pettenkofer, 'The Value of Health to a City', *Bulletin of the History of Medicine*, 10 (1941), pp. 473–503, 593–613, especially p. 609.

12. De Swaan, *In Care of the State: Health Care, Education and Welfare in Europe and the USA in the Modern Era* (Oxford: Oxford University Press, 1988), especially pp. 252 ff.

13. Oesterlen, *Handbuch der Hygiene, der privaten und öffentlichen*, 3. verm. Aufl. (Tübingen, 1876), p. 1, Pettenkofer, 'Einleitung' to Pettenkofer and H. von Ziemsen (eds), *Handbuch der Hygiene und der Gewerbekrankheiten*, 1. Theil: Individuelle Hygiene (Leipzig, 1882), p. 3 and Pettenkofer, 'The Value of Health to a City', p. 487.

14. Reclam, 'Die heutige Gesundheitspflege und ihre Aufgaben', *Deutsche Vierteljahrsschrift für öffentliche Gesundheitspflege*, 1 (1869), pp. 1–5, citation p. 2.

15. On the development of bacteriology, see S. Berger, *Bakterien in Krieg und Frieden: Eine Geschichte der medizinische Bakteriologie in Deutschland 1890–1933* (Göttingen: Wallstein, 2009), P. Sarasin et al. (eds), *Bakteriologie und Moderne: Studien zur Biopolitik des Unsichtbaren, 1870–1920* (Frankfurt: Suhrkamp, 2006), A. Mendelsohn, 'Cultures of Bacteriology: Formation and Transformation of a Science in France and Germany, 1870–1914' (Dissertation, Princeton University, 1996) and A. Hüntelmann, *Hygiene im Namen des Staates: Das Reichsgesundheitsamt 1876–1933* (Göttingen: Wallstein, 2008).

16. Koch, 'Die Bekämpfung der Infektionskrankheiten insbesondere der Kriegsseuchen', cited in Berger, *Bakterien in Krieg und Frieden*, pp. 57–8.

17. There is a widespread tendency to misuse the term 'social hygiene' to describe both the hereditarian and the social-economic-environmental possibilities of post-bacteriological thought. Andrew Mendelsohn provides a much more acute analysis of the analytical function of the 'social' in '"Typhoid Mary" Strikes Again: The Social and the Scientific in the Making of Modern Public Health', *Isis*, 86 (1995), pp. 268–77.

18. Hueppe, *Handbuch der Hygiene* (Berlin, 1899), p. 11.

19. On the German social hygiene movement, see A. Labisch, *Homo Hygienicus. Gesundheit und Medizin in der Neuzeit* (Frankfurt: Campus Verlag, 1992), pp. 164ff., G. Rosen, 'What is Social Medicine?', *Bulletin of the History of Medicine*, 21 (1947), pp. 675–733, D. Nadav, *Julius Moses (1868–1942) und die Politik der Sozialhygiene in Deutschland* (Gerlingen: Bleicher Verlag, 1985) and S. Stöckel, *Säuglingsfürsorge zwischen sozialer Hygiene und Eugenik: Das Beispiel Berlins im Kaiserreich und in der Weimarer Republik* (Göttingen: De Gruyter, 1996).

20. M. Mosse und G. Tugendreich (eds), *Krankheit und soziale Lage* (Munich, 1913) and A. Gottstein, 'Die Soziale Hygiene, ihre Methoden, Aufgaben und Ziele', *Zeitschrift für soziale Medizin*, 2 (1907), pp. 3–36, 100–35, especially p. 14 and Gottstein, 'Die Entwicklung der Hygiene im letzten Vierteljahrhundert', *Zeitschrift für Sozialwissenschaft*, 12 (1909), pp. 65–82, especially pp. 76–7.

21. Grotjahn, *Soziale Pathologie: Versuch einer Lehre von den sozialen Beziehungen der menschlichen Krankheiten als Grundlage der sozialen Medizin* (2. Aufl., Berlin,1915), citations on pp. 9–18, Grotjahn, *Soziale Hygiene* (=*Weyl's Handbuch der Hygiene*, 2. Aufl., Ergänzungsband, Berlin, 1918), pp. 392–4 and Grotjahn, 'Was ist und wozu treiben wir soziale Hygiene?', *Hygiensiche Rundschau*, Beilage to 14:20 (15 October 1904), pp. 1017–32. On the abstraction of the individual from the social world, see Gottstein, 'Die Entwicklung der Hygiene im letzten Vierteljahrhundert', p. 76.

22. Gottstein, 'Die Regelung des Gesundheitswesens in den deutschen Großstädten', *Deutsche medizinische Wochenschrift*, 34 (19 March 1908), pp. 512–15, on p. 513.

23. Gottstein, 'Die Soziale Hygiene, ihre Methoden, Aufgaben und Ziele', p. 135.

24. The following pages summarize the arguments that I developed at length in 'Prevention, Welfare and Citizenship'.

25. Weindling, *Health, Race and German Politics* and S. Fehlemann, 'Armutsrisiko Mutterschaft: Mütter- und Säuglingsfürsorge im Deutschen Reich, 1890–1924' (Dissertation, Düsseldorf Univesity, 2004).

26. Frohman, *Poor Relief and Welfare in Germany*, pp. 186–200.

27. G. Steinmetz, *Regulating the Social: The Welfare State and Local Politics in Imperial Germany* (Princeton, NJ: Princeton University Press, 1993).

28. It should also be noted that in other areas the dominance of conservative industrialists in the city council gave municipal social policies, as well as those sponsored by the employers themselves, an entirely different cast. See D. Sweeney, *Work, Race and the Emergence*

of Radical Right Corporatism in Imperial Germany (Ann Arbor, MI: University of Michigan Press, 2009) and P. Brandmann, *Leipzig zwischen Klassenkampf und Sozialreform: Kommunale Wohlfahrtspolitik zwischen 1890 und 1929* (Vienna: Böhlau, 1995).

29.   For three such examples, see J. Rabnow, *Bekämpfung der Tuberkulose in Berlin-Schöneberg* (Berlin, 1913), pp. 7ff.; Oberin v. Gordon, 'Die Organisation der Säuglingsfürsorge in der Stadt Darmstadt', *Mutter und Kind*, 4:8 (May 1912), pp. 6–10; and W. Kade, *Die communale Säuglingsfürsorge in Halle (Saale) bis zum Ausbruch des Weltkrieges* (Maschinenschrift, o.D.), pp. 9ff.

30.   Stadtrat Sieblist, 'Praktische Durchführung der Lungenkrankenfürsorge in der Mittelstadt und auf dem Lande', *Tuberkulose-Fürsorge-Blatt*, 1:3 (September 1913), pp. 28–30.

31.   Dr Wendenburg, 'Die westfälischen Tuberkulose-Fürsorgestellen', in *Tuberkulose und Tuberkulosefürsorge* (=*Beiträge zur sozialen Fürsorge*, Heft 9 [1927]), pp. 67–83, on p. 67.

32.   Schlossmann, 'Vorwärts?', *Mutter und Kind*, 2:5 (May 1910), pp. 2–3.

6 Elliot, 'From Tobacco in the War to the War on Tobacco: Smoking in Britain and Germany from *c.* 1900 to 1945'

1.   See http://www.who.int/fctc/en/ [accessed 1 November 2011].

2.   P. Brown, 'Europe Moving at the Speed of its Slowest Member in Controlling Tobacco', *British Medical Journal*, 324 (2002), p. 382.

3.   R. Proctor, *The Nazi War on Cancer* (Princeton, NJ: Princeton University Press, 1999), pp. 173–242, 226–7; C. Merki, 'Die Nationasozialistische Tabakpolitik', *Vierteljahresheft für Zeitgeschichte*, 46 (1998), pp. 19–42; A. Gilmore, E. Nolte, M. McKee and J. Collin, 'The Continuing Influence of the Tobacco Industry in Germany', *Lancet*, 360 (2002), p. 1255; G. Frankenberg, 'Between Paternalism and Voluntarism: Tobacco Consumption and Tobacco Control in Germany', in E. A. Feldman and R. Bayer (eds), *Unfiltered: Conflicts Over Tobacco Policy and Public Health* (Cambridge, MA: Harvard University Press, 2004), pp. 161–89.

4.   Proctor, *The Nazi War on Cancer*, pp. 176–8.

5.   R. Elliot, 'Smoking for Taxes: the Triumph of Fiscal Policy over Health in Post-war West Germany', *Economic History Review*, 65 (2012), pp. 1450–74.

6.   M. Hilton, *Smoking in British Popular Culture 1800–2000* (Manchester: Manchester University Press, 2000); J. Rudy, *The Freedom to Smoke: Tobacco Consumption and Identity* (Montreal: McGill-Queens Press, 2005).

7.   *Lancet*, 4 April 1857, p. 354.

8.   J. Parton, *Smoking and Drinking* (London, 1888) p. 2; R. L. Carpenter, *A Lecture on Tobacco* (London: National Temperance Publication Department, 1882), p. 25.

9.   'Baneful Effects of Excessive Smoking', *Lancet*, 4 April 1857, pp. 345–6; J. G. Schneider, *Lancet*, 31 January 1857, p. 127.

10.   R. Elliot, *Women and Smoking since 1890* (London/New York: Routledge, 2007), pp. 15–18.

11.   W. MacDonald, Letter, *Lancet*, 28 February 1857, p. 232.

12.   M. Lander, *The Tobacco Problem* (Boston, MA, 1886), p. 1.

13.   M. C. Enke, *Über die Bedeutung des Tabaks in der europäischen Medizin vom 16. bis ins 20. Jahrhundert* (Berlin: Verlag für Wissenschaft und Forschung, 1998), pp. 284–6.

14.   Elliot, *Women and Smoking*, p. 19.

15. Ibid., pp. 32–3; B. Kosta, 'Cigarettes, Advertising and the Weimar Republic's Modern Woman', in G. Finney (ed.), *Visual Culture in Twentieth Century Germany* (Bloomington, IN: Indiana University Press, 2006), pp. 134–5.

16. P. Weindling, *Health, Race and German Politics between National Unification and Nazism, 1870–1945* (Cambridge: Cambridge University Press, 1989), p. 100.

17. Hilton, *Smoking in British Popular Culture*.

18. Elliot, *Smoking and Women*.

19. D. Heater, *Citizenship in Britain: A History* (Edinburgh: Edinburgh University Press, 2006).

20. K. Grieves, *The Politics of Manpower, 1914–1918* (Manchester: Manchester University Press, 1988).

21. R. Barker, *Conscience, Government and War: Conscientious Objection in Great Britain, 1939–45* (London and Boston, MA: Routledge and Kegan Paul, 1982).

22. T. Nipperdey, *Deutsche Geschichte 1866–1918 vol. 2: Machtstaat vor der Demokratie* (Munich: Beck, 1992), pp. 230–8.

23. S. O. Rose, *Which People's War? National Identity and Citizenship* (Oxford: Oxford University Press, 2003).

24. Elliot, *Women and Smoking*, pp. 45–6.

25. *Tobacco Trade Review*, 1 January 1915, p. 7.

26. J. W. Spearman to editors, *BAT Bulletin*, 15 May 1915, p. 3.

27. Letter from Private A. Jay, *BAT Bulletin*, 1 May 1915, p. 1.

28. Nottingham Record Office (hereafter NRO), DD PL 6/18/10, R.W. Horne to John Players and Sons, 29 July 1918; DD PL 7/19/2, William Rushton to John Players and Sons, 8 August 1916.

29. NRO DD PL 6/18/1G. Dowell to John Players and Sons, 8 December 1914.

30. NRO, DD PL 6/18/2, W.W. to John Players and Sons, 18 December 1916.

31. NRO, DD PL 6/17/7 Harry Collins, 22 January 1918, to British American Tobacco, 22 January 1918; also DD PL 6/18/8–17.

32. *Tobacco Trade Review*, 1 September 1915, p. 308.

33. *Glasgow Herald*, 14 December 1915, p. 9; 15 December 1914, p. 9.

34. *Tobacco Trade Review*, 1 September 1915, p. 307.

35. B. W. E Alford, *W. D. & H. O. Wills and the Development of the U.K. Tobacco Industry* (London: Methuen, 1973).

36. 'All the men and women merely Wills', *Weekly Dispatch*, 25 November 1917, p. 4.

37. 'The Cigarette Hoarders: Women Smoking as Many as Usual', *Weekly Dispatch*, 9 December 1917, p. 3; 'More Smokers, less Tobacco', *Daily News*, 31 August 1918, p. 5; 'Women's Life in Hutments: YWCA replies to 'Gay Time' Criticism, *Daily News*, 3 August 1918, p. 2.

38. M. Weisser, *Über die Kunst Blauen Dunst zu Verkaufen: Die Geschichte der Zigarette, ihrer Industrie und ihrer Werbung von 1860 bis 1930* (Bassum: Doell Verlag, 2002).

39. Advertising brochure for Da Capo cigarettes, 1909, Hamburger Institut für Sozialforschung, PFR, 404, 20.

40. Ibid. p. 49.

41. Landesarchiv Baden-Württemberg, Hauptstaatsarchiv Stuttgart (hereafter Stuttgart) M77/1 Bü 1111, Abschrift, Königl. Württ. Ministerium des Innern, 31 December 1915.

42. M. Stieg, 'The 1926 German Law to Protect Youth Against Trash and Dirt: Moral Protectionism in a Democracy', *Central European History*, 23 (1990), pp. 22–56.

43. Stuttgart, E151/52 Bü 15, Aufruf an die deutschen Frauen und Mädchen, Bund Deutscher Tabakgegner, undated but archived with material from the 1920s.

44. W. Perti, 'Zur Beurteilung des Nicotingehaltes der Tabake', *Zeitschrift für Lebensmitteluntersuchung und Forschung*, 60 (1930), pp. 448.

45. Stuttgart, E151/52 Bü 15, G. von Bunge, Die Tabakvergiftung, Bund Deutscher Tabakgegner, undated, archived with material from the 1920s.

46. 'Wir Tabakgegner und das neue Reich', *Deutscher Tabakgegner*, 2–3 (1933), p. 18.

47. F. Lickint, 'Tabak und gesunde Jugenderziehung', *Deutscher Tabakgegner*, 2 (1933), p. 21.

48. Proctor, *The Nazi War on Cancer*; S. Zimmermann, M. Egger and U. Hossfield, 'Commentary: Pioneering Research into Smoking and Health in Nazi Germany' – the 'Wissenschaftliches Institut zur Erforschung der Tabakgefahren', in Jena, *International Journal of Epidemiology*, 30 (2001), pp. 35–7.

49. Zimmermann and Hossfield, 'Pioneering Research into Smoking'.

50. Lickint, *Tabak Und Organismus*, p. 884. The term 'germ plasm' comes originally from Weissmann's now obsolete theory of hereditary, which argued that germ cells, passed from parents to infant, have a hereditary substance capable of development. This was limited and divided amongst the offspring. In Nazi Germany, the germ plasm was configured at the racial level.

51. Ibid. My translation.

52. Proctor, *The Nazi War on Cancer*.

53. Hamburger Institut für Sozialforschung, PFR 140–01, Letter from Phillip F. Reemstma to Berchard Köhler, Kommission für Wirtschaftspolitik der NSDAP, 28 February 1939.

54. C. Merki, 'Die Nationalsozialistische Tabakpolitik', *Vierteljahresheft für Zeitgeschichte*, 46:1 (1998), pp. 19–42.

55. Elliot, 'Smoking for Taxes'.

56. R. Elliot, 'From Youth Protection to Individual Responsibility: Addressing Smoking among Young People in Post-War West Germany, *Medizinhistorisches Journal*, 45:1 (2010), pp. 79–87.

57. Rose, *Which People's War?*

58. Ibid.

59. *The Times*, 13 April 1943, p. 8, col. F; Mrs. H.7.P (born 1916), *Social Life in Preston 1890–1940*, Elizabeth Robert's Archive, University of Lancaster.

60. J. Costello, *Love, Sex and War: Changing Values 1939–1945* (London: Guild Publishing, 1985).

61. S. Kiryluk and N. Wald, *UK Smoking Statistics* (Oxford: Oxford University Press, 1987); Letter from Geoffrey Howard, *The Times*, 2 November 1944, p. 5, col. 5.

62. National Archives, WO 32/10801War Office Ration Scales Committee minutes.

63. *The Times*, 4 October 1939, p. 5.

64. Bristol Record Office, hereafter BRO, Wills 38169/HAF/18(k) Gift Parcels for British and Allied Prisoners of War In Europe – price list, 15 November 1943.

65. National Archives, London WO 32/10801 (30) Minutes of meeting of ration scales (Overseas theatres), Part One, matters relating to Prisoners of War, 7 December 1943.

66. BRO 38169/HAF/18k Letter to travellers about zoning scheme, 12 November 1943; National Archives, BT 131/51 *Tobacco Control*.

67. National Archives, BT 131/51 *Tobacco Control*.

68. 'Fewer cigarettes', *The Times*, 2 September 1944, p. 2.

69. '6/– a lb on tobacco', *The Times*, April 1943, p. 5.

70. 'All Square', *The Times*, 24 April 1943, p. 5.

71. National Archives, BT 131/51 *Tobacco Control*.
72. Imperial War Museum, D18234, 'Leisure and Entertainment during World War Two'.
73. Bodleian Library, Oxford, John Johnson Collection, Tobacco Box 1 'Tobacco Whiffs for the Smoking Carriage', 1874; oral history interviews carried out by the author recalled the opprobrium which 'Pasha' cigarettes aroused in the Second World War – Interview with Alex, 11 October, 2002; Interview with Rory, 12 November 2002 (names have been changed).
74. 372 HC Deb 5s, 17 June 1941, col. 469–70; 'Woman's Outlook – London Diary – Women's War Work', *Scotsman*, 13 June 1941, p. 7.
75. 'The War Resumed', *Clean Air: The National Society of Non-smokers Review*, no. 17, 17 October 1939; Letter from Maurice Cassidy, *The Times*, 17 April 1942, p. 7, col. e; Letter from Marie Stopes, *The Times*, 30 December 1942, p. 6, col. g; 393 HC Deb 5s, 9 November 1943, col. 1083–4.
76. Letter from J. Wardale, *The Times*, 13 August 1942, p. 8, col. a; Alfred Dunhill, *The Times*, 20 December, 1943, p. 8, Col. A. Dunhill was a tobacco merchant.
77. 'Jews blamed for teaching Germans to smoke', *Scotsman*, 8 November 1938, p. 9.
78. 'Against alcohol and tobacco', *The Times*, 14 July 1939, p. 13.
79. 'The Tobacco Problem', *British Medical Journal*, 23 October 1937, p. 822.
80. J. H. Wodehouse, *The Smoking Habit: Its Dangers and its Cure* (London: W. H. Jacklen, 1924, repr. 1930, 1936), pp. 7–8.
81. *British Medical Journal*, 12 September 1931, p. 517.

7 Oosterhuis, 'Mental Health and Civic Virtue: Psychiatry, Self-Development and Citizenship in the Netherlands, 1870–2005'

1. These models of self-development are borrowed from J. W. Duyvendak, *De planning van ontplooiing: Wetenschap, politiek en de maakbare samenleving* (The Hague: Sdu, 1999) and E. Tonkens, *Het zelfontplooiingsregime: De actualiteit van Dennendal en de jaren zestig* (Amsterdam: Bert Bakker, 1999).
2. S. Stuurman, 'Het einde van de productieve deugd', *Bijdragen en Mededelingen betreffende de geschiedenis der Nederlanden*, 106 (1991), pp. 610–24; I. de Haan, 'Burgerschap, sociale stratificatie en politieke uitsluiting in de negentiende eeuw', in J. Kloek and K. Tilmans (eds), *Burger: Een geschiedenis van het begrip 'burger' in de Nederlanden van de Middeleeuwen tot de 21ᶜ eeuw* (Amsterdam: Amsterdam University Press, 2002), pp. 231–75.
3. H. te Velde, *Gemeenschapszin en plichtsbesef. Liberalisme en nationalisme in Nederland, 1870–1918* (The Hague: Sdu, 1992); H. te Velde, 'How High did the Dutch Fly? Remarks on Stereotypes of Burger Mentality', in A. Galema, B. Henkes and H. te Velde (eds), *Images of the Nation: Different Meanings of Dutchness 1870–1940* (Amsterdam and Atlanta: Rodopi, 1993), pp. 59–79; H. te Velde, 'Zedelijkheid als ethiek en seksueel fatsoen: De geschiedenis van een Nederlands begrip', in R. Aerts and K. van Berkel (eds), *De Pijn van Prometheus: Essays over cultuurkritiek en cultuurpessimisme* (Groningen: Historische Uitgeverij, 1996), pp. 198–218.
4. A. de Regt, *Arbeidersgezinnen en beschavingsarbeid: Ontwikkelingen in Nederland 1870–1940; een historisch-sociologische studie* (Meppel and Amsterdam: Boom, 1984); P. Koenders, 'Tussen christelijk réveil en seksuele revolutie: Bestrijding van zedeloosheid in Nederland, met nadruk op de repressie van homoseksualiteit' (PhD dissertation, University of Leiden, 1996); D. J. Noordam, 'Getuigen, redden en bestrijden: De

ontwikkeling van een ideologie op het terrein van de zedelijkheid, 1811–1911', *Theoretische Geschiedenis*, 23:4 (1996), pp. 494–518; H. Nijenhuis, *Volksopvoeding tussen elite en massa: Een geschiedenis van de volwasseneneducatie in Nederland* (Amsterdam and Meppel: Boom, 1981); W. A. W. de Graaf, *De zaaitijd bij uitnemendheid: Jeugd en puberteit in Nederland 1900–1940* (Leiden: Academisch Boekencentrum, 1989); S. Karsten, *Op het breukvlak van opvoeding en politiek: Een studie naar socialistische volksonderwijzers rond de eeuwwisseling* (Amsterdam: Sua, 1986); W. Krul, 'Volksopvoeding, nationalisme en cultuur: Nederlandse denkbeelden over massa-educatie in het Interbellum', *Comenius*, 9:36 (1989), pp. 386–94.

5. H. Oosterhuis and M. Gijswijt-Hofstra, *Verward van geest en ander ongerief: Psychiatrie en geestelijke gezondheidszorg (1870–2005)* (Houten: Nederlands Tijdschrift voor Geneeskunde and Bohn Stafleu Van Loghum, 2008), pp. 64–70, 207–21; H. Oosterhuis and J. Slijkhuis, *Verziekte zenuwen en zeden: De opkomst van de psychiatrie in Nederland (1870–1920)* (Rotterdam: Erasmus Publishing), pp. 57–81, 187–206.

6. T. E. D. van der Grinten, *De vorming van de ambulante geestelijke gezondheidszorg: Een historisch beleidsonderzoek* (Baarn: Ambo, 1987); L. de Goei, *De psychohygiënisten: Psychiatrie, cultuurkritiek en de beweging voor geestelijke volksgezondheid in Nederland, 1924–1970* (Nijmegen: SUN, 2001); H. Oosterhuis, 'Insanity and Other Discomforts: A Century of Outpatient Psychiatry and Mental Health Care in the Netherlands 1900–2000', in M. Gijswijt-Hofstra et al. (eds), *Psychiatric Cultures Compared. Psychiatry and Mental Health Care in the Twentieth Century: Comparisons and Approaches* (Amsterdam: Amsterdam University Press, 2005), pp. 73–102.

7. R. van Ginkel, *Op zoek naar eigenheid: Denkbeelden en discussies over cultuur en identiteit in Nederland* (The Hague: Sdu, 1999), pp. 86–98.

8. See for example: K. H. Bouman, 'Psychische Hygiëne', in J. van der Hoeve et al. (eds), *Praeventieve geneeskunde* II (Groningen and Batavia: J. B. Wolters Uitgevers-Maatschappij, 1938), pp. 439–62.

9. J. C. H. Blom, 'Jaren van tucht en ascese: Enige beschouwingen over de stelling in Herrijzend Nederland 1945–1950', *Bijdragen en Mededelingen betreffende de Geschiedenis der Nederlanden*, 96:2 (1981), pp. 300–33; H. Galesloot and M. Schrevel (eds), *In fatsoen hersteld: Zedelijkheid en wederopbouw na de oorlog* (Amsterdam: Sua, 1986); Van Ginkel, *Op zoek naar eigenheid*, pp. 177–205; I. de Haan, *Zelfbestuur en staatsbeheer: Het politieke debat over burgerschap en rechtsstaat in de twintigste eeuw* (Amsterdam: Amsterdam University Press), p. 92.

10. P. Luykx and P. Slot (eds), *Een stille revolutie? Cultuur en mentaliteit in de lange jaren vijftig* (Hilversum: Verloren, 1997); K. Schuyt and E. Taverne, *1950. Welvaart in zwartwit* (The Hague: Sdu, 2000).

11. T. de Vries, *Complexe consensus: Amerikaanse en Nederlandse intellectuelen in debat over politiek en cultuur 1945–1960* (Hilversum: Verloren, 1996); Van Ginkel, *Op zoek naar eigenheid*, pp. 207–44.

12. M. Gastelaars, *Een geregeld leven. Sociologie en sociale politiek in Nederland, 1925–1968* (Amsterdam, Sua, 1985); E. Jonker, *De sociologische verleiding. Sociologie, sociaaldemocratie en de welvaartsstaat* (Groningen: Wolters-Noordhoff, 1988); De Goei, *De psychohygiënisten*; I. de Haan and J. W. Duyvendak, *In het hart van de verzorgingsstaat: Het ministerie van Maatschappelijk Werk en zijn opvolgers (CRM, WVC, VWS) 1952–2002* (Zutphen: Walburg Pers, 2002), pp. 27, 76–83.

13. A. Dercksen and L. Verplanke, *Geschiedenis van de onmaatschappelijkheidsbestrijding in Nederland, 1914–1970* (Meppel and Amsterdam: Boom, 1987); F. W. van Wel, *Gezinnen onder toezicht: De stichting volkswoningen te Utrecht 1924–1975* (Amsterdam: Sua, 1988).

14. F. J .J. Buytendijk, *De zin van de vrijheid in het menselijk bestaan* (Utrecht and Antwerpen: Uitgeverij Het Spectrum, 1958); F. J. J. Buytendijk, *Gezondheid en vrijheid* (Utrecht and Antwerpen: Uitgeverij Het Spectrum, 1950); H. M. M. Fortman, *Een nieuwe opdracht: Poging tot historische plaatsbepaling en tot taakomschrijving van de geestelijke gezondheidszorg in het bijzonder voor het katholieke volksdeel in ons land* (Utrecht and Antwerpen: Uitgeverij Het Spectrum, 1955); De Goei, *De psychohygiënisten*, pp. 154, 194–7.

15. See for example: G. Brillenburg Wurth et al. (eds), *Geestelijke Volksgezondheid: Nederlands Gesprekcentrum Publicatie No. 17* (Kampen, Utrecht, Antwerpen and The Hague: J. H. Kok, Het Spectrum and W. P. van Stockum en Zoon, 1959).

16. J. Kennedy, *Nieuw Babylon in aanbouw: Nederland in de jaren zestig* (Amsterdam and Meppel: Boom, 1995); H. Righart, *De eindeloze jaren zestig: Geschiedenis van een generatieconflict* (Amsterdam and Antwerpen: De Arbeiderspers, 1995).

17. J. A. Weijel, *De mensen hebben geen leven: Een psychosociale studie* (Haarlem: Bohn, 1970); J. van den Bergh et al., *Verbeter de mensen, verander de wereld: Een verkenning van het welzijnsvraagstuk vanuit de geestelijke gezondheidszorg* (Deventer: Kluwer, 1970); G. van Beusekom-Fretz, *De demokratisering van het geluk* (Deventer: Van Loghum Slaterus, 1973).

18. D. Ingleby, 'The View from the North Sea', in M. Gijswijt-Hofstra and R. Porter (eds), *Cultures of Psychiatry and Mental Health Care in Postwar Britain and the Netherlands* (Amsterdam and Atlanta: Rodopi, 1998), pp. 295–314; G. Blok, *Baas in eigen brein: 'Antipsychiatrie' in Nederland, 1965–1985* (Amsterdam: Uitgeverij Nieuwezijds, 2004).

19. F. M. J. Lemmens and P. Schnabel, 'Vestiging en ontwikkeling van de psychotherapie', in C. P. F. van der Staak, A. P. Cassee and P. E. Boeke (eds), *Oriëntatie in de psychotherapie* (Houten and Zaventem: Bohn Stafleu Van Loghum, 1994), pp. 9–26; W. J. de Waal, *De geschiedenis van de psychotherapie in Nederland* ('s-Hertogenbosch: De Nijvere Haas, 1992), p. 126; P. van Lieshout and D. de Ridder (eds), *Symptomen van de tijd. De dossiers van het Amsterdamse Instituut voor Medische Psychotherapie (IMP), 1968–1977* (Nijmegen: SUN, 1991).

20. Weijel, *De mensen hebben geen leven*.

21. Van den Bergh et al., *Verbeter de mensen*; Van Beusekom-Fretz, *De demokratisering van het geluk*.

22. I. de Haan, *Na de ondergang: De herinnering aan de Jodenvervolging in Nederland 1945–1995* (The Hague: Sdu, 1997); J. Withuis, *Erkenning: Van oorlogstrauma naar klaagcultuur* (Amsterdam: De Bezige Bij, 2002); J. Kennedy, *Een weloverwogen dood: Euthanasie in Nederland* (Amsterdam: Uitgeverij Bert Bakker, 2002); E. Ketting, *Van misdrijf tot hulpverlening: Een analyse van de maatschappelijke betekenis van abortus provocatus in Nederland* (Alphen aan den Rijn: Samson Uitgeverij, 1978), pp. 82–3; J. V. Outshoorn, 'De politieke strijd rondom de abortuswetgeving in Nederland 1964–1984' (PhD dissertation, University of Amsterdam, 1986), pp. 123, 139, 179–80; M. de Kort, 'Tussen patiënt en delinquent: Geschiedenis van het Nederlandse drugsbeleid' (PhD dissertation, Erasmus University Rotterdam, 1995).

23. R. H. van den Hoofdakker, *Het bolwerk van de beterweters: Over de medische ethiek en de status quo* (Amsterdam: Van Gennep, 1971), p. 50.

24. H. Achterhuis, *De markt van welzijn en geluk: Een kritiek van de andragogie* (Baarn: Ambo, 1980); De Haan and Duyvendak, *In het hart van de verzorgingsstaat*, pp. 121–2, 182, 352–3.

25. A. K. Oderwald and J. Rolies, 'De psychiatrie als morele onderneming', *Tijdschrift voor Psychiatrie*, 32 (1990), pp. 601–15; P. Schnabel, *Het recht om niet gestoord te worden: Naar een nieuwe sociologie van de psychiatrie* (Utrecht: Nederlands centrum Geestelij-

ke Volksgezondheid, 1992); G. van Loenen, 'Van chronisch psychiatrische patiënt naar brave burger: Over de moraal van psychiatrische rehabilitatie', *Maandblad Geestelijke volksgezondheid*, 52 (1997), pp. 751–61; G. A. M. Widdershoven, R. I. P. Berghmans and A. C. Molewijk, 'Autonomie in de Psychiatrie', *Tijdschrift voor Psychiatrie*, 6 (2000), pp. 389–98; D. Kal, *Kwartiermaken: Werken aan ruimte voor mensen met een psychiatrische achtergrond* (Amsterdam: Boom, 2001); J. Pols, *Good Care: Enacting a Complex Ideal in Long-term Psychiatry* (Utrecht: Trimbos-instituut, 2004).

26. M. H. Kwekkeboom, 'Sociaal draagvlak voor de vermaatschappelijking in de geestelijke gezondheidszorg: Ontwikkelingen tussen 1976 en 1997', *Tijdschrift voor Gezondheidswetenschappen*, 78:3 (2000), pp. 165–71.

27. J. Droës, 'De metamorfose van de GGZ', *Maandblad Geestelijke volksgezondheid*, 57 (2002), pp. 143–5; E. Borst-Eilers, *Brief Geestelijke Gezondheidszorg aan de Tweede Kamer der Staten-Generaal* (Rijswijk: Ministerie van Volksgezondheid, Welzijn en Sport, 1997), p. 9.

28. R. V. Bijl, G. van Zessen and A. Ravelli, 'Psychiatrische morbiditeit onder volwassenen in Nederland: het NEMESIS-onderzoek. II. Prevalentie van psychiatrische stoornissen', *Nederlands Tijdschrift voor Geneeskunde*, 141:50 (1997), pp. 2453–60; R. V. Bijl and A. Ravelli, 'Psychiatrische morbiditeit, zorggebruik en zorgbehoefte: Resultaten van de Netherlands Mental Health Survey and Incidence Study (NEMESIS)', *Tijdschrift voor gezondheidswetenschappen*, 76 (1998), pp. 446–57.

29. Scenariocommissie Geestelijke Volksgezondheid en Geestelijke Gezondheidszorg en Onderzoeksteam van het Nederlands centrum Geestelijke volksgezondheid, *Zorgen voor geestelijke volksgezondheid in de toekomst: Toekomstscenario's geestelijke volksgezondheid en geestelijke gezondheidszorg 1990–2010* (Utrecht and Antwerpen: Bohn, Scheltema en Holkema, 1990); M. Gastelaars et al., *Vier gevaarlijke kruispunten: Een voorzet voor een geestelijk volksgezondheidsbeleid* (Utrecht and Amsterdam: Centrum voor Beleid en Management, 1991); P. Schnabel, R. Bijl and G. Hutschemaekers, *Geestelijke volksgezondheid in de jaren '90: Van ideaal tot concrete opgave* (Utrecht: Nederlands centrum Geestelijke volksgezondheid, 1992); Landelijke Commissie Geestelijke Volksgezondheid, *Zorg van velen: Eindrapport van de Landelijke Commissie Geestelijke Volksgezondheid* (The Hague: Landelijke Commissie Geestelijke Volksgezondheid, 2002).

30. Nationaal Fonds Geestelijke Volksgezondheid, *Manifest van het Nationaal Fonds Geestelijke Volksgezondheid: Verontrustende ontwikkelingen* (Utrecht: NGHV, 1998), pp. 3, 8.

31. H. Wigbold, *Bezwaren tegen de ondergang van Nederland* (Amsterdam and Antwerpen: De Arbeiderspers, 1995); H. Vuijsje, *Correct: Weldenkend Nederland sinds de jaren zestig* (Amsterdam and Antwerpen: Uitgeverij Contact, 1997); J. van der Stel, 'Individualisering, zelfbeheersing en sociale integratie', in P. Schnabel (ed.), *Individualisering en sociale integratie* (Nijmegen: SUN, Nederlands Gesprek Centrum, 1999), pp. 126–58; H. Beunders, *Publieke tranen: De drijfveren van de emotiecultuur* (Amsterdam and Antwerpen: Uitgeverij Contact, 2002); D. Pessers, *Big Mother: Over de personalisering van de publieke sfeer* (The Hague: Boom Juridische uitgevers, 2003); R. Diekstra, M. van den Berg and J. Rigter (eds), *Waardenvolle of waardenloze samenleving? Over waarden, normen en gedrag in samenleving, opvoeding en onderwijs* (Uithoorn: Karakter, 2004); G. van den Brink, *Schets van een beschavingsoffensief: Over normen, normaliteit en normalisatie in Nederland* (Amsterdam: Amsterdam University Press, 2004).

32. M. Thomson, 'Before Anti-Psychiatry: "Mental Health" in Wartime Britain', in Gijswijt-Hofstra and Porter (eds), *Cultures of Psychiatry and Mental Health Care*, pp. 43–59; M. Thomson, 'Constituting Citizenship: Mental Deficiency, Mental Health and Human

Rights in Inter-war Britain', in C. Lawrence and A. K. Mayer (eds), *Regenerating England: Science, Medicine and Culture in Inter-war Britain* (Amsterdam and Atlanta: Rodopi, 2000), pp. 231–50; J. C. Pols, 'Managing the Mind: The Culture of American Hygiene, 1910–1950' (PhD dissertation University of Pennsylvania, 1997); F. W. Kersting (ed.), *Psychiatrie als Gesellschaftsreform: Die Hypothek des Nationalsozialismus und der Aufbruch der sechziger Jahre* (Paderborn, Munich and Vienna: Ferdinand Schönigh, 2004).

33. Van Lieshout and De Ridder, *Symptomen van de tijd*; H. Oosterhuis, *Homoseksualiteit in katholiek Nederland: Een sociale geschiedenis 1900–1970* (Amsterdam: Sua, 1992).

34. H. Oosterhuis, 'Outpatient Psychiatry and Mental Health Care in the Twentieth Century: International Perspectives', in Gijswijt-Hofstra et al. (eds), *Psychiatric Cultures Compared*, pp. 248–74.

35. C. Brinkgreve and M. Korzec, *'Margriet weet raad': Gevoel, gedrag, moraal in Nederland 1938–1978* (Utrecht and Antwerpen: Het Spectrum, 1978); W. Zeegers, *Andere tijden, andere mensen. De sociale representatie van identiteit* (Amsterdam: Bert Bakker, 1988); C. Wouters, *Van minnen en sterven. Informalisering van omgangsvormen rond seks en dood* (Amsterdam: Bert Bakker, 1990); R. Abma et al., *Het verlangen naar openheid. Over de psychologisering van het alledaagse* (Amsterdam: De Balie, 1995).

36. L. Halman et al., *Traditie, secularisatie en individualisering: Een studie naar de waarden van Nederlanders in een Europese context* (Tilburg: Tilburg University Press, 1987).

37. H. Knippenberg and B. de Pater, *De eenwording van Nederland: Schaalvergroting en integratie sinds 1800* (Nijmegen: SUN, 1990), pp. 128–30; C. J. M. Schuyt, 'Sociaal-culturele golfbewegingen in de twintigste eeuw', in C. van Eijl, L. Heerma van Voss and P. de Rooy (eds), *Sociaal Nederland: Contouren van de twintigste eeuw* (Amsterdam: Aksant, 2001); Beunders, *Publieke tranen*, pp. 61, 125–6.

8 Powell, 'Neo-Republican Citizenship and the British National Health Service since 1979'

1. C. Webster, *The NHS: A Political History* (Oxford: Oxford University Press, 2002); M. Powell, *Evaluating the National Health Service* (Buckingham: Open University Press, 1997). The position of Minister of Health was changed to Secretary of State for Health in the 1970s.

2. R. Blank and V. Burau, *Comparative Health Policy* (Basingstoke: Palgrave, 2007).

3. Powell, *Evaluating the NHS*; I. Greener, *Healthcare in the UK* (Bristol: Policy Press, 2009).

4. G. Esping-Andersen, *The Three Worlds of Welfare Capitalism* (Cambridge: Polity Press, 1990), p. 21.

5. See for example, Greener, *Healthcare in the UK*; M. Moran, *Governing the Health Care State* (Manchester: Manchester University Press, 1999); B. Salter, *The New Politics of Medicine* (Basingstoke: Palgrave Macmillan, 2004).

6. S. Pickard, 'Citizenship and Consumerism in Health Care: A Critique of Citizens' Juries', *Social Policy and Administration*, 32:3 (1998), pp. 226–44; T. Milewa, J. Valentine and M. Calnan, 'Managerialism and Active Citizenship in Britain's Reform Health Service', *Social Science and Medicine*, 47:4 (1998), pp. 507–17; T. Milewa, Community Participation and Citizenship in British Health Care Planning, *Sociology of Health and Illness*, 21:4 (1999), pp. 445–65; T. Milewa, 'Local Participatory Democracy in Britain's

Health Service', *Social Policy and Administration*, 38:3 (2004), pp. 240–52; D. Porter, *Health, Civilization and the State* (London: Routledge, 1999).

7. Greener, *Healthcare in the UK*, pp. 187–8.
8. Salter, *New Politics of Medicine*, p. 2.
9. D. Marquand, *The Unprincipled Society* (London: Jonathan Cape, 1988), pp. 29–30.
10. M. Moran, 'The Frontiers of Social Citizenship: The Case of Health Care Entitlements', in U. Vogel and M. Moran (eds), *The Frontiers of Citizenship* (Basingstoke: Macmillan, 1991), pp. 32–57 on p. 35.
11. Moran, *Governing the Healthcare State*, pp. 32, 61.
12. E. Isin and B. Turner, *Handbook of Citizenship Studies* (London: Sage, 2002); T. Janoski, *Citizenship and Civil Society: A Framework of Rights and Obligations in Liberal, Traditional and Social Democratic Regimes* (Cambridge: Cambridge University Press, 1998).
13. C. Hogg, *Patients, Power and Politics: From Patients to Citizens* (London: Sage, 1999); C. Hogg, *Citizens, Consumers and the NHS* (Basingstoke: Palgrave Macmillan, 2009); M. Powell and I. Greener, 'The Healthcare Consumer', in R. Simmons, M. Powell and I. Greener (eds), *The Consumer in Public Services* (Bristol: Policy Press, 2009), pp. 99–117.
14. J. Le Grand, *The Other Invisible Hand* (Princeton, NJ: Princeton University Press, 2007).
15. S. Henderson and A. Petersen (eds), *Consuming Health: The Commodification of Health Care* (London: Routledge, 2002).
16. Greener, *Healthcare in the UK*; Powell and Greener, 'The Healthcare Consumer'; C. Needham, *The Reform of Public Services under New Labour* (Basingstoke: Palgrave, 2007); J. Clarke, J. Newman, N. Smith, E. Vidler and L. Westmarland, *Creating Citizen-Consumers* (London: Sage, 2007); Le Grand, *The Other Invisible Hand*.
17. C. Williamson, *Whose Standards? Consumer and Professional Standards in Health Care* (Buckingham: Open University Press, 1992). Cf. Clarke et al., *Creating Citizen-Consumers*.
18. S. Harrison and R. McDonald, *The Politics of Healthcare in Britain* (London: Sage, 2008), p. 105.
19. The term 'classic NHS' is broadly associated with Charles Webster, the official historian of the NHS and draws on the term 'classic welfare state'. It refers to the period of 'Butskellite' consensus in the period 1948–79 before the election of the Thatcher Conservative Government in 1979. See Webster, *The NHS*. At the time of writing, a coalition Conservative–Liberal Democrat government was in power after the 2010 general election.
20. G. Finlayson, *Citizen, State and Social Welfare in Britain, 1830–1990* (Oxford: Clarendon Press, 1994); D. Marquand, *The Progressive Dilemma* (London: Heinemann, 1992), pp. 214–16; Greener, *Healthcare in the UK*, pp. 187–8.
21. T. H. Marshall, *Sociology at the Crossroads* (London: Heinemann, 1963), pp. 108–9.
22. T. H. Marshall, *The Right to Welfare* (London: Heinemann, 1981), pp. 65–6.
23. Moran, *Governing the Health Care State*, p. 61.
24. Moran, 'The Frontiers of Citizenship', p. 35.
25. Marshall, *Sociology at the Crossroads*, p. 109.
26. Marshall, *The Right to Welfare*, p. 87.
27. The term is associated with M. Lipsky, *Street-Level Bureaucracy* (New York: Russell Sage Foundation, 1980). See A. Coulter, *The Autonomous Patient: Ending Paternalism in Medical Care* (London: Stationery Office, 2002), p. 106; C. Smee, *Speaking Truth to Power* (Oxford: Radcliffe Publishing, 2005), p. 131.
28. For example, M. Brazier, 'Rights and Health Care', in R. Blackburn (ed.), *Rights of Citizenship* (London: Mansell, 1983), pp. 56–74; D. Woodhouse, 'The Judiciary in the 1990s: Guardians of the Welfare State?', *Policy and Politics*, 26:4 (1998), pp. 457–70.

29. Brazier, *Rights and Health Care*, pp. 56–7, 60, 69–70.
30. Greener, *Healthcare in the UK*.
31. Marquand, *The Progressive Dilemma*, pp. 214–16.
32. In Pickard, 'Citizenship and Consumerism', p. 228.
33. See Powell, *Evaluating the NHS*.
34. Powell and Greener, 'The Healthcare Consumer'.
35. For more details, see for example Greener, *Healthcare in the UK*; R. Klein, *The New Politics of the National Health Service* (Abingdon: Radcliffe Publishing, 2006); C. Ham, *Health Policy in Britain* (Basingstoke: Palgrave Macmillan, 2009).
36. Powell, *Evaluating the NHS*.
37. Department of Health, *Working for Patients* (London: HMSO, 1989), para 1.8.
38. Department of Health, *The Patient's Charter* (London: HMSO, 1991).
39. Department of Health, *The Health of the Nation* (London: HMSO, 1992).
40. Department of Health, *The New National Health Service* (London: Stationery Office), p. 10.
41. The 'postcode lottery' is a term given to a situation where patients living in different areas are eligible for different treatments and drugs. In other words, despite a 'national' service, people's treatment varies by postcode.
42. Department of Health, *The NHS Plan* (London: Stationery Office, 2000).
43. A. Pollock, *NHS Plc: The Privatization of Our Health Care* (London: Verso, 2004); Le Grand, *The Invisible Hand*; Greener, *Healthcare in the UK*.
44. Pollock, *NHS Plc*; Greener, *Healthcare in the UK*, pp. 216–19.
45. J. Glasby and R. Littlechild, *Direct Payments and Personal Budgets*, 2ND edn (Bristol: Policy Press, 2009).
46. D. Hunter, *The Health Debate* (Bristol: Policy Press, 2008).
47. Department of Health, *Our NHS, Our Future*. NHS Next Stage Review – Interim Darzi Report (London: DH, 2007); Department of Health, *High Quality Care for All*. NHS Next Stage Review – Final Darzi Report (London: DH, 2008).
48. M. Powell, 'Quasi Markets in British Health Policy: a Longue Durée Perspective', *Social Policy and Administration*, 37:7 (2003), pp. 725–41.
49. Pollock, *NHS Plc*.
50. *With Respect to Old Age*, Report of the Royal Commission on Long Term Care (Chair: Sir S. Sutherland) (London: Stationery Office, 1999); J. Horton, 'Council Spending on Free Personal Care at Home up by 21%', *Herald*, 27 August 2008.
51. Secretary of State for Health, *Shaping the Future of Care Together* (London: Stationery Office). A White Paper was promised for 2010 – if New Labour was returned at the General Election. The new Conservative–Liberal Coalition set up the Dilnot Commission on Funding of Care and Support to review of the funding system for care and support in England, which reported in July 2011.
52. Department of Health Press Release, Personal Care at Home Bill introduced to Parliament, 25 November 2009.
53. K. Devlin, 'Millions could be given Legal Right to see an NHS Dentist', *Daily Telegraph*, 11 November 2009.
54. Ham, *Health Policy in Britain*; M. Richards, *Improving Access to Medicine for NHS Patients* (Richards Review) (London: Department of Health, 2008).
55. Powell, 'Welfare State Reforms in the UK'.
56. Ibid.
57. Le Grand, *The Invisible Hand*; Pollock, *NHS Plc*.

58. For example, J. Laurence, 'The Hospital of Death', *Independent*, 18 March 2009; C. Man-thorp, 'Can Gerry Robinson Fix Care Homes?', *Guardian*, 15 December 2009.

59. Harrison and McDonald, *The Politics of Healthcare in Britain*, p. 114; Perri 6, 'Giving Consumers of British Public Services More Choice: What Can be Learned from Recent History?', *Journal of Social Policy*, 32:2 (2003), pp. 239–70, on p. 248.

60. The term is associated with Klein, *New Politics of the NHS*; Needham, *The Reform of Public Services under New Labour*, p. 61.

61. In Powell, 'Quasi-Markets in Health Policy'.

62. Brazier, *Rights and Health Care*, pp. 56–7.

63. Needham, *The Reform of Public Services under New Labour*, 2007, p. 58; Powell, *Evaluating the NHS*, p. 83; Coulter, *The Autonomous Patient*, p. 90.

64. Salter, *The New Politics of Medicine*, pp. 2–5.

65. Le Grand, *The Invisible Hand*.

66. Ham, *Health Policy in Britain*, pp. 63–4; R. Gauld, *The New Health Policy* (Maidenhead: Open University Press, 2009), p. 31; Harrison and McDonald, *The Politics of Healthcare in Britain*, p. 94.

67. See for example, Le Grand, *The Invisible Hand*; Clarke et al., *Creating Citizen Consumers*, Needham, *The Reform of Public Services under New Labour*; Powell and Greener, 'The Healthcare Consumer'.

68. E. Stopp, *Complementary Therapies in the NHS* (PhD, Bath University, 2002).

69. King's Fund, *Choice at the Point of Referral* (London: King's Fund, 2009).

70. N. Prarities, 'Experts Attack Ill-Conceived Plans for Patients to Buy Homeopathy on the NHS', *Pulse*, 26 November 2009.

71. Coulter, *The Autonomous Patient*, p. 1; Bristol Royal Infirmary Inquiry, *Learning from Bristol: The Report of the Public Inquiry into Children's Heart Surgery at the Bristol Royal Infirmary 1984–1995*, Cm 5207 (Chairman: Ian Kennedy), (London: Stationery Office, 2001).

72. Department of Health (2013), NHS Constitution for England, London: Stationery Office.

73. Department of Health, New legal rights for NHS patients, Press Release, 10 November 2009; N. Timmins, 'No Guarantee in Right to NHS Waiting Times', *Financial Times*, 10 November 2009.

74. Department of Health, *The Health of the Nation*.

75. Department of Health, *Our Healthier Nation*; Department of Health, *The NHS Plan*.

76. House of Commons Health Committee, *Report on Health Inequalities* (London: Stationery Office, 2009).

77. Ham, *Health Policy in Britain*, p. 307; D. Hunter, *The Health Debate* (Bristol: Policy Press, 2008).

78. M. Powell, 'How Uniform are Uniform Services?', in S. Greer (ed.), *Devolution and Social Citizenship in the UK* (Bristol: Policy Press, 2009), pp. 161–73.

79. 'Cancer Postcode Lottery is Killing Thousands', *The Times*, 1 December 2009.

80. D. Birrell, *The Impact of Devolution on Social Policy* (Bristol: Policy Press, 2009); S. Greer, *Devolution and Social Citizenship in the UK* (Bristol: Policy Press, 2009).

81. Le Grand, *The Invisible Hand*; Clarke et al., *Creating Citizen-Consumers*; Needham, *The Reform of Public Services under New Labour*.

82. Klein, *The New Politics of the NHS*, pp. 225–6.

83. R. Klein, 'Acceptable Inequalities?', in D. Green (ed.), *Acceptable Inequalities* (London: IEA, 1988), pp. 3–20; Powell, *Evaluating the NHS*; Powell, 'How Uniform are Uniform Services?'
84. Klein, 'Acceptable Inequalities?'
85. Hogg, *Patients, Power and Politics*; Harrison and McDonald, *The Politics of Healthcare in Britain*; R. Baggott, 'A Funny Thing Happened on the Way to the Forum? Reforming Patient and Public Involvement in the NHS in England', *Public Administration*, 83:3 (2005), pp. 533–51. I was briefly a member of a CHC. To continue the dog example, the public were invited to CHC meetings, but they often consisted of two people and a dog, with the dog appearing to have the greatest interest in proceedings.
86. Powell, *Evaluating the NHS*.
87. NHSME, *Local Voices*.
88. The meanings of the acronyms are not vital to the argument, but see Hogg, *Patients, Power and Politics*.
89. Hogg, *Patients, Power and Politics*; Baggott, Harrison and McDonald, *The Politics of Healthcare in Britain*, ch. 5; Gauld, *The New Health Policy*, pp. 95–101.
90. P. Dwyer, *Welfare Rights and Responsibilities* (Bristol: Policy Press, 2000); P. Dwyer, *Understanding Social Citizenship* (Bristol: Policy Press, 2004).
91. See the views of focus groups in Dwyer, *Welfare Rights and Responsibilities*.
92. M. Lalonde, *A New Perspective on the Health of Canadians* (Ottawa: Minister of Supply and Services, 1974); D. Hunter, *Public Health Policy* (Cambridge: Polity, 2003), pp. 38–42.
93. A. Petersen and D. Lupton, *The New Public Health: Health and Self in the Age of Risk* (London: Sage, 1996), p. 13; WHO, *European Charter on Environment and Health* (1990), pp. 29–31.
94. Gauld, *The New Health Policy*, p. 110; M. Fitzpatrick, *The Tyranny of Health: Doctors and the Regulation of Lifestyle* (London: Routledge, 2001), pp. 79–81. Cf. J. Le Fanu, *The Rise and Fall of Modern Medicine* (London: Abacus, 2000).
95. Fitzpatrick, *The Tyranny of Health*, p. 72; Department of Health and Social Security, *Prevention and Health: Everybody's Business. Discussion Document* (London: DHSS, 1976), p. 95; Department of Health and Social Security, *Prevention and Health: Everybody's Business*. Cmnd 7047 (London, HMSO, 1977), p. 39.
96. DH, *Our Healthier Nation*, para 3.1.
97. Hunter, *The Health Debate*, p. 142; Department of Health, *Choosing Health* (London: Stationery Office, 2004).
98. In Fitzpatrick, *The Tyranny of Health*, p. 71.
99. For 'workfare', see Dwyer, *Welfare Rights and Responsibilities*; Fitzpatrick, *The Tyranny of Health*, p. 85.
100. Sky News, 'Binge-drink Teen Left Hospital Bed for Pub', 25 August 2009.
101. J. Oldham, 'Criticism Grows of Best Liver Decision', *Scotsman*, 14 July 2003.
102. 'Attack in NHS Hospital "Every Three Minutes"', *Daily Telegraph*, 4 November 2009.
103. T. McVeigh, 'Who's to Blame for Britain's Obesity Epidemic?', *Observer*, 25 October 2009.
104. The term can be found in Porter, *Civilization, Health and the State*.

9 Horstman, 'Struggling with Science and Democracy: Public Health and Citizenship in the Netherlands'

1. W. Bijker, R. Bal, R. Hendriks, *The Paradox of Scientific Authority: The Role of Scientific Advice in Democracies* (Cambridge: MIT Press, 2009); M. Callon, P. Lascoumes and Y. Barthe, *Acting in an Uncertain World: An Essay on Technological Democracy* (Cambridge: MIT Press, 2009).
2. E. Aarden, I. van Hoyweghen, K. Horstman and R. Vos, 'Learning for the Co-Evolution of Policy and Technology: Different PGD's in the Netherlands, Germany and Britain', *Journal of Comparative Policy Analysis*, 10:2 (2008), pp. 191–206. S. Jasanoff, *Designs on Nature: Science and Democracy in Europe and the United States* (Princeton, NJ: Princeton University Press, 2005). K. Horstman and K. Finkler (eds), 'Genetics, Health Care, Family and Citizenship in a Global Perspective: Situated Processes of Co-Construction' (special issue), *Social Science and Medicine*, 72 (2011) pp. 1739–42.
3. D. Lupton, *The Imperative of Health: Public Health and the Regulated Body* (London: Sage, 1995).
4. S. E. Kooiker, *Hoe denken Nederlanders over gezondheid en gezond leven*. Achtergrondrapport bij de VTV 2010 Van Gezond naar Beter (Bilthoven/Den Haag: RIVM, 2011). P. Allmark and A. Todd, 'How Should Public Health Professionals Engage with Lay Epidemiology', *Journal of Medical Ethics*, 32 (2006), pp. 460–3.
5. K. Horstman and R. Houtepen, *Worstelen met gezond leven: Ethiek in de preventie van hart – en vaatziekten* (Amsterdam: Het Spinhuis, 2005).
6. P. Bourdieu, *Distinction: A Social Critique of the Judgement of Taste* (Cambridge, MA: Harvard University Press, 1984).
7. L. Prior, 'Belief, Knowledge and Expertise: The Emergence of the Lay Expert in Medical Sociology', *Sociology of Health and Illness*, 25:3 (2003), pp. 41–57.
8. U. Beck, *Risk Society: Towards a New Modernity* (London: Sage, 1992).
9. U. Beck, A.Giddens and S. Lash (eds), *Reflexive Modernization: Politics, Tradition and Aesthetics in the Modern Social Order* (Cambridge: Polity Press, 1994).
10. J. Zeh, '*Corpus Delicti: A Ttrial*' (Frankfurt am Main: Schoeffling & Co., 2009).
11. For instance the chair of the Dutch Covenant Overweight Rosenmuller suggested the link between overweight children and child abuse in an interview in the newspaper *De Pers*, 23 November 2009.
12. C. Prins, 'Heeft digitale jeugdzorg de toekomst?', in M. van den Berg, C. Prins and M. Ham (eds), *In de greep van de technologie: Nieuwe toepassingen en het gedrag van de burger* (Amsterdam, Van Gennip, 2008). P. M. Garret, 'The Electronic Eye: Emerging Surveillance Practices in Social Work with Children and Families', *European Journal of Social Work*, 7:1 (2004), pp. 57–71.
13. I. Lecluize, B. Penders, F. Feron and K. Horstman, 'Innovation and Justification in Public Health: The Introduction of the Child Index in the Netherlands', in D. Strech, I. Hirschberg and G. Marckmann (eds), *Ethics in Public Health and Health Policy: Concepts, Methods, Case Studies* (Berlin: Springer, forthcoming).
14. M. de Winter, 'Hoedt U voor het evidence beest', *Facta*, 16:4 (2010), p. 17.
15. S. White, C. Hall and S. Peckover, 'The Descriptive Tyranny of the Common Assessment Framework: Technologies of Categorization and Professional Practice in Child Welfare', *British Journal of Social Work* (2008), pp. 1–21. S. Peckover, S.White and C.

Hall, 'Making and Managing Electronic Children: E-assessment in Child Welfare', *Information, Communication & Society*, 11:3 (2008), pp. 375–94.

16. A. Meershoek, Y. Bartholomee and K. Horstman, 'Vitaal en bevlogen: Economisering van gezondheid van werknemers', *Beleid en Maatschappij*, 37:3 (2010), pp. 232–45.

17. A. de Swaan, R. van Gelderen and V. Kense, *Het spreekuur als opgave: Sociologie van de psychotherapie 2* (Utrecht/Antwerpen: Het Spectrum, 1979).

18. See www.tno.nl [accessed 9 May 2010]. See also A. Meershoek, Y. Bartolomee, E. Aarden, I. van Hoyweghen and K. Horstman, *Vitaal en bevlogen: Vermarkting van gezondheid van werknemers* (Den Haag: Voorstudie WRR, 2010), p. 25.

19. See www.achmeavitale.nl [accessed 9 May 2010].

20. See www.maastrichtuniversity.nl [accessed 9 May 2010]. See also Meershoek et al., *Vitaal en bevlogen*, p. 26.

21. A. Mooij, *Geen paniek: Aids in Nederland* (Amsterdam: Bert Bakker, 2004).

22. S. Blume, 'Anti-Vaccine Movements and their Interpretation', *Social Science and Medicine*, 62 (2006), pp. 628–42.

23. Gezondheidsraad, *Vaccinatie tegen baarmoederhalskanker* (Den Haag: Gezondheidsraad, 2008). I. M. C. M. de Kok, J. D. F.Habbema, M. J. Mourits, J. W. W. Coebergh and F. E. van Leeuwen, 'Onvoldoende gronden voor opname van vaccinatie tegen Humaan papillomavirus in het Rijksvaccinatieprogramma', *Nederlands Tijdschrift voor Geneeskunde*, 152 (2008), pp. 2001–4.

24. E. van Rijswoud, 'Flu: Weighing up Conflicting Expert Information', *Nature*, 460 (2009), p. 571; E. van Rijswoud, 'Virology Experts in the Boundary Zone between Science, Policy and the Public: A Biographical Analysis', *Minerva*, 48:2 (2010), pp. 145–67.

25. R. Bunton, S. Nettleton and Burrows (eds), *The Sociology of Health Promotion: Critical Analyses of Consumption, Lifestyle and Risk* (London: Routlegde, 1995); J. Greenl and R. Labonte (eds), *Critical Perspectives in Public Health* (London: Routledge, 2008).

26. M. Minkler and N. Wallerstein (eds), *Community-Based Participatory Research for Health: From Process to Outcomes* (San Fransisco, CA: Jossey-Bass, John Wiley and Sons, 2008).

27. I. Kickbusch (ed.), *Policy Innovation for Health* (New York: Springer, 2009).

28. D. R. Buchanan, *An Ethic for Health Promotion: Rethinking the Sources of Human Wellbeing* (Oxford: Oxford University Press, 2000).

29. H. Zwart and A. Nelis, 'What is ELSA Genomics?', *EMBO Reports*, 10 (2009), pp. 540–4. P. Penders, K. Horstman and R. Vos, 'A Ferry Between Cultures: Crafting a Profession at the Intersection of Science and Society', *EMBO Reports* 9:8 (2008), pp. 709–13.

30. H. Nowotny, P. Scott and M. Gibbons, *Re-thinking Science: Knowledge and the Public in an Age of Uncertainty* (Cambridge: Polity Press, 2001); H. Nowotny (ed.), *Cultures of Technology and the Quest for Innovation* (New York: Berghahn Books, 2006).

31. T. Porter, *Trust in Numbers: The Pursuit of Objectivity in Science and Public Life* (Princeton, NJ: Princeton University Press, 1995).

32. J. W. Duyvendak, T. Knijn and M. Kremer, *Policy, People and the New Professional: De-professionalszation and Re-professionalisation in Care and Welfare* (Amsterdam: Amsterdam University Press 2006); M. Power, *The Audit Society: Rituals of Verification* (Oxford: Oxford University Press, 1999). See also T. Dehue, *Changing the Rules: Psychology in the Netherlands 1900–1985* (Cambridge: Cambridge University Press, 1995).

33. Power, *Audit Society*.

34. R. Rorty, *Consequences of Pragmatism: Essays: 1972–1980* (Brighton: Harvester Press, 1982); R. Rorty, *Contingency, Irony and Solidarity* (Cambridge: Cambridge University Press, 1989); H. R. van Gunsteren, *A Theory on Citizenship: Organizing Plurality in*

Contemporary Societies (Boulder: Westview Press, 1998); J. Keulartz, M. Korthals, M. Schermer, T. Swierstra (eds), *Pragmatist Ethics for a Technological Culture* (Dordrecht: Kluwer, 2002).

35. Van Gunsteren, *Theory on Citizenship*; Z. Bauman, *Life in Fragments: Essays in Postmodern Morality* (Oxford: Blackwell, 1995); M. Callon, P. Lascoumes and Y. Barthe, *Acting in an Uncertain World: An Essay on Technological Democracy* (Cambridge: MIT Press, 2009).

36. The Cochrane Collaboration is an organization producing systematic reviews about the effectiveness of interventions in health care. It started in 1972 as a critical research practice and developed into a basis for evidence based health care, thereby ranking different kinds of evidence about the quality of interventions in such a way that evidence produced in a RCT is considered to be of more value than evidence produced by other methodologies.

37. G. de Vries and K. Horstman (eds), *Genetics from Laboratory into Society: Societal Learning as an Alternative to Regulation* (Basingstoke: Palgrave MacMillan, 2008).

38. B. Latour and P. Weibel (eds), *Making Things Public: Atmospheres of Democracy* (Cambridge: MIT Press, 2005); N. Marres, 'The Issues Deserve More Credit: Pragmatist Contributions to the Study of Public Involvement in Controversy', *Social Studies of Science*, 37:5 (2007), pp. 759–80.

39. Van Gunsteren, *Theory on Citizenship*.

40. S. Jasanoff, 'Technologies of Humility: Citizen Participation in Governing Science', *Minerva*, 41 (2003), pp. 223–44.

41. M. Fricker, *Epistemic Injustice: Power and the Ethics of Knowing* (Oxford: Oxford University Press, 2007).

10 Van Hoyweghen, 'Underwriting Citizenship: The Introduction of Predictive Medicine in Private Insurance'

1. Cited in N. N., 'De preventieve geneeskunde in verband met de belangen der onvolwaardigen', *Geneeskundig tijdschrift der Rijksverzekeringsbank*, 22:7 (1937), pp. 217–19, on 219 (my translation).

2. K. Horstman, *Public Bodies Private Lives: The Historical Construction of Life Insurance, Health Risks and Citizenship in the Netherlands, 1880–1920* (Rotterdam: Erasmus Publishing, 2001); T. M. Porter, 'Life Insurance, Medical Testing and the Management of Mortality', in L. Daston (ed.), *Biographies of Scientific Objects* (Chicago, IL: University of Chicago Press, 2000), pp. 226–46.

3. See for example, M. Dean, 'Risk, Calculable and Incalculable', *Soziale Welt*, 49 (1998), pp. 25–42; N. Rose, 'Governing Liberty', in R. Ericson and R. Stehr (eds), *Governing Modern Societies* (Toronto: University of Toronto Press, 2000), pp. 141–76; N. Rose, *The Politics of Life Itself: Biomedicine, Power and Subjectivity in the Twenty-First Century* (Princeton, NJ: Princeton University Press, 2007).

4. R. Ericson, A. Doyle and B. Dean, *Insurance as Governance* (Toronto: University of Toronto Press, 2003); R. Ericson and A. Doyle, *Risk and Morality* (Toronto: University of Toronto Press, 2003); T. Baker and J. Simon, 'Embracing Risk: The Changing Culture of Insurance and Responsibility', in T. Baker and J. Simon (eds), *Embracing Risk: The Changing Culture of Insurance and Responsibility* (Chicago, IL and London: University of Chicago Press, 2002), pp. 1–25; D. Stone, 'The Struggle for the Soul of Health Insurance', *Journal of Health Politics, Policy and Law*, 18:2 (1993), pp. 287–317.

5. F. Ewald, *L'Etat-Providence* (Paris: Bernard Grasset, 1986).

6. D. Stone, 'Beyond Moral Hazard: Insurance as Moral Opportunity', in Baker and Simon (eds), *Embracing Risk*, pp. 52–79, on p. 74.

7. V. A. R. Zelizer, *Morals and Markets: The Development of Life Insurance in the United States* (New Brunswick, NJ: Transaction Books, 1983); T. Baker, 'Risk, Insurance and the Social Construction of Responsibility', in Baker and Simon (eds), *Embracing Risk*, pp. 33–51.

8. I. Van Hoyweghen, *Risks in the Making: Travels in Life Insurance and Genetics* (Amsterdam: Amsterdam University Press, 2007).

9. A. Strauss, *Continual Permutations of Action* (New York: Aldine de Gruyter, 1993).

10. B. Latour and S. Woolgar, *Laboratory Life: The Construction of Scientific Facts* (Chichester: Princeton University Press, 1979).

11. P. L. Bernstein, *Against the Gods: The Remarkable Story of Risk* (New York: Wiley, 1998).

12. R. D. C. Brackenridge and W. J. Elder, *Medical Selection of Life Risks* (New York: Stockton Press, 1996).

13. M. Foucault, *Surveiller et punir: Naissance de la prison* (Paris: Gallimard, 1975).

14. Stone, 'The Struggle', p. 299.

15. D. Haraway, *Cimians, Cyborgs and Women: The Reinvention of Nature* (New York: Routledge, 1991).

16. Porter, 'Life Insurance', p. 227.

17. Ibid., p. 228.

18. R. Jureidini and K. White, 'Life Insurance, the Medical Examination and Cultural Values', *Journal of Historical Sociology*, 13:2 (2000), pp. 190–214; Zelizer, *Morals and Markets*; M. W. Dupree, 'Other than Healing: Medical Practitioners and the Business of Life Assurance During the Nineteenth and Early Twentieth Centuries', *Society for the Social History of Medicine*, 10:1 (1997), pp. 79–103; B. J. Glenn, 'The Shifting Rhetoric of Insurance Denial', *Law & Society Review*, 34:3 (2000), pp. 779–808.

19. This method, designed for calculating premium rates for people who normally would not qualify for life insurance, was first described in 1919 by a physician, Oscar Rodgers and an actuary, Arthur Hunter.

20. A. de Swaan, *Zorg en de staat. Welzijn, onderwijs en gezondheidszorg in Europa en de Verenigde Staten in de nieuwe tijd* (Amsterdam: Berk Bakker, 1989); Ewald, *L'Etat-Providence*.

21. Between 1970 and 1980, insurers introduced the use of biochemical testing in their business. Since the mid-1980s, urine and blood testing have been further expanded and refined, while more advanced urine testing also resulted in the development of tests for tobacco (codeine testing). Since the 1990s, the insurance industry has been exploring the usefulness of 'alternative fluids', such as simple urine samples used for testing for disorders that previously could only be diagnosed via blood tests (Hoyweghen, *Risks in the Making*). In the introduction of the third edition of *Medical Selection of Life Risks*, Brackenridge and Elder explain the addition of a chapter on laboratory screening with reference to the increasing importance of laboratory screening in risk selection. In these chapters on laboratory-derived data for risk selection one can read: 'Multi phasic screening as a laboratory tool has grown enormously in the past few decades due to technical advances, entrepreneurial enthusiasm and the need to screen for HIV disease' (p. 177).

22. Quoted from http://www.hannoverlifere.com/prod-sol/uw-services/lifestyle/index. html [accessed 14 September 2013].

23. Interview case 1, underwriter K.

24. R. Swiss, *Life Risk Selection at a Fair Price: Reinforcing the Actuarial Basis* (Zurich: Swiss Re., 2007), p. 14.

25. Note that this tendency is also apparent in epidemiology. See, for example, on the construction of cholesterol, K. Garrety, 'Social Worlds, Actor-Networks and Controversy: The Case of Cholesterol, Dietary Fat and Heart Disease', *Social Studies of Science*, 27 (1997), pp. 727–73; on the overweight and obedsity D. Davies, 'Health and the Discourse of Weight Control', in A. Petersen and C. Waddell (eds), *Health Matters: A Sociology of Illness, Prevention and Care* (Buckingham: Open University Press, 1998), pp. 141–55; and on the 'hypotensive' patient, G. Hatt, 'Uncertainty in Medical Decision-Making', in Petersen and Waddell (eds), *Health Matters*, pp. 223–39.

26. Interview case 1, underwriter B.

27. Whereas research on the link between smoking and lung cancer has been applied in clinical medicine since the sixties, it took the insurance business some decades more to begin differentiating between smokers and non-smokers. The smoking case illustrates well how insurers take into account the level of social acceptability when pondering the introduction of a new risk classification factor. For a long time, insurance companies believed that society would not be prepared to tolerate differentiation based on smoking. In the 1960s, for example, as this handbook of life insurance suggests, life insurance companies were 'well-aware that smoking had deleterious effects on health and longevity but *intentionally* chose not to include it as a rating factor': S. S. Huebner and K. Black Jr, *Life Insurance* (New York: Appleton-Century-Crofts, 1969), p. 477.

28. R. Swiss, *Life Underwriting Experience Study 2000: Mortality Investigation Based on Data from the Medical Statistics of Swiss Re Zurich 1965–1996* (Zürich: Swiss Re., 2002), p. 4.

29. Interview case 1, manager K.

30. B. Wilkinson, 'When a Desired Rating is Undesirable', *Reinsurance Reporter*, 153:1 (1998). http://www.lincolnre.com/eprise/main/lre/publications/Reporter/Issues/153/153_01.htm [accessed 15 March 2001].

31. A. Chuffart, *Genetics and Life Insurance: A Few Thoughts* (Zürich: Swiss Re., 1997), p. 23.

32. Interview case 1, underwriter K.

33. Note that this idea of 'managing death' was exactly the philosophical foundation of the development of insurance (Ewald, *L'Etat-Providence*). By calculating risks and framing death into *risk*, the governmentality of death became visible.

34. LVO (Wet van 25 juni op de Landverzekeringsovereenkomst), *Belgisch Staatsblad*, 20 August 1992 (18283–18333).

35. See for example, A. Lippman, 'Prenatal Genetic Testing and Geneticization: Mothers Matter for All', *Fetal Diagnosis and Therapy*, 8:1 (1993), pp. 175–88; P. Kitcher, *The Lives to Come: The Genetic Revolution and Human Possibilities* (London: Penguin, 1996).

36. I. Van Hoyweghen, K. Horstman and R. Schepers, 'Genetic "Risk Carriers" and Lifestyle "Risk Takers": Which Risks Deserve our Legal Protection in Insurance?', *Health Care Analysis*, 15:3 (2007), pp. 179–93.

37. J. N. Shklar, *The Faces of Injustice* (New Haven, CT and London: Yale University Press, 1990).

38. See for example, D. Carmelli, A. C. Heath and D. Robinette, 'Genetic Analysis of Drinking Behavior in World War II Veteran Twins', *Genetic Epidemiology*, 10 (1993), pp. 201–13.

39. See for example, R. E. Straub, P. F. Sullivan, Y. Ma and M. V. Myakishev et al. (eds), 'Susceptibility Genes for Nicotine Dependence: A Genome Scan and Follow-up in an Independent Sample Suggest that Regions on Chromosomes 2, 4, 10, 16, 17, 18 Merit Further Study', *Molecular Psychiatry*, 4 (1999), pp. 129–44.

40. Hoyweghen, *Risks in the Making*.

41. A. A. Dicke, 'Discussion after Chambers 1999', *North American Actuarial Journal*, 3 (1999), pp. 31–3.

INDEX

Milton Keynes UK
Ingram Content Group UK Ltd.
UKHW031144141024
449569UK00024B/1069